# HOSPITALS, CLINICS, and HEALTH CENTERS

# HOSPITALS, CLINICS, and HEALTH CENTERS

*AN ARCHITECTURAL RECORD BOOK*

MCGRAW-HILL BOOK COMPANY, INC.

*New York    Toronto    London*

HOSPITALS, CLINICS, AND HEALTH CENTERS

IV

# FOREWORD

Few people take illness or accidents lightly, least of all the doctors, administrators, and others who are directly charged with the responsibility for the care and treatment of the ill or injured. The men and women of the medical professions take their responsibilities seriously. They have won a reputation for their dedication to the prevention and healing of diseases and injury.

Architecture is serious, too. And architects are serious about it, for the most part. Many are just as dedicated, in their own way, as the members of the medical professions. For some reason, hospital architects seem to be possessed of an even higher sense of obligation or dedication than usual. They tend to become involved not only with the purely architectural and engineering aspects of their buildings, but with the relationships of the architecture to all of human life and death.

When planning hospitals or other medical buildings, architects seem to be driven to study more deeply, with broader scope. They travel extensively, in pursuit of the newest, the best, the most effective ways of doing things. They visit medical buildings, questioning, measuring, analyzing. They spend as much time as they can in the study of materials such as those discussed in this book.

There is, therefore, an important reason for the book. It is intended for architects, hospital administrators and consultants, and all others responsible for the planning of medical buildings. It is intended to be a source book of information and, it is hoped, enlightenment.

All of the discussions and presentations in the book originally appeared in the pages of ARCHITECTURAL RECORD. They have been carefully chosen for their value, variety, and lasting interest. There is a considerable amount of background information on the problems of planning medical buildings. A number of medical buildings are shown, some in great detail. Widely varied in size and complexity, these give some indication of the means that have been used by architects for solving some of the problems.

The book is divided into four sections, covering almost the entire range of medical building types. One section deals with hospitals, another with special facilities, a third with rehabilitation centers, the fourth with health centers, clinics, and offices. Included are articles on the planning of such specific elements as surgical suites, X-ray suites, and pediatric units. There are technical articles on air distribution, electrical systems, and the like.

All who are concerned with the planning of medical buildings should find something of value here, a lesson or two, some useful ideas. It is hoped that the book will form another link in the chain of medical building evolution, and contribute in some measure to the growing efficiency of medical facilities. It should help those who are responsible for planning and constructing medical buildings to create an environment that is more comfortable for both staff and patients. Finally, it may help medical architecture to make more positive contributions to the successful treatment of human maladies.

WILLIAM DUDLEY HUNT, JR., A.I.A.
*Senior Editor, Architectural Record*

# CONTENTS

SECTION I

HOSPITAL BUILDINGS

Hospital Planning Starts with Circulation, by Emerson Goble . . . . . . . . 2
Evaluation of a Hospital . . . . . . . . . . . . . . . . 8
Small Hospital Has Three Zones . . . . . . . . . . . 20
Core Plan Is Efficient for Small Hospital . . . . . . . . . . . . 23
A Clean Little Hospital for an Air Force Base . . . . . . . . 26
Small Hospital for a Rural Community . . . . . . . 32
Centralized Supply System Permits Logical Plan . . . . . . . . . 36
Hospital Plan Based on Supply System Organization . . . . . . . . . . 40
Improved Supply System for Better Patient Care . . . . . . . . . . 43
General Hospital Planned for Expansion . . . . . . . . . . . 49
Hospital Planned for Unusual Emergency Requirements in Industrial Area . . 52
Large Hospital for Military and Civilian Use in Alaska . . . . . . . . . 61
Large Hospital with Imaginative Plan . . . . . . . . 68
Hospital Based on Research . . . . . . . . . . . 72
Pavilion for a Large Hospital . . . . . . . . . . . . . . . 78
Large General Hospital with Several Innovations . . . . . . . . . 86
Limited Site Size, Extreme Grade Help Determine Hospital Plan . . . . . . 94
An Efficient Hospital on a Rural Site . . . . . . . . . . . . 100
Psychiatric Unit for a General Hospital . . . . . . . . . . . 103
Pleasant and Open Plan for Psychiatric Patients . . . . . . . . . . 107


SECTION II

SPECIAL FACILITIES

Planning the Surgical Suite, by Aaron N. Kiff and Mary Worthen . . . . . . 114
A New Approach to Air Distribution in Operating Rooms,
    by Edward DeVan . . . . . . . . . . . . . . . . . . 134
Planning the Pediatric Nursing Unit . . . . . . . . . . . . . . . . 137
Diagnostic X-ray Suites for the General Hospital, by Wilbur R. Taylor,
    Clifford E. Nelson, and William W. McMaster . . . . . . . . . . 140
Design of Teletherapy Units, by Wilbur R. Taylor, William A. Mills, and
    James G. Terrill, Jr. . . . . . . . . . . . . . . . . . . 147
A Reference Guide to Hospital Electrical Facilities . . . . . . . . . . 152

Section III

REHABILITATION CENTERS

Rehabilitation Facilities for Multiple Disability . . . . . . . . . . . . . 158
Chronic Disease Hospital . . . . . . . . . . . . . . . . . . 161
Nursing Home Connected with a Hospital . . . . . . . . . . . 164
Hospital with Emphasis on Chronic Cases . . . . . . . . . 166
Planning the Physical Therapy Department . . . . . . . 173
First Complete Facilities for Paraplegics . . . . . . . . . . 178
General Hospital Combined with Rehabilitation Center . . . . . . . . 181
Rehabilitation Hospital School for Children . . . . . . . . . . . . 186
Hearing and Speech Center . . . . . . . . . . . . . . . 190
Comprehensive Rehabilitation Center . . . . . . . . . . . 192
Rehabilitation Center with Research Facilities . . . . . . . . . . . . 196
Rehabilitation Center for a Small Community . . . . . . . . . . . . 201


Section IV

HEALTH CENTERS, DOCTORS' OFFICES, AND CLINICS

Planning the Public Health Center . . . . . . . . . . . . 204
Check List on Health Center Planning . . . . . . . . . . . . . . 206
Mechanical and Electrical Systems for Health Centers . . . . . . . . . . . 207
Type Plans for Health Centers . . . . . . . . . . . . . . . . 208
Tulsa Builds Several Health Centers . . . . . . . . . . . . . . 213
Two Public Health Centers for Counties in the South . . . . . . . . . 214
Small Health Center for a Rural Town . . . . . . . . . . . . . 216
Medium-Sized Health Center for the South . . . . . . . . . . . 217
65-Bed General Hospital and County Health Center . . . . . . . . . 218
Health Insurance and Outpatient Clinic . . . . . . . . . . . . 224
Medical Clinic with Non-Medical Look . . . . . . . . . . . . . 226
Prestige Values in a Dental Clinic . . . . . . . . . . . . . . . 228
Large Clinic Screened from Traffic Noise . . . . . . . . . . . . 230
Doctors' Collaboration for Investment . . . . . . . . . . . . . 232
Doctors' Offices for Group Practice . . . . . . . . . . . . . . 234
Examination and Treatment Center for a Union . . . . . . . . . . . . 242
Pediatric Clinic for Four Doctors . . . . . . . . . . . . . . . 245
Pleasant Atmosphere for Group Medicine . . . . . . . . . . . . 248
Medical Building with Rental Offices . . . . . . . . . . . . . 250
Dental Offices Combined with Apartments . . . . . . . . . . . . 252
Co-op Medical Building for Eight Practices . . . . . . . . . . . . 254
Small Medical Building on a Sloping Site . . . . . . . . . . . . 256
INDEX . . . . . . . . . . . . . . . . . . . . . . . . . 259

# HOSPITAL BUILDINGS

# Hospital Planning Starts with Circulation

*Separate all departments, yet keep them all close together; separate types of traffic, yet save steps for everybody: that's all there is to hospital planning*

*by Emerson Goble*

For the architect not already familiar with modern hospital planning, the principal subject for study will be circulation — the proper integration of the many departments so that different types of traffic through the building will be separated as much as possible, traffic routes will be short, and important functions protected against intrusion. Needless to say, the skill with which circulation is handled will determine the efficiency of the hospital for all of the years of its use. If nurses have to walk too far (according to hospital administrators all nurses are old and have varicose veins) curses will be heaped on the architect's name, day and night, for fifty years.

## Principles of Planning

Protection of the patient (despite the nurses' beefing) is the primary principle of circulation schemes. Too much traffic in the nursing unit corridor will disturb the patient, will involve excessive risk of contamination, or at least of confused and inefficient care. Any unwanted traffic in the surgical suite means dilution of the effectiveness of aseptic technique. Assured protection against contamination is the very heart of good patient care, and is the basis of hospital planning.

Short traffic routes, with as much separation as is feasible, assist in assurance of asepsis. For another reason, however, they become the second principle of circulation; obviously short routes save steps for everybody concerned with hospital care. Nurses, doctors, patients, service and office personnel — all have a share in the patient's welfare. All must work fast at times, and all are subject to fatigue. Their steps take time and cost money, more money each year. Hospital planning is increasingly concerned with labor saving in all possible ramifications.

Separation of dissimilar activities is another principle, for the reasons stated and for other reasons. Separate the "clean" and "dirty" operations. Separate different types of patients. Separate quiet and noisy operations. Separate different types of traffic outside the building as well as inside. Separate pleasant and unpleasant functions. Separate types of workers.

Control is a fourth general objective. No matter how much control may be inherent in good separation, in good disposition of functions, there are places where control must be still more positive. So the nurses' station must involve some supervision of patients' corridors; the infants must be protected against germs brought in by visitors, or even by doctors; the surgical suite must be protected similarly. And so it goes.

Separate everything. Yet have everything close together. That's all there is to it.

If it begins to sound impossible, well, it is. Yet it is still possible to do very well or very poorly. Accordingly is the architect's reputation established. This article will state, as quickly as possible, the major factors in circulation, with reasons for the most urgent requirements. The individual hospital plans presented in the following pages will give practical demonstrations of the theories.

## Separate Exterior Traffic

It is customary to start separating traffic before it even gets within the building; in fact it is necessary to separate it outside in order to do it inside. The key flow chart, Figure 1, offers a general guide to circulation lines in the building, and thus also to exterior traffic.

Usually there are separate entrances for these main traffic lines: 1) Inpatients and visitors; 2) Outpatients; 3) Emergency patients (or ambulance cases); 4) Supplies and fuel.

The main entrance would usually serve for ambulant inpatients arriving for admission, or leaving after their stay. They would proceed through main lobby to admitting desk, possibly with a stop at a social service office. Visitors would also use the main entrance, largely for reason of control of visitor traffic by the receptionist.

The main entrance can also be used by doctors, so that they may be clocked in or out, or possibly so that the records clerk may catch them for a task the doctors always seem to find onerous. On the other hand, doctors frequently prefer a separate entrance, so that they will

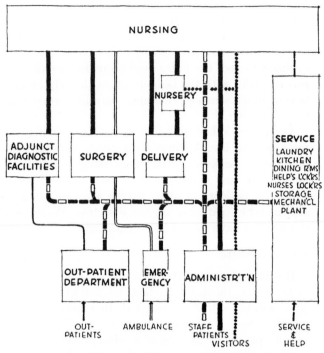

Figure 1: Key Flow Chart, Acute General Hospital

not be button-holed by visitors or relatives or just friends. Another consideration is that usually the doctors have a separate parking area, and another entrance may be much more convenient.

The ambulance or emergency entrance is presumed to be convenient to elevators for inpatients who must be brought in by ambulance or private car. The emergency entrance is principally intended, however, for real emergency cases, who might arrive in some unsightly condition and who would require instant attention in the emergency suite. The "emergency" patient might even be a drunk, or a criminal arriving with full escort. Also the emergency case might be a medically "dirty" patient, not to be taken any farther than necessary until he can be given some preparation.

This same entrance is usually designed also to offer an unobtrusive means of removing the dead.

A separate entrance is desirable for outpatients since any volume of them would soon confuse the main entrance and the departments nearby. Moreover, there is the need to control the movements of outpatients, to keep them out of principal corridors, to confine them to certain areas. Merely from the standpoint of unpleasantness it is desirable to shield the main hospital from a constant parade of sufferers coming and going.

Separate entrance for service and employees seems to have obvious advantages. An especial point is that deliveries are usually a fairly noisy operation, sometimes unpleasant in other respects, and should be iso-lated and screened as much as practicably possible.

Parking space is usually grouped roughly according to entrances. At the least there should be separate and convenient parking space for doctors, who should not be expected to fight a traffic jam at each visit. Perhaps hospital workers should have a separate parking area. Clearly any separation that can be arranged for parking areas will help to maintain separations of types of traffic both within and without the building.

**Interior Traffic Streams**

Figure 1, the key flow chart, shows the main streams of traffic within the hospital to and from principal departments. It does not, of course, show all of the comings and goings up and down these lanes; these are indicated in more detail in departmental charts. The key chart is reliable for indicating the major departmental separations, nevertheless, and this is of course the first step in traffic control.

Architects have developed notable ingenuity in schematics designed to control traffic. The cruciform plan is an old favorite, providing a central traffic and service core and a goodly number of cul de sac locations in the wings.

The T form is another favorite. Again there is a central core, with various medical departments isolated in bases of the T, floor by floor, and nursing units facing south in the top of the T.

Variations are found, literally by the dozen, with wings added on to isolate departments, particularly on the lower floors. Sometimes a wing is sent out, only to be folded back again against the building.

Double corridors have been extensively used, and often they serve to shorten horizontal travel in ingenious ways.

Always the intent is to separate departments yet keep horizontal travel to a minimum. It is worth noting, and quite healthful, that "standard" schemes do not seem to do very well against the wide variety of individual conditions and sites. And against the ever-changing display of originality that architects have exhibited.

**Nursing Department**

As seen in Figure 2, the nursing unit corridor is really a traffic highway. The main streams indicated are endlessly repeated throughout the day and possibly the night. Obviously, then, any possible saving in steps can be multiplied many times over, especially for the nursing staff.

The first point, then, is the location of the nurses' station, as this is the starting and finishing line for all their little footraces. Modern practice usually puts their station roughly in the center of their group of patients. It is generally assumed that the maximum travel distance should be about 80 ft. This almost automatically places a reasonable limit of 25 to 30 patients in one nursing unit, though practice varies in this respect.

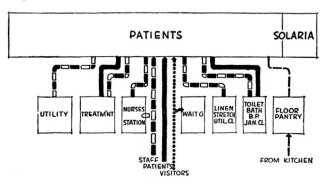

**Figure 2: Nursing Department Flow Chart**

There is some clash of objectives in the placing of the nurses' station, as the central location, it is argued, might weaken the element of control. The central location within the nursing unit might not be quite so good, as to control, as some other location nearer the elevators or stairs where the nurse can keep a weather eye out for the unauthorized visitor or the wandering employee, or can assume the role of policeman as may be required.

Present thinking nevertheless tends in the direction of the central location, where nurses' patient duties are most readily and most quickly performed. The control, it is said, is tenuous at best, for the nurses are usually busy with running for the patients, and cannot always stand with a billy club in their hand. That is, control of the exceptional incident would be tenuous — control of most matters, such as visitors, would be almost automatic anyway, since there is so much going on through most hours that anything untoward would be quickly spotted.

Where the control argument takes on more substance is in the matter of night hours. Then there might be but a single nurse, and she might even have to handle two different nursing units. This consideration might be the prevailing one, depending on such factors as size of nursing units, their relation to each other, or any of many layout factors affecting the need for control.

Elements that group themselves around the nurses' station are utility rooms, baths, floor pantries, drug cabinets, possibly a flower room, maybe also a treatment room. The location and convenience of these facilities can make the nurses' tasks relatively easy or very difficult. If there is one bedpan closet poorly located,

this error alone can drive the nurses to distraction. Good practice puts two bedpan closets in each nursing unit, each centrally located in one half of the unit.

Recent practice also is to put private toilets in as many patient rooms as possible. When the patient is confined to bed, the nurse need go no farther than the private toilet with the bedpan. Or, with early ambulation so much stressed, the nurse may be needed much less frequently.

There are other step-saving devices coming into more general use. An important one is two-way communication between patient and nurse, so that the nurse is at least saved the trip down the hall just to learn the patient's want — maybe she can bring the aspirin tablet with her on the first trip. Many times she will not have to make the trip at all.

### Surgical Suite

It is important that the operating suite be completely isolated from the rest of the hospital, and so located that there will be no traffic through it. In a large hospital it might occupy a separate floor; in a smaller one it is usually placed at the end of a wing. Operating rooms and associated areas must, of course, be protected against unwanted persons, mostly to minimize the risk of contamination, but also to prevent interruptions and confusion.

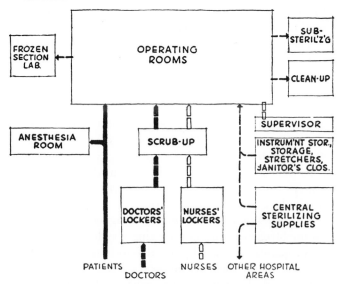

**Figure 3: Surgery Flow Chart**

*Note: Since first publication of this material the prevailing practice has been to include recovery rooms in most surgical suites.*

The suite ought to be close to elevators, or to the surgical nursing unit. It has some relationship also to the emergency department, as emergency cases might require major operating procedures. Or, in case of a general emergency (railroad wreck or fire) the whole

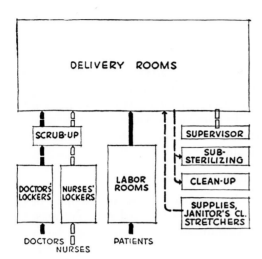

**Figure 4: Obstetrics Department**

operating department might be taken over temporarily for emergency use.

The surgical suite also has an obvious relationship to the x-ray department. The fracture room-x-ray relationship is especially close, and radiographic work is done also in cystoscopy, though portable x-ray equipment might solve this problem. The fracture room, incidentally, is sometimes placed in the emergency suite, especially if a large volume of accident cases may be expected, but it is usually considered part of the operating department and so placed.

Modern practice tries to put the central sterilizing department either adjacent to or within the surgical suite. This arrangement naturally makes it convenient to supply the sterile packs and so on needed in the operating rooms with minimum risk of contamination after sterilizing. It also puts the sterilizing operation more or less under control of the surgical nursing staff. In many hospitals this staff actually does the sterilizing in free time when operations are not in progress. The sterilizing department would be arranged also, of course, to dispense supplies to the rest of the hospital without involving outside traffic within the surgical department itself.

Figure 3 is useful in showing the main elements of the operating department and their relationships to each other.

## Obstetrics Department

The delivery suite is very much like the operating department, and the same general considerations of location and control hold here. The obstetrical suite is given a similar location, though its primary relationship is to the maternity nursing unit, not to emergency or x-ray facilities.

Special consideration should be given to separating the suite from the nursery itself, since the newborn infants attract a great deal of visitor traffic. On the contrary, however, a long distance means that much more risk in the moving of newborn from delivery suite to nursery. The separation, then, should ideally be a matter of control, not distance.

Some of the newer hospital plans show the delivery suite actually adjacent to the surgical department, especially in small buildings. There are obvious advantages, and some disadvantages. The two departments require the same isolation, the same type of nursing service, same cleaning, air conditioning, sterile supplies and so on. Nevertheless, intertraffic between the two is undesirable, and the possibility of cross-contamination is ever-present. If the two departments are nearby, then, especially good control is required.

Figure 4 shows the units of the delivery department and their interrelationships.

## Nurseries

The nursery is designed to keep traffic to an absolute minimum, for nothing worries the hospital administrator quite as much as the possibility of an epidemic in the nursery, especially the dread infant diarrhea. The nursery is closed off from the corridor, entered only through the nurse's work room. The usual arrangement permits only the nurse — not even the doctor — to enter the nursery itself. The baby is taken by the nurse to the examination room, off the work room, for the doctor.

Frequently each nursery is limited to eight bassinets, representing the number of babies a single nurse can handle. Thus each infant is normally in contact with only one person; that is, in the nursery. The baby is taken to the mother, of course, and that necessity imposes some requirements on the location of the nursery.

It should be centrally located within the maternity nursing unit, to keep distances as short as possible and again minimize risk of infection. The central location is good also to keep down delivery routes for linen, bottles and medication.

## Adjunct Diagnostic and Treatment Facilities

In general all of adjunct diagnostic facilities have about the same traffic conditions, and the same type of uses. So they are grouped together.

From the circulation standpoint the main point is that diagnostic facilities are used both by inpatients and outpatients. The natural location, then, is on the street floor, for convenience of outpatients, but near elevators or main corridor for convenience of inpatients and staff (see Figures 5 and 6).

As previously mentioned, the outpatient department

usually has a separate entrance and waiting room, to keep the department self-contained, and to keep outpatients from wandering about the hospital. Thus it is desirable, on the inside, to maintain some isolation of the diagnostic facilities. Access to the department by inpatients, therefore, while it should be convenient, should be susceptible to positive control, not for the hospital patients themselves but for the outpatients.

In some hospitals there may be a public health department, which will have use for the diagnostic facilities, for their own patients, and this relationship may

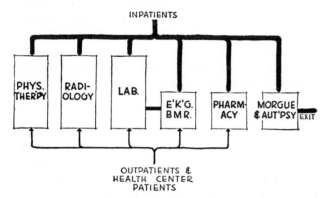

**Figure 5: Adjunct Diagnostic Facilities**

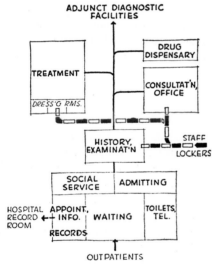

**Figure 6: Outpatient Department**

have to be separately planned. There may occasionally also be doctors' offices in connection with the hospital, and the doctors will have use for diagnostic facilities. Even if the hospital does not maintain a normal outpatient department, there will be some use of these facilities by doctors attached to the hospital and by their patients needing x-ray diagnosis or treatment.

It is worth noting that modern medicine places increasing reliance on diagnostic and laboratory procedures. There are some staffing problems in these departments, and some hospital administrators don't particularly like them, especially in rural areas. But in just those areas the diagnostic facilities may be most appreciated; they might be necessary to induce young doctors to practice there, and thus they are very important to the hospital's community service. The point is that it is not safe to plan on the basis of having no outpatient department, or of keeping the diagnostic facilities to a minimum.

### Administration Department

The administrative offices are grouped in the area adjoining the main lobby and main entrance (see Figure 7). Certain sub-groupings should be considered, so that each unit within a sub-group will be conveniently located with reference to each other unit in that sub-group.

For example, the administrator's office, the director of nurses' office, the general business offices, the secretary's office and the toilet facilities for the administrative staff form one sub-group of the administrative facilities, each unit of which should be convenient to each other unit.

Other sub-groups include: the main lobby and waiting room, the information desk, the cashier's window alcove and the public toilets; the admitting office, the social service office; the medical record room and that section of the staff room intended for the record study; and the staff room, locker room, library and conference or board room.

Many hospitals have found it desirable to provide a separate small retiring room in this area for the use of distraught relatives.

The medical record room should be accessible from the admitting office and the outpatient department. It may well adjoin and control the entrance to the staff locker room, and should have convenient access to the inactive record storage room below, possibly by a spiral staircase. Space should be available either in the record room or in the staff room for staff members to use while completing their medical records and for reviewing microfilmed records if that system is contemplated. In larger hospitals it may be necessary to provide a pneumatic tube or other device to convey records to and from the nurses' stations, admitting room, outpatient department and emergency room.

In the larger hospitals, a separate library and conference room should be provided. It is advantageous if this can adjoin the medical record room, thus serving the double purpose of furnishing a control for the library books and space for staff members to consult records without removing them from the control of the medical record librarian. If interns are to be trained at the hospi-

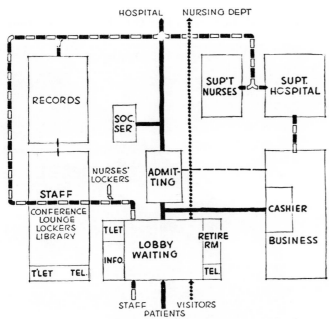

Figure 7: Administration Department

the building. This is usually accomplished by a tray service system, with individually prepared trays or bulk food sent from kitchen to nursing units. Floor pantries may or may not enter into the operation, usually not for regular meals. But they serve for bedtime or between-meal snacks or for certain peculiar dietary situations.

Storage problems are always harassing in a hospital. It's a chronic complaint that there is never enough storage area, and that it's never in the right place. Just the same, the central storage system is preferred, for reasons of control. A hospital stores an infinite variety of commodities, from foods to furniture. Some of it is quite valuable, or at least very subject to disappearance, so control is a strong need. Storage problems might be said to compare with those of a hotel, and so require more than ordinary attention in planning.

**More Detail**

This has been the quickest possible introduction to the circulation problems involved in hospital schematics.

tal, a library is required. The library should have adequate shelving and provisions for unbound periodicals. In smaller hospitals a combination board room, staff conference room and medical library may be arranged in conjunction with the administrator's office by the use of accordion doors, thus enabling the total space to be made available for large meetings.

**Service Departments**

Figure 8 outlines the flow of activities in the kitchen and other service departments. These are not too different from similar facilities in other types of buildings, but there are a few notable points in hospital operation.

One is to maintain if possible a more than normal isolation of these areas, largely because there is much noisy bustle about them which would disturb the quiet of a hospital or interfere with concentration in the departments where people do critical things. A basement location is frequently given them, yet it is often pointed out that a great many people work in these departments, or eat in staff dining rooms, and these busy and underpaid souls should not be asked to struggle in basement space. A change of grade is useful in this problem, giving ground level delivery access and windows for dining rooms. A principle is to point delivery entrances, say, to the rear — at any rate in the opposite direction from the patients' rooms — to screen the less pleasant, noisier activities.

A complicating factor as to kitchens is that food must be delivered to patients in their rooms, so that the food operation must reach into most corners of

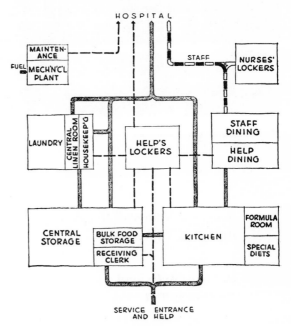

Figure 8: Service Department

If the review seems to deal mainly in principles, they are principles most frequently neglected. Those who have studied hundreds of hospital plans say they are violated by experts as well as beginners, and that when you find a bad hospital scheme the trouble usually goes back to these basic worries about circulation.

They have been treated in considerably more detail in various publications of the U. S. Public Health Service.

# Evaluation of a Hospital

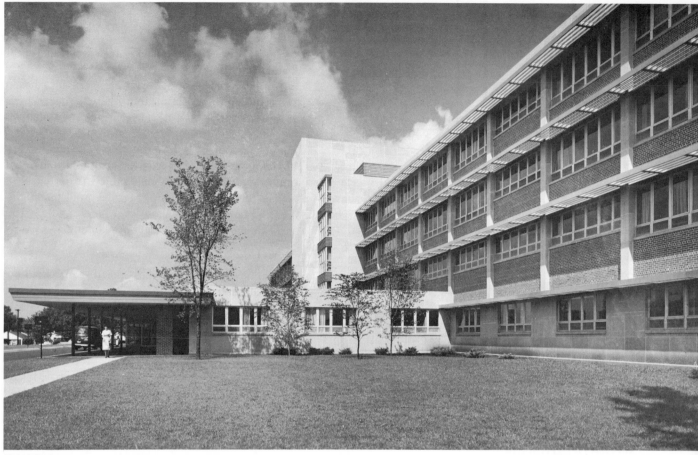

Hedrich-Blessing

*Rockford Memorial Hospital*
*Rockford, Illinois*

*Hubbard & Hyland*
*Perkins & Will*
*Associated Architects*
*and Engineers*

*Hendrik P. Maas*
*Hospital Consultant*

*E. R. Gritschke & Associates*
*Mechanical Engineers*

*Paul F. Griffenhagen*
*Structural Engineer*

*Review panel, led by Everett W. Jones of The Modern Hospital, included representatives of the architects, John L. Brown, director of the hospital, Paul J. Connor, Jr., associate director, George B. Caldwell, administrative resident, and virtually all department heads and supervisors*

PLANNING OF THIS HOSPITAL was intensively studied both before it was built and after it was put in operation. This presentation will touch lightly on the pre-construction planning, and treat in more detail the findings of a review committee which studied plan and equipment features as tested in actual operation.

After a full year of operation the review committee held exhaustive interviews with hospital personnel to get criticisms and suggestions. Reports included major and minor items alike: plan features, equipment details, operating methods; altogether a fairly rough test of hospital planning after the fact. There were some compliments, some complaints, and a great many constructive comments. And a photographer was present to record it visually; these pages are largely devoted to a picture-and-caption report of the investigation.

Original planning began when Hendrik P. Maas was

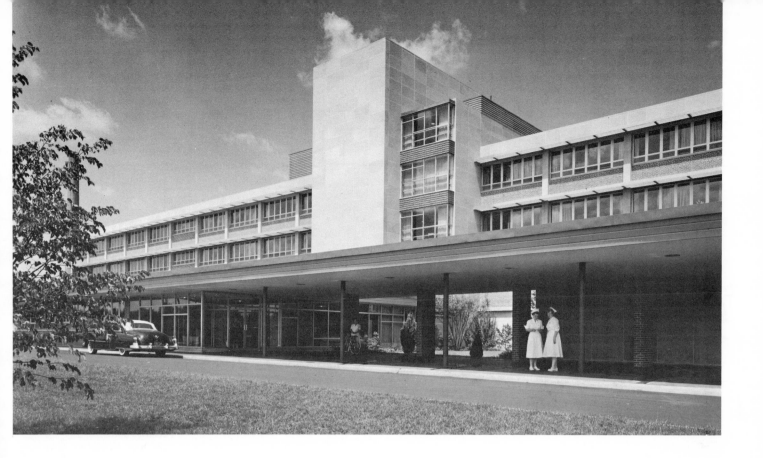

retained as architectural consultant and the determination was made to start with a fresh site and build a new plant. Two architectural firms teamed together. Hubbard and Hyland had performed many odd tasks in connection with the older buildings, were familiar with the hospital's problems, and Perkins and Will joined up to contribute a fresh approach, "not inhibited by previous tenets." Their work together started with the basic hospital room in the effort to design "a hotel for people who are ill."

After primary research into room units and plan types the architects settled on a high percentage of private rooms, with two-bed rooms arranged with the longer dimension paralleling the window wall. Thus each of the two patients has a like share in the daylight and the view and in the facilities of the room. There is a private toilet for each double room, a connecting one for the single rooms; lavatories are in the rooms.

A T-shaped, four-story building resulted when all elements were accounted for, with each wing or unit offset to avoid transmission of sound and long tunnel-

Hedrich-Blessing

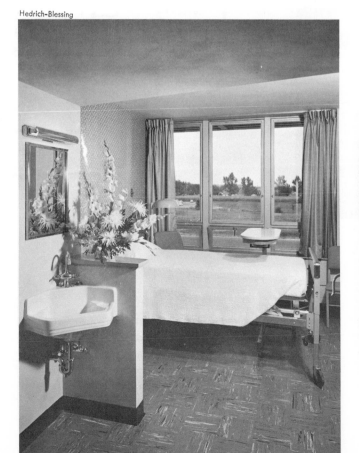

*Out-patient waiting room, looking out on entrance court*

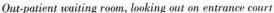

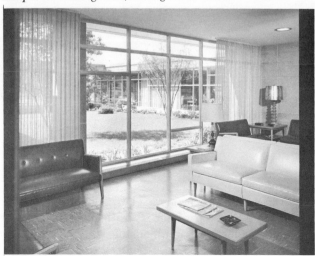

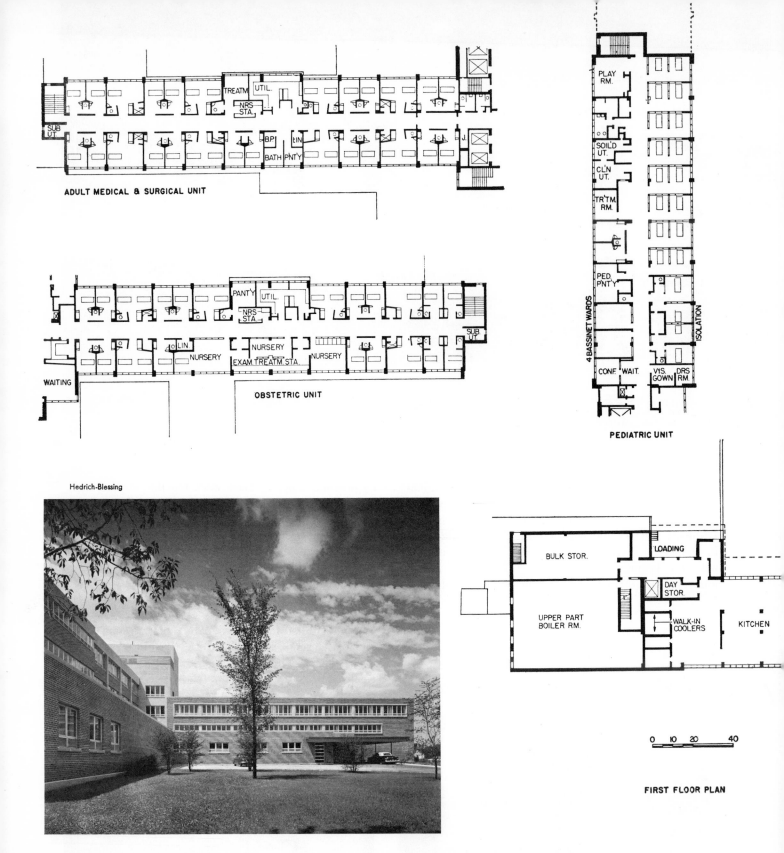

ADULT MEDICAL & SURGICAL UNIT

OBSTETRIC UNIT

PEDIATRIC UNIT

Hedrich-Blessing

FIRST FLOOR PLAN

like views down corridors. Two individual nursing units form the top of the T, with other facilities or special nursing units forming the base. Ground floor and basement are of course enlarged to house principal departments, which in the T form are easily expanded should that prove necessary in the future.

The rather free arrangement of first floor separates departments and their traffic patterns quite well, but does manage to establish relationships between complementary elements. There is an exceptionally large radiology department, with double-corridor scheme to shorten travel distances, located near a large out-patient department and laboratory. The emergency unit has its own entrance, and is located close by the

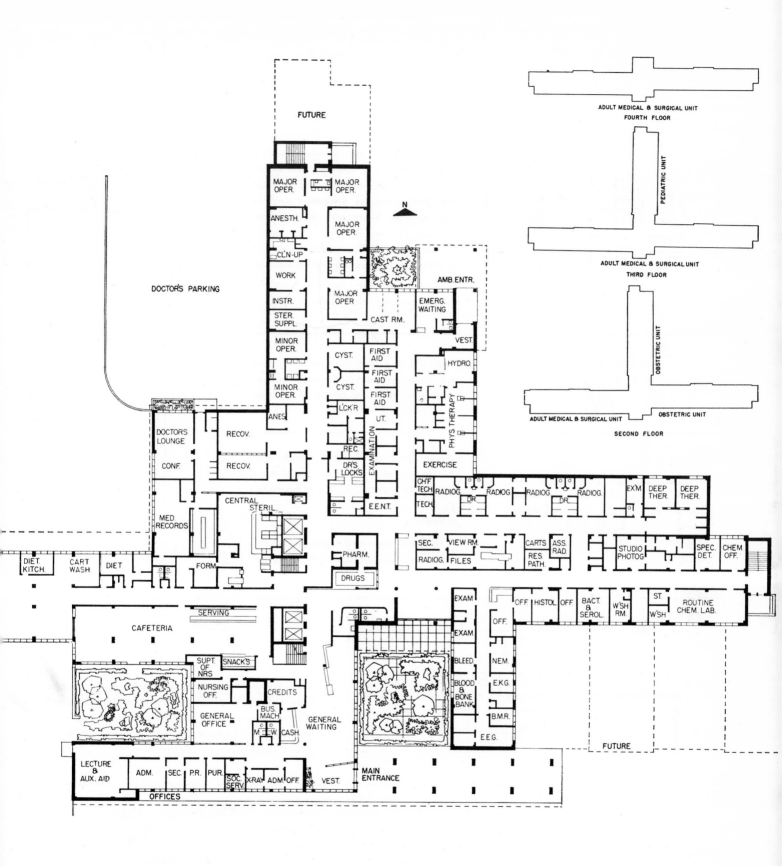

FUTURE

MAJOR OPER.

MAJOR OPER.

ANESTH.

MAJOR OPER.

DOCTOR'S PARKING

CL'N-UP

WORK

INSTR.

STER. SUPPL.

MINOR OPER.

MINOR OPER.

ANES.

DOCTORS LOUNGE

RECOV.

CONF.

RECOV.

CENTRAL STERIL.

MED. RECORDS

CYST.

CYST.

L'CK'R

REC.

DR'S LOCK'S

EXAMINATION

E.E.N.T.

U.T.

FIRST AID

FIRST AID

FIRST AID

CAST RM.

AMB. ENTR.

EMERG. WAITING

VEST.

HYDRO.

PHYS. THERAPY

EXERCISE

CH'F TECH

TECH

RADIOG.

DR.

RADIOG.

RADIOG.

DR.

RADIOG.

EX'M.

DEEP THER.

DEEP THER.

STUDIO PHOTOG.

SPEC. DET.

CHEM. OFF.

SEC.

RADIOG.

VIEW RM.

FILES

CARTS

RES. PATH.

ASS. RAD.

PHARM.

DRUGS

OFF.

EXAM

EXAM

BLEED

BLOOD & BONE BANK

E.E.G.

HISTOL

OFF.

NEM.

E.K.G.

B.M.R.

BACT. & SEROL.

W'SH RM.

W'SH

ST.

W'SH

ROUTINE CHEM. LAB.

FUTURE

DIET. KITCH.

CART WASH

DIET

FORM

CAFETERIA

SERVING

SUPT. OF NRS

SNACK'S

NURSING OFF.

CREDITS

GENERAL OFFICE

BUS. MACH

M E W

CASH.

GENERAL WAITING

LECTURE & AUX. AID

ADM.

SEC.

P.R.

PUR.

SOC. SERV.

X-RAY

ADM. OFF.

VEST.

MAIN ENTRANCE

OFFICES

ADULT MEDICAL & SURGICAL UNIT
FOURTH FLOOR

PEDIATRIC UNIT

ADULT MEDICAL & SURGICAL UNIT
THIRD FLOOR

OBSTETRIC UNIT

ADULT MEDICAL & SURGICAL UNIT    OBSTETRIC UNIT
SECOND FLOOR

operating suite; notice that the cast room serves to tie these two departments together. If this large floor begins to look a bit complicated, it will be seen that traffic routes for the public are kept simple and direct. The public also is treated to landscaped court yards which are bound to do much to alleviate any institutional feeling.

The new hospital has a 15-acre site at the edge of the city. Ultimately the rest of the site will be developed with nurses' residence, nurses' school, medical arts building, and some expansion of the main building.

In the initial phase, at 200 beds, the building was estimated to cost approximately $4,000,000; working out to $20,000 per bed. When the full plan of 268 beds is realized, per bed cost will come down to $16,000.

*Rockford Memorial Hospital*

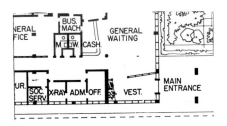

Room for chest X-ray at admittance not used as such — still some question of best procedure. X-ray room now used as admitting office; rooms so designated used for other purposes. X-ray room (now admitting office) should have glass partition looking into waiting area. May need more space for admitting, as hospital approaches full load.

Would appreciate room near admitting offices to keep two wheel chairs

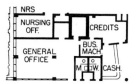

Originally no private office for credit manager; has taken space for business machine. Needed this space for private credit interviews; space still too small

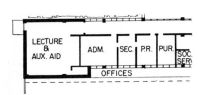

Original program did not provide office for administrative assistant, nor for administrative resident. These two have taken offices designated for public relations and purchasing.

The combined board room and meeting room near administrator's office was considered very good

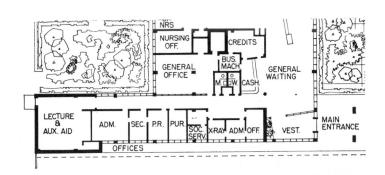

Relationships between admitting office, cashier's counter and cage, credit officer were considered excellent. Close proximity of these is important. Especially good is location of general accounting and business office near cashier's cage and across from administrator and his assistant

Hedrich-Blessing

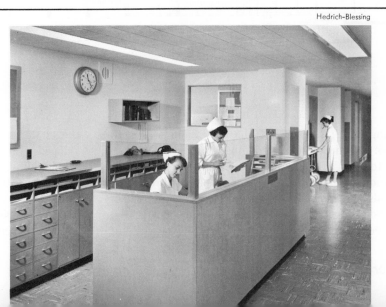

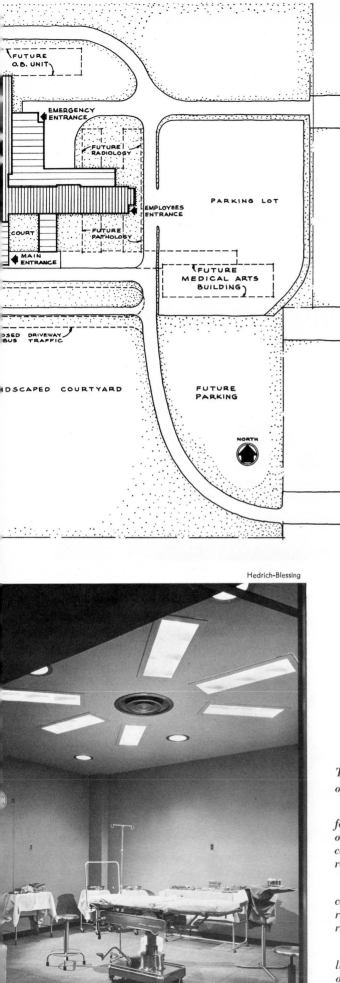

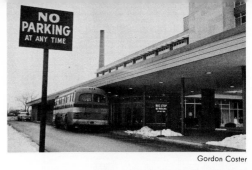

*Main entrance area considered well planned. Good turn-around drive at entrance; good parking areas elsewhere. But later problem was buses coming to door: bus company insisted no parking at all near entrance. Really need space for short parking time for few cars; so suggest turn-around be enlarged. May then need doorman to control this new parking space*

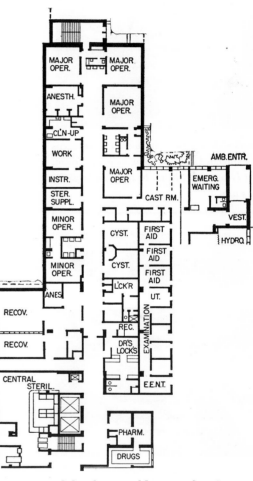

*The chief of surgical department said that the general layout and equipment of operating suite was excellent.*

*Appreciation expressed for ten-foot corridors in operating suite: if occasionally patients need be left in corridor on stretcher, no congestion results.*

*Some question of sufficient miscellaneous storage space in operating rooms: it would be nice to have separate room for equipment storage.*

*Would also appreciate separate linen chute for laundry from the operating rooms.*

*Doors should be installed to close off recovery room from operating cor-*

*ridor: some patients scream when coming out of anesthesia.*

*There was criticism of location of air intake immediately over operating table.*

*Room intended for anesthesia induction not used for that purpose, but proves ideal for storage of anesthesia equipment.*

*General area around emergency entrance, cast room, operating suite considered very good. Main emergency room might have been a bit larger, and needs telephone.*

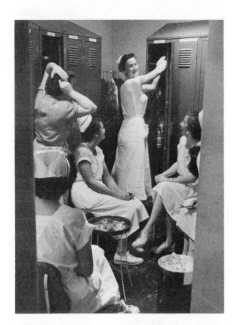

Nurses' locker room in operating area was not intended as a smoking or lounge room, but is so used. Should be twice as large for this use.

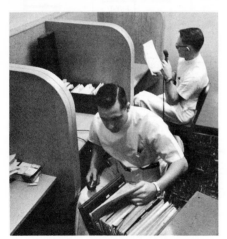

Gordon Coster

Appreciation expressed for dictating booths in medical records department. Portable file keeps records available to doctors at odd hours.

Medical records librarian needs a private office; five clerks work here.

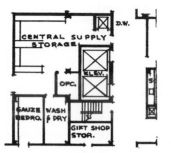
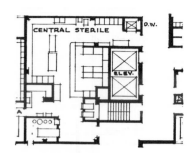

Lower level                    Upper level

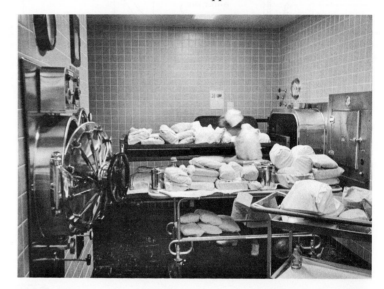

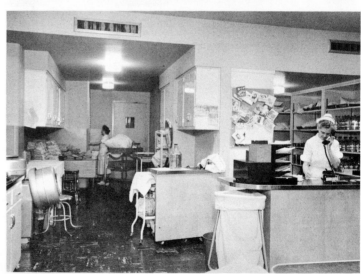

Two-level operation (ground and first floor) of central sterile supply department is most unusual. At this date nobody was sure how it came about. No real study of its feasibility yet made, but is yet to come. Meanwhile only one level now used, and certain troubles have arisen: No "retail storage area" to store few cases of materials right in room. Dumbwaiter presently overloaded, and is not well located. Inadequate loading space at the large sterilizer; bundle wrapping area too far from sterilizers. Need an office area for the supervisor. A sterilizer manufacturer is now studying plans for this area, hoping for a new layout which might yield a more efficient operation.

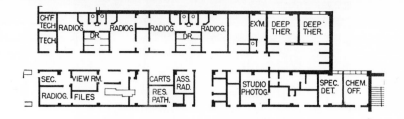

In radiology suite, technicians would appreciate a sub-corridor behind X-ray rooms, as in out-patient department. Here there were some of the usual expressions by the hospital personnel that certain rooms are too small, the toilet room doors are too confined. Most serious seems to be that one or two of the radioscopic rooms are too small, and the stretcher parking area too tight. They would have liked more storage area.

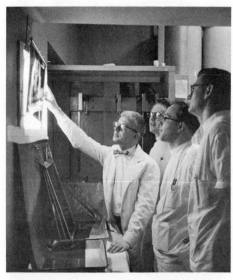

*Maybe a sliding door?*

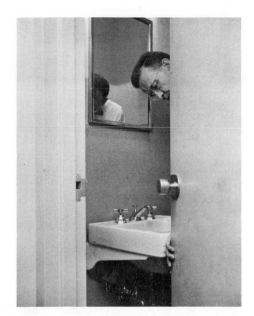

*Designed for one — four's a crowd; viewing area in X-ray film developing area. Sometimes several want a quick look at a wet plate. Also, a small dark room for individual processing would be a nice idea.*

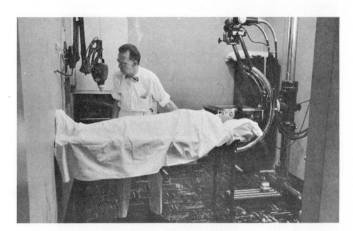

*Head radioscopic room is too narrow*

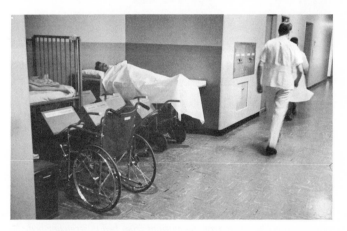

*More parking space needed in X-ray corridor*

*Everybody concerned felt the cast room "was perfect"*

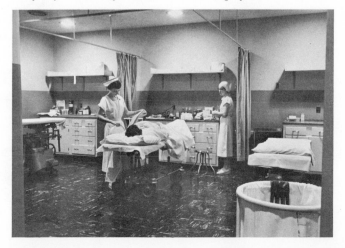

*Rockford Memorial Hospital*

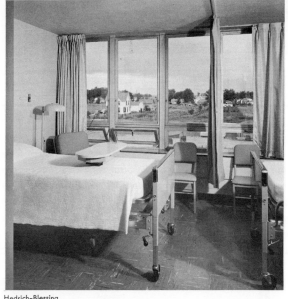

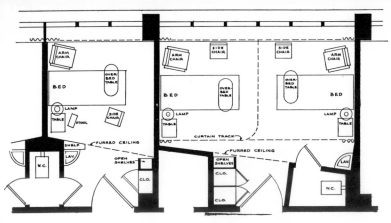

Hedrich-Blessing

*How did patients like the large window area? Reactions were mixed: 70 per cent liked them; 30 per cent said the light hurt their eyes*

Gordon Coster

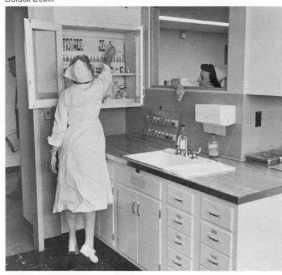

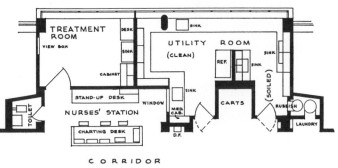

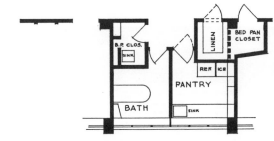

*Location of medicine cabinet over sink board in nurses station utility room is awkward — also needs better light.*

*A change in the architects' plans made a problem about bed pans. It was decided during construction not to include bed pan* *washing equipment in patients' toilets as planned; thus bed pan closets were afterthought, are poorly located and take space from linen room where space is at a premium*

*If the bedrooms were just a little larger, it would be easier to move patient's bed out into corridor, or to transfer patient from bed to stretcher-bed. Nurses have to move other furniture around to accomplish either method of moving patient*

*Nurses are always too small*

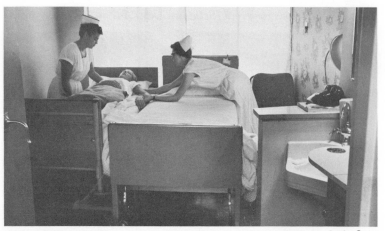

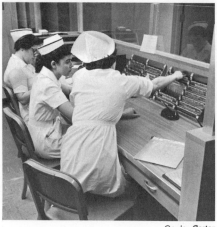

Gordon Coster

Gordon Coster

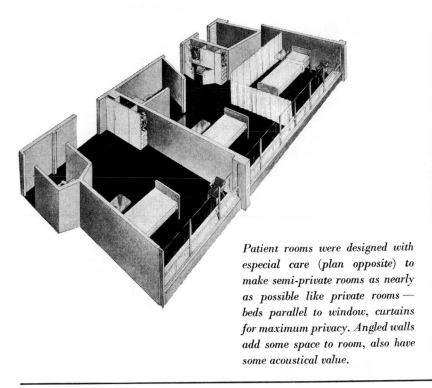

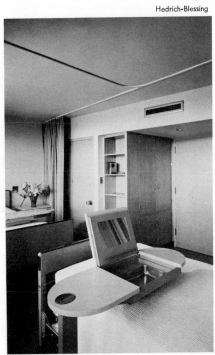

Hedrich-Blessing

*Patient rooms were designed with especial care (plan opposite) to make semi-private rooms as nearly as possible like private rooms — beds parallel to window, curtains for maximum privacy. Angled walls add some space to room, also have some acoustical value.*

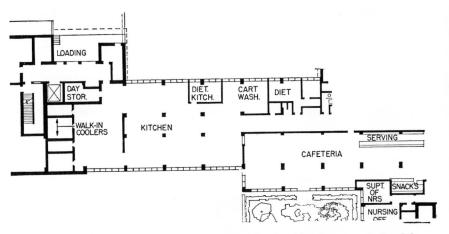

LOADING

DAY STOR.

WALK-IN COOLERS

KITCHEN

DIET. KITCH.

CART WASH.

DIET

SERVING

CAFETERIA

SUPT. OF NRS

SNACKS

NURSING

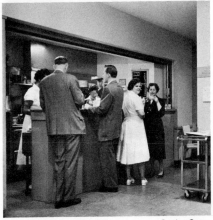

Gordon Coster

*General arrangement of cafeteria and snack bar considered very good. Snack bar appreciated — might be larger, also needs more storage space*

*Kitchen employees think everything here is well laid out. Refrigerator boxes are well located for deliveries, as are bulk food storage and ice boxes. The assembly line for hot-pack type of meal service is working well. Patients gave their praise for the food service, and that is a rugged test in a hospital*

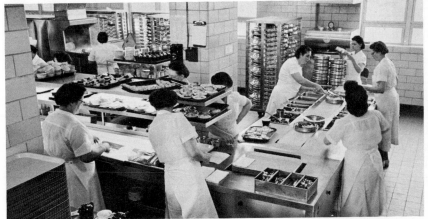

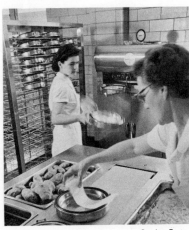

Gordon Coster

Gordon Coster

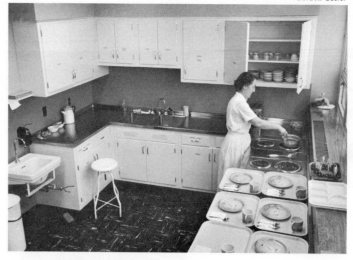

*Nurses in the pediatrics department were well pleased with their suite and arrangements. They were especially pleased with the special diet kitchens, where all meals for youngsters are prepared, and with the pediatrics play room*

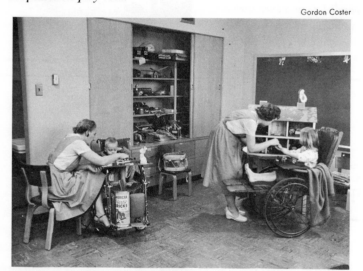

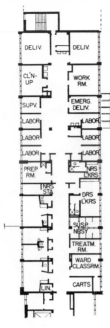

OBSTETRIC UNIT

*Standard hospital doors in obstetrical department proved a bit narrow for moving labor room beds in and out, for here the labor room beds go right into delivery room for transfer of patients.*

*Patient rooms in this suite were designed for mothers whose babies were in suspect nursery; rooms not yet used for this purpose, might not ever be. Rooms might be assigned for normal use. Now being used for sleeping rooms for male nurses, doctors or residents on call*

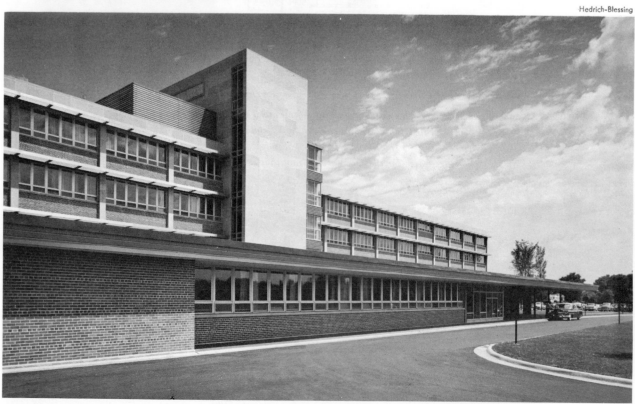

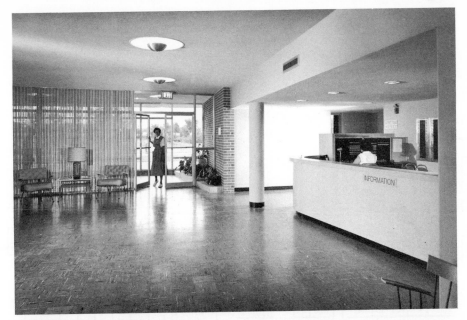

*Two views of main floor lobby; gift shop in background, below*

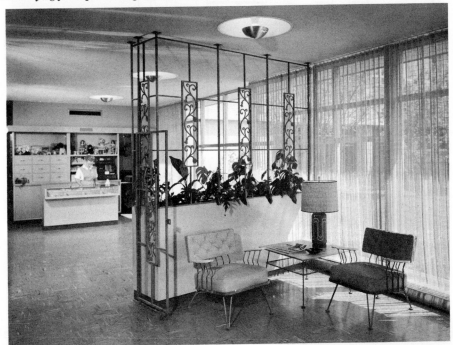

*Below: secretary's desk and waiting room on upper floor*

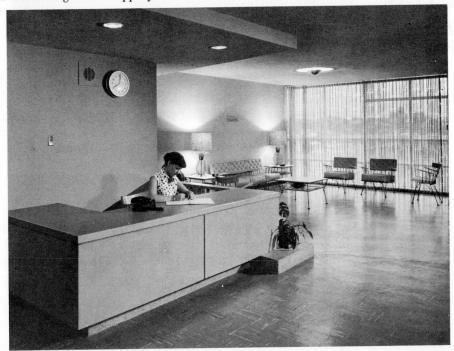

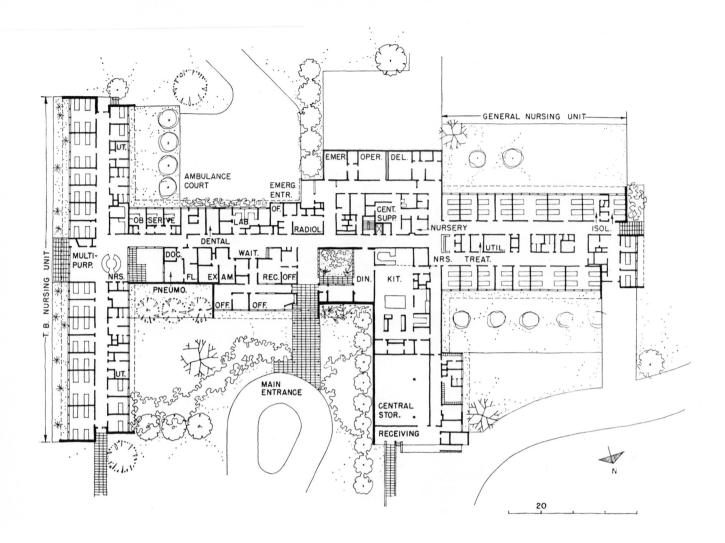

# Small General Hospital Has Three Zones

*Mendocino County Hospital, Mendocino County, Ukiah, California; Stone, Marracini & Patterson, Architects; Art Smith, Structural Engineer; Buonaccorsi & Murray, Mechanical and Electrical Engineers; Utah Construction Company, Contractor*

For this 80-bed county hospital, the architects worked out a simple and flexible plan, zoned for the present needs of the people in this area. Because these ends are not exactly the same as those which might be found elsewhere, the hospital becomes quite special in some ways. For example, there are two main nursing zones (with the beds equally divided between them), a wing for patients who require general nursing care and one for tuberculosis patients. In addition, there is a small three-bed psychiatric unit. One of the program requirements considered very important was the provision for fairly large numbers of outpatients. If a case can be made for the special features of the medical service to be rendered here, an equally strong one might be prepared for the design as a vehicle for general hospital care. The tuberculosis ward may be converted to general nursing either in part or in its entirety with little effort. This change would cause the hospital to be more similar to other general hospitals, though with rather more complete facilities than most others of this same size.

The overall layout of the hospital is unusually well defined into four major areas, the tuberculosis wing at the left, general nursing wing at

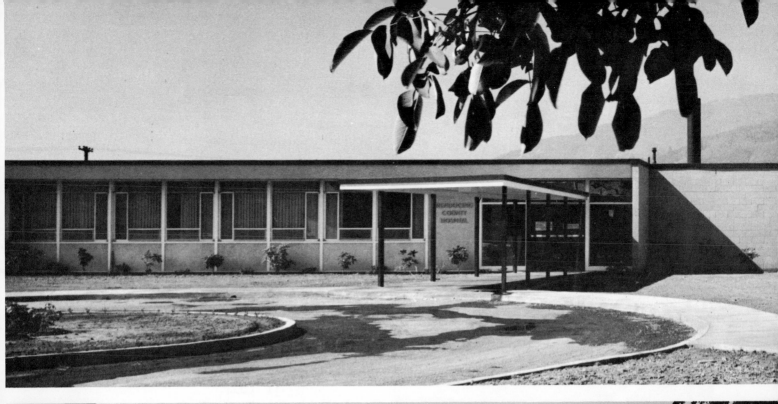

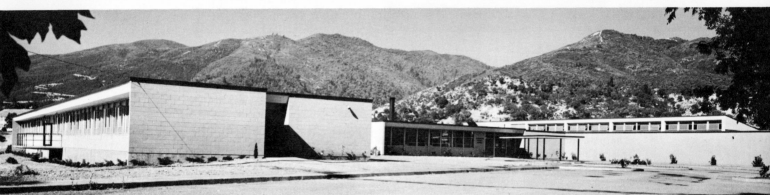

Phil Fein

the right, the link between the two which houses all of the medical, diagnostic, surgical, and outpatient facilities, and the service wing which projects out from the front. The TB wing is a selfcontained unit zoned away from the remainder of the facilities. This area contains special observation rooms and very complete facilities of all types needed for treatment of tubercular patients. As may be seen from the plan, the wing may be completely cut off from the rest of the hospital. The general nursing wing is planned as a double corridor arrangement around a central core. Its position is such that it is shielded from outpatient and other types of traffic which are not directly related to the functions of the department. A unique arrangement in this wing permits the inclusion of two isolation rooms and three psychiatric rooms so placed that these patients are segregated from the general nursing cases, yet are accessible enough to be cared for by nurses in the general wing. Each of these small special departments has its own entrance. Central sterile supply is in a convenient location for serving the operating, delivery, and emergency rooms, yet can also handle its other demands. The emergency room is well-located with respect to the ambulance entrance and emergency court. It is completely separated from other elements of the hospital by a private corridor, yet conveniently located in respect to surgery and other important areas. The outpatient department has complete clinic facilities zoned away from other hospital activities, yet located with respect to the laboratories and the radiographic suite.

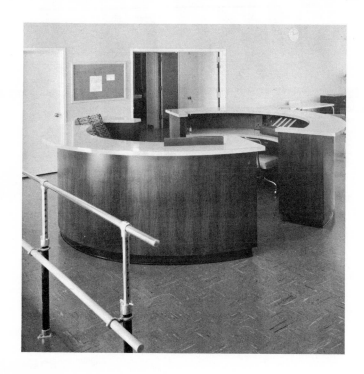

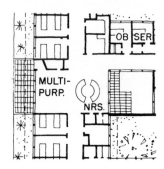

The plan and photographs give some indication of the relationships worked out in the tuberculosis wing to simplify procedures. The nurses' center shown here is located between the two sections of this wing. One of the sections is now used for men, the other for women. Through the use of a central nurses' station, visual control of both sections from one location has been made possible. In addition, considerable flexibility has been gained, since at some later time when the expected decline in TB patients occurs, the function of one of the sections may be changed to some other necessary purpose

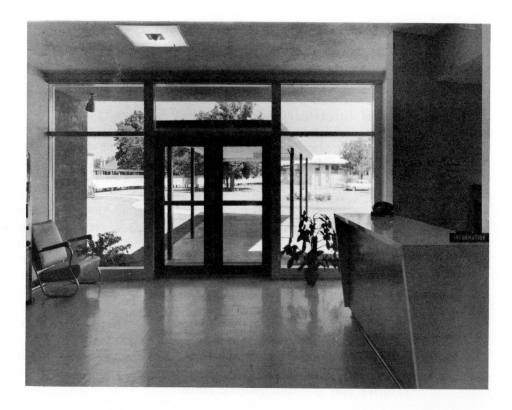

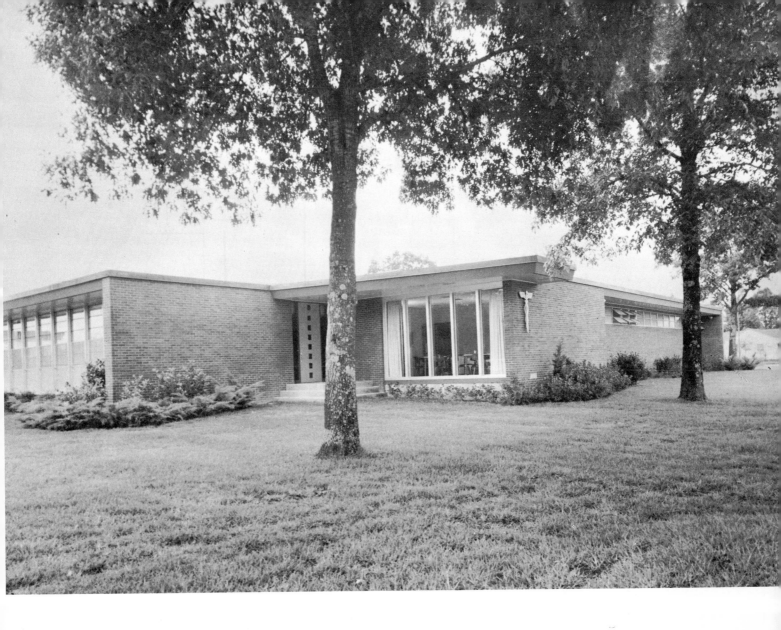

# Core Plan Is Efficient for Small Hospital

*Little River Memorial Hospital, Ashdown, Arkansas; Reinheimer & Cox, Architects; Rawland E. Blaylock & Associates, Consulting Engineers; Texarkana Construction Co., Contractors*

This little 30-bed hospital was designed for expansion to 50 beds. All facilities needed for the expanded size have been provided. The additional beds may be obtained very easily by extending the patient wings. Located in a small community, the hospital provides complete general facilities for the population of the county and surrounding trade area. The major planning problem was the achievement of a design which could be built within the budget and could pay its own way. Quality could not be sacrificed since the hospital would be required to compete with larger institutions in neighboring towns. In order to provide a plant of the quality required and at economical first and long-run costs, the architects spent a great deal of time studying means which would permit efficient operation with a minimum number of personnel and with the lowest possible overhead expenses. The resulting structure has been successful in this respect. The friendly residential-like atmosphere is well received by patients and staff members. The plan functions well and adds greatly to the success of the building.

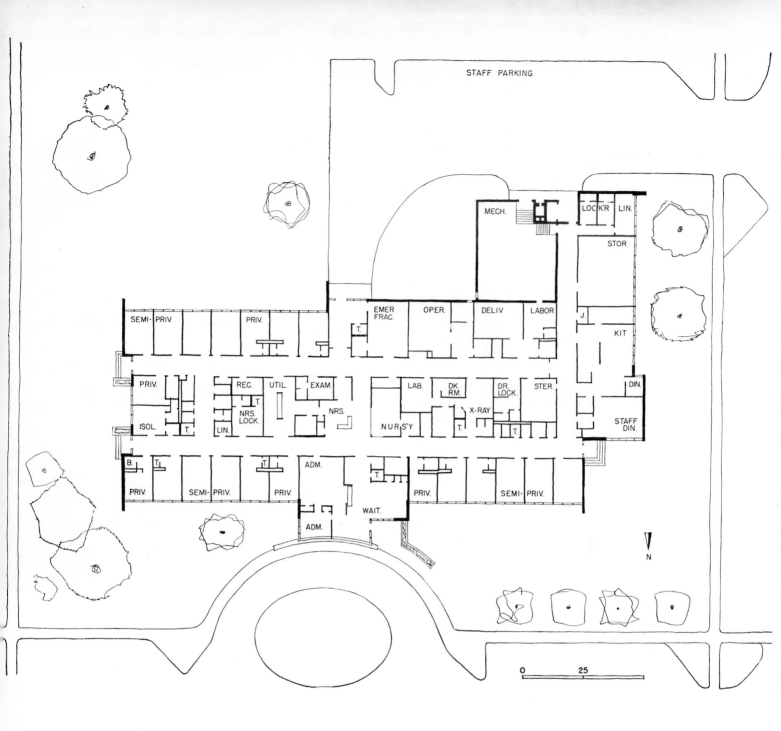

STAFF PARKING

MECH.    LOCK'R   LIN.

STOR

SEMI-PRIV.    PRIV.    EMER FRAC.    OPER.    DELIV    LABOR    J.

KIT

T.

PRIV.    REC.    UTIL.    EXAM.    LAB.    DK. RM.    DR. LOCK.    STER.    DIN.

T.

NRS. LOCK.    NRS.    X-RAY

ISOL.    LIN.    NURS'Y    T.    STAFF DIN.

T.

B.    T.    T.    ADM.    T.

PRIV.    SEMI-PRIV.    PRIV.    PRIV.    SEMI-PRIV.

WAIT.

ADM.

N

0      25

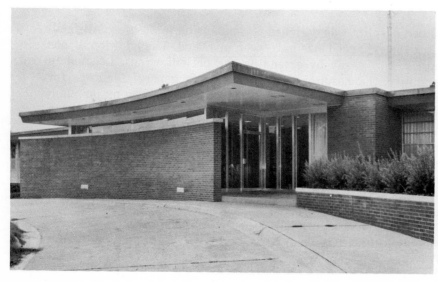

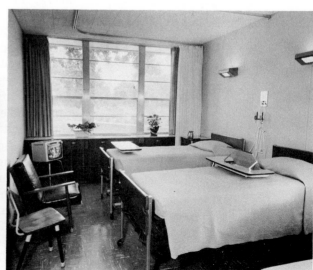

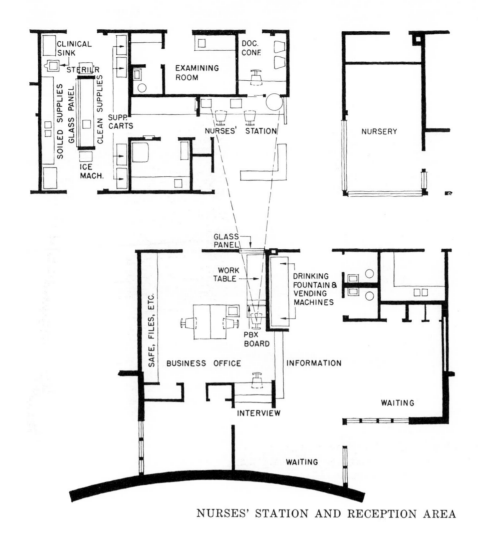

NURSES' STATION AND RECEPTION AREA

The major problem in designing this hospital for operation by a minimum number of personnel resulted in the selection by the architects of a core type design. This plan, often used for larger hospitals, seems especially successful here. Nursing and diagnostic facilities are grouped in the core. Patient room and related facilities are ranged around the outside. The nurses' station is located near the geographical center of the core. By these means, the travel required of nurses to care for the patients and perform other duties, has been reduced to a minimum. From the nurses' station, visual control of the waiting room, emergency entrance, and the nursery, has been provided for. This is particularly important during the later hours of the night when only two to four people are on duty in the hospital. During these late hours, entry to the hospital is confined to the emergency doors of the main entrance. All other doors are locked from the outside. In this way, one nurse seated at the desk can control all incoming traffic. Without leaving the desk, a nurse may attend to paper work, consult patients' charts, consult with doctors in the adjacent room (through a sliding glass panel), use the telephone (and take incoming calls through the night when the switchboard is closed), make calls on the paging system, talk with patients on the nurse call system, and observe warning lights for failure of boilers, piped oxygen, and other systems. In addition, the nurse may talk to doctors in their automobiles via two-way short wave radio. The business office is located to allow nurses and office personnel to cooperate fully and aid each other.

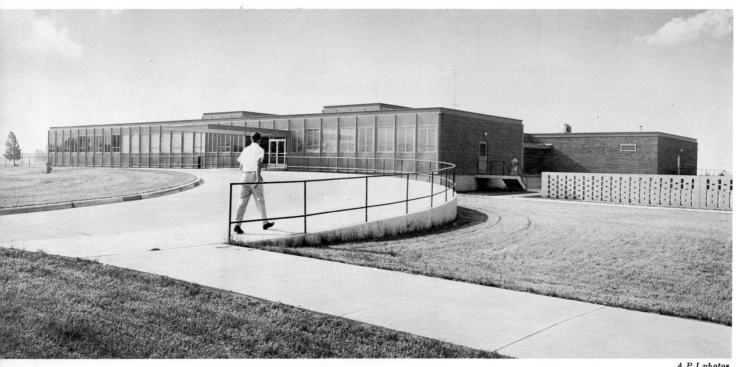

# A Clean Little Hospital for an Air Force Base

*Hospital for Blytheville Air Force Base, Memphis, Tenn.*
*A. L. Aydelott and Associates, Architects and Engineers*

Here is an exceptionally clean little hospital, clean architecturally as well as medically. As an air force base hospital it is not, of course, substantially different from any general hospital of comparable size, since it serves a total community at the base. Present capacity is 25 beds, its chassis being large enough for expansion of the hospital to a 50-bed capacity. The expansion would be accomplished by just filling in the outlines of the plan at 25-bed stage; most of the additional bed capacity would be in eight-bed wards added onto the present ward unit. Main plan of the hospital portion would not be changed importantly, if at all, most of the rest of the growth needed being in offices, dining facilities, storage and so on.

Architecturally the design makes much of a system of wall panels, with essentially two types of materials. Main window wall panels are prefabricated of enameled iron; end walls are of cavity wall construction, outside wythe of 4-in. hard burned clay brick; inside wythe lightweight concrete block.

The building is set on concrete footings and suspended concrete slab on concrete piers, beams and grade beams. Interior partitions are of metal lath over steel studs and glazed structural facing units. The roof is 3-in. vermiculite slab over steel joists supported by steel column and beam frame.

Inside the typical floor and base is of vinyl plastic, the walls and ceilings are plastered, with noncombustible acoustical tile on many of the ceilings. Special floors, bases and wainscots are of ceramic tile. Doors have metal bucks and wood doors.

The building is air conditioned throughout. The central core area has a combination forced warm air heating and air conditioning system supply ducts above furred ceiling, returns in crawl space below the floor. Outside rooms have unit ventilators below the windows at outside wall with a system of hot water, chilled water piping providing hot water for heating in winter and chilled water for cooling in summer weather.

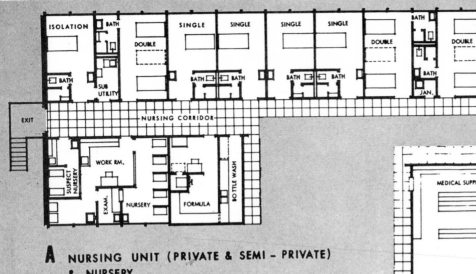

## A NURSING UNIT (PRIVATE & SEMI - PRIVATE) & NURSERY

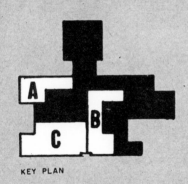

KEY PLAN

Above is the nursing unit of the 25-bed scheme, that is, the private and semi-private rooms and the nursery; there is also, in the top wing of the diagrammatic plan, the start of the ward wing, containing at present two four-bed wards and one eight-bed. At the right is the administration and service wing of the 25-bed scheme; and at the bottom the out-patient and adjunct facilities section, also of the 25-bed stage. Operating suite and delivery suite, plus central sterilizing, take up the space between the out-patient department and the nursing unit shown above

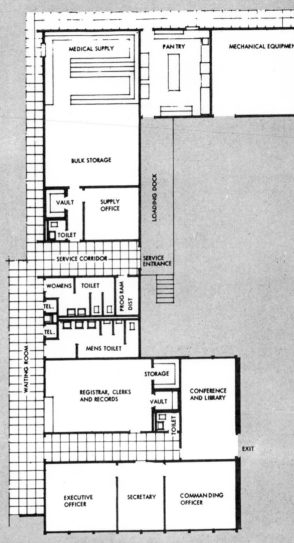

## B ADMINISTRATION AND SERVICE 25 BED STAGE

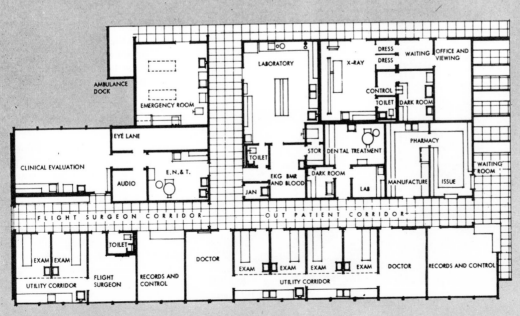

## C OUTPATIENT AND ADJUNCT FACILITIES

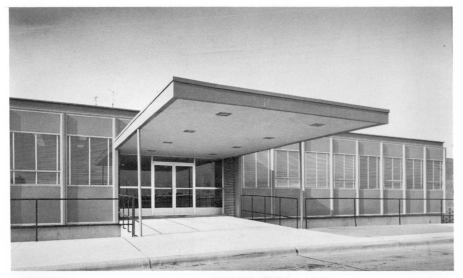

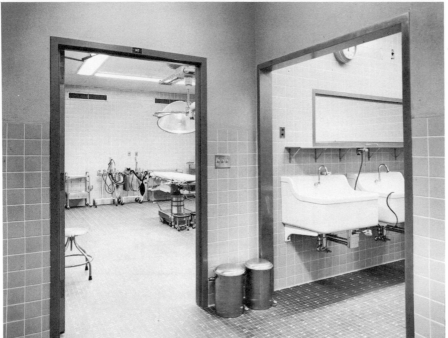

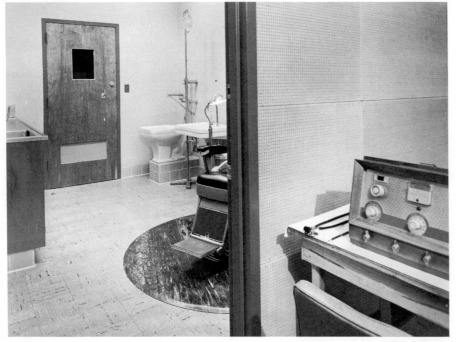

*Upper left:* main window walls are of prefabricated enameled iron panels set in steel sash frames. View shows main entrance, which opens in bottom of the plan diagram at outpatient department. *Center view* looks into main operating room, also into scrubup alcove. *Lower view at left* shows the ear, nose, and throat operating room, audio room at right of the photograph

*Opposite page:* plans at upper part show the ward section of the plan at both the 25- and 50-bed stages. The three eight-bed wards to be added in the expansion would virtually double the capacity of the hospital. Plan at bottom shows an interesting scheme to combine the operating suite and the delivery suite in one unit and yet to keep them isolated from each other for aseptic control

*A P I photos*

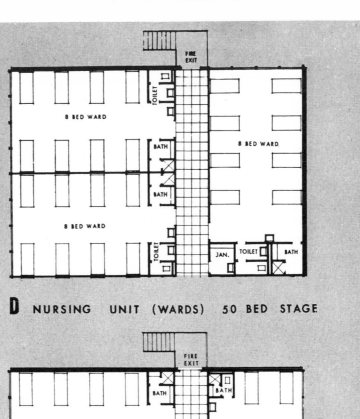

**D** NURSING UNIT (WARDS) 50 BED STAGE

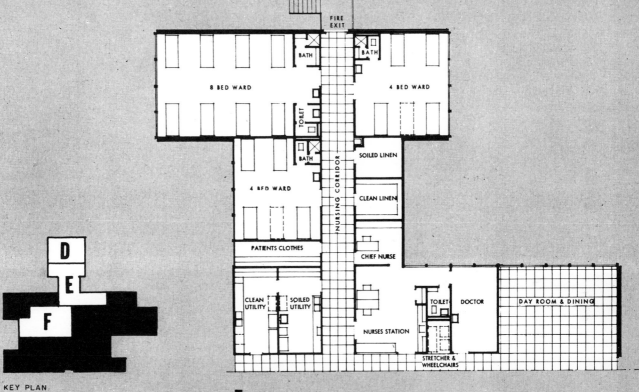

KEY PLAN

**E** NURSING UNIT (WARDS) 25 BED STAGE

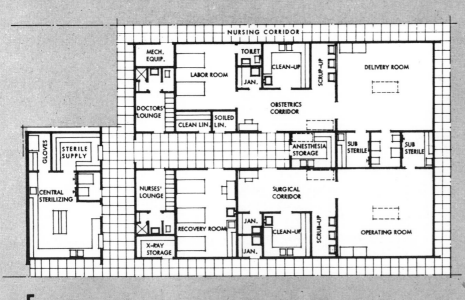

**F** SURGICAL AND OBSTETRICAL SUITES

5

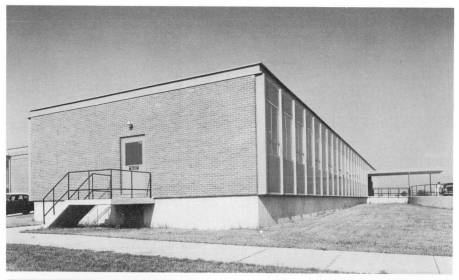

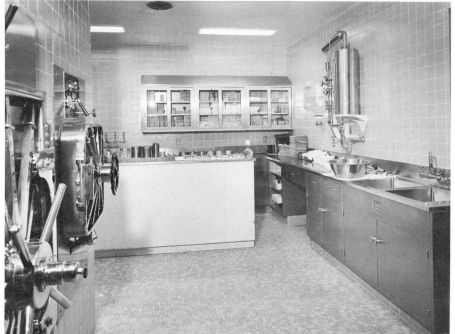

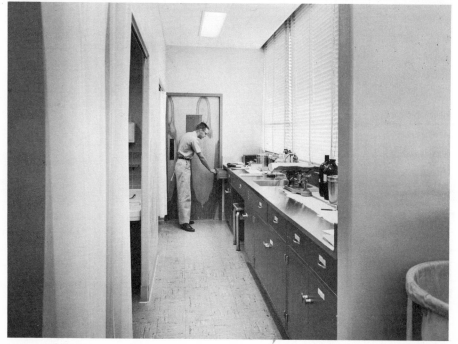

*Upper left:* end walls are of cavity wall construction, exterior panels of hard burned brick. They are neatly enclosed by enameled iron fascia and end of panel walls, to join well with window wall panels. *Left center:* view of central sterilizing room, shown in plan on preceding page. View in lower left shows utility corridor behind examining rooms in the flight surgeons suite

*Opposite page:* the plans shown here take a couple of the service areas to the 50-bed stage. The dining room fills in an area of the earlier stage plan left empty and involves some arrangement of the boiler room for the kitchen. The new office portion at the bottom of the page represents a considerable expansion of offices, addition of the library-conference room, plus morgue and record storage

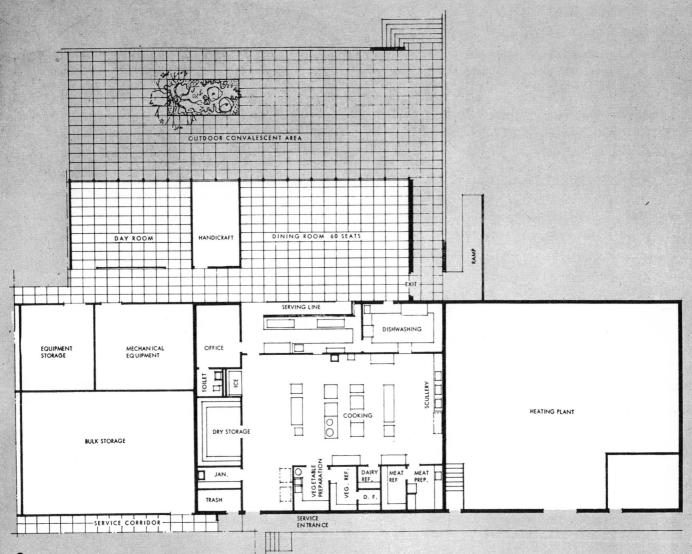

**G** SERVICE FACILITIES 50 BED STAGE

Labels within image 1:
OUTDOOR CONVALESCENT AREA
DAY ROOM · HANDICRAFT · DINING ROOM 60 SEATS · RAMP
EXIT · SERVING LINE · DISHWASHING
EQUIPMENT STORAGE · MECHANICAL EQUIPMENT · OFFICE · TOILET · ICE · SCULLERY · HEATING PLANT
BULK STORAGE · DRY STORAGE · COOKING
JAN. · VEGETABLE PREPARATION · VEG. REF. · DAIRY REF. · MEAT REF · MEAT PREP.
TRASH · D. F.
SERVICE CORRIDOR · SERVICE ENTRANCE

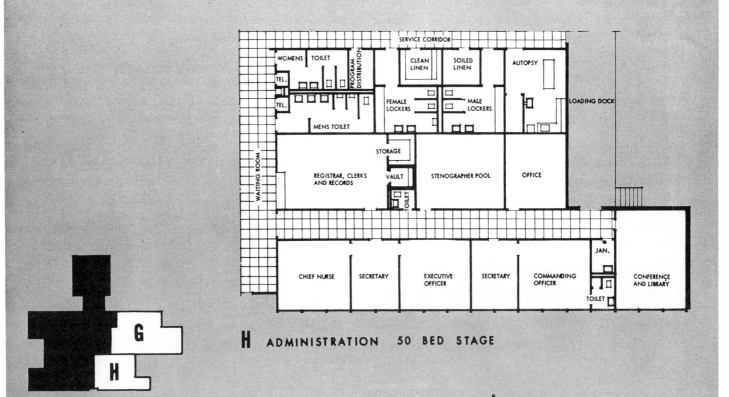

**H** ADMINISTRATION 50 BED STAGE

Labels within image 2:
SERVICE CORRIDOR
WOMENS TOILET · PROGRAM DISTRIBUTION · CLEAN LINEN · SOILED LINEN · AUTOPSY
TEL. · FEMALE LOCKERS · MALE LOCKERS · LOADING DOCK
TEL. · MENS TOILET
WAITING ROOM · STORAGE
REGISTRAR, CLERKS AND RECORDS · VAULT · STENOGRAPHER POOL · OFFICE
TOILET
CHIEF NURSE · SECRETARY · EXECUTIVE OFFICER · SECRETARY · COMMANDING OFFICER · JAN. · CONFERENCE AND LIBRARY
TOILET

KEY PLAN
G
H

5

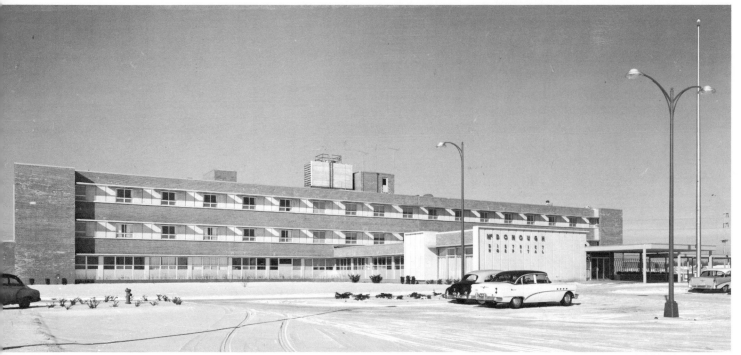

# Small Hospital for a Rural Community

*McDonough District Hospital, Macomb, Ill. Lankton-Ziegele-Terry and Associates, Architects; Gerhard Hartman, Ph.D., Hospital Consultant; Beling Engineering Consultants, Mechanical Engineers; Alfred Benesch and Associates, Structural Engineers; S. Patti Construction Co., General Contractors*

One of the heavily stressed objectives of the Hill-Burton program of the federal government is to get better hospital facilities in outlying districts. This hospital is the direct result of such purpose, following creation of a hospital district to build and operate a hospital in an area not previously served.

The architects make much of the fact that both they and the hospital consultant were named long before the selection of a site, and that the administrator was on the job a year and a half before completion of the building.

The hospital is a nominal 50-bed hospital, but all its basic facilities—kitchen and dining, operating, delivery, adjunct facilities, and so on—are adequate for a much larger building. Though present size should be sufficient for the next ten years or so, vertical expansion could add bedrooms at any time without disturbance to the working of the hospital.

Moreover, on the nursing floors the nurses' station and other facilities are so placed that wings can be sent out horizontally to complete the same cruciform plan as on the lower floors.

"It will be noted," say the architects, "that the plan of the hospital indicates that all patient rooms are semi-private rooms; in other words, one or two beds can be installed in each room. Each has its own toilet room, clothes locker, drawers and built-in vanity. Wallpaper was used on one wall of each patient room to add to the decorative effect. All patients' bathrooms are tiled, both floor and side wall. An extensive communication system between nurses' stations and patient rooms provides for good communication between these points. A great deal of attention was given during the planning to make the patient rooms as comfortable and cheerful as possible.

The building is completely air conditioned throughout. Costs are given as $24.42 per sq ft, for 87,942 sq ft; and $1.958 per cu ft, for 1,096,474 cu ft. These costs include all construction costs, built-in equipment such as sterilizers, kitchen equipment, built-in refrigerators, mortuary refrigerator and so on.

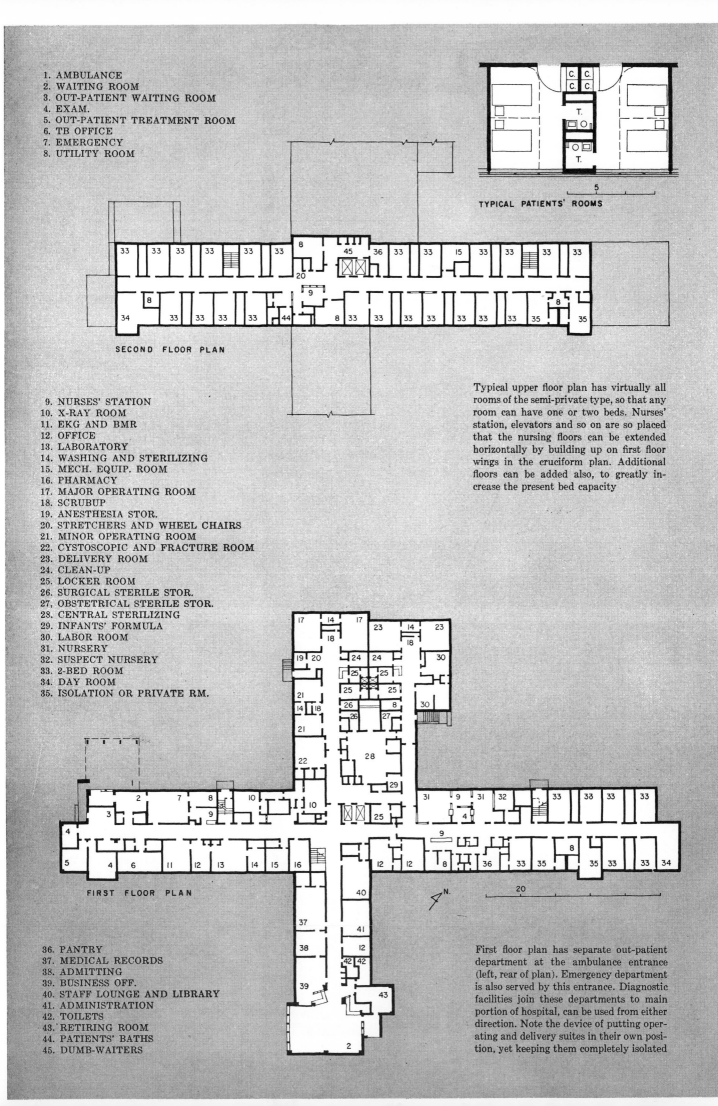

1. AMBULANCE
2. WAITING ROOM
3. OUT-PATIENT WAITING ROOM
4. EXAM.
5. OUT-PATIENT TREATMENT ROOM
6. TB OFFICE
7. EMERGENCY
8. UTILITY ROOM

TYPICAL PATIENTS' ROOMS

SECOND FLOOR PLAN

9. NURSES' STATION
10. X-RAY ROOM
11. EKG AND BMR
12. OFFICE
13. LABORATORY
14. WASHING AND STERILIZING
15. MECH. EQUIP. ROOM
16. PHARMACY
17. MAJOR OPERATING ROOM
18. SCRUBUP
19. ANESTHESIA STOR.
20. STRETCHERS AND WHEEL CHAIRS
21. MINOR OPERATING ROOM
22. CYSTOSCOPIC AND FRACTURE ROOM
23. DELIVERY ROOM
24. CLEAN-UP
25. LOCKER ROOM
26. SURGICAL STERILE STOR.
27. OBSTETRICAL STERILE STOR.
28. CENTRAL STERILIZING
29. INFANTS' FORMULA
30. LABOR ROOM
31. NURSERY
32. SUSPECT NURSERY
33. 2-BED ROOM
34. DAY ROOM
35. ISOLATION OR PRIVATE RM.

Typical upper floor plan has virtually all
rooms of the semi-private type, so that any
room can have one or two beds. Nurses'
station, elevators and so on are so placed
that the nursing floors can be extended
horizontally by building up on first floor
wings in the cruciform plan. Additional
floors can be added also, to greatly increase the present bed capacity

FIRST FLOOR PLAN

N

36. PANTRY
37. MEDICAL RECORDS
38. ADMITTING
39. BUSINESS OFF.
40. STAFF LOUNGE AND LIBRARY
41. ADMINISTRATION
42. TOILETS
43. RETIRING ROOM
44. PATIENTS' BATHS
45. DUMB-WAITERS

First floor plan has separate out-patient
department at the ambulance entrance
(left, rear of plan). Emergency department
is also served by this entrance. Diagnostic
facilities join these departments to main
portion of hospital, can be used from either
direction. Note the device of putting operating and delivery suites in their own position, yet keeping them completely isolated

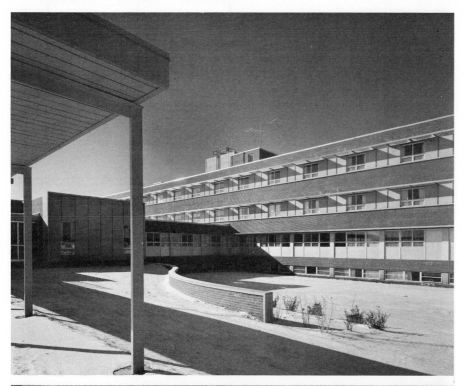

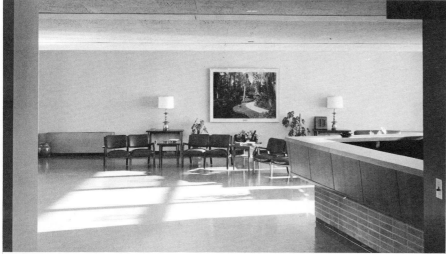

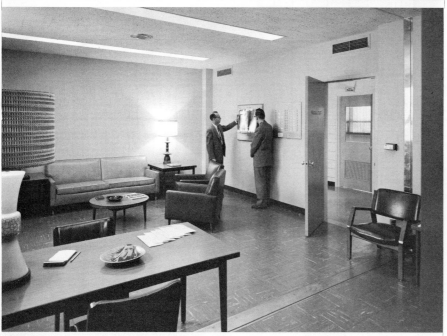

Hedrich-Blessing

*Left above:* although the site was flat Illinois farm land, considerable grading was done to permit access to the front of the hospital without steps, and to provide loading dock at the basement level in the rear. *Left, center:* view of the main lobby. *Left, bottom:* view of medical staff lounge and library

*Opposite page:* nurseries are in a corner location between delivery suite and maternity nursing unit, in corridor closed off from main hospital traffic. *Bottom, opposite page:* view into main operating room, with scrubup sinks shown at the right

*McDonough District Hospital*

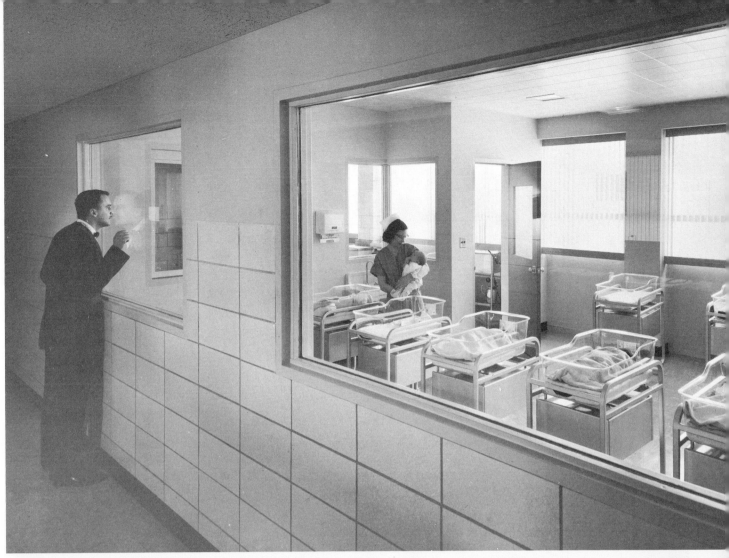

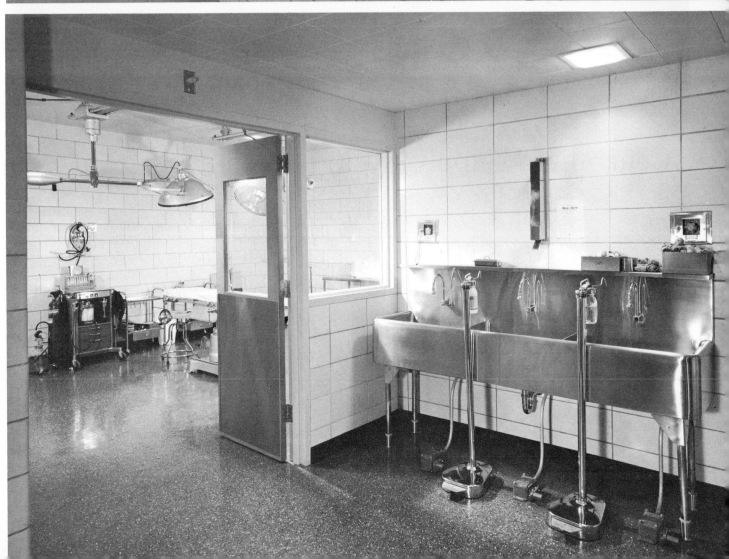

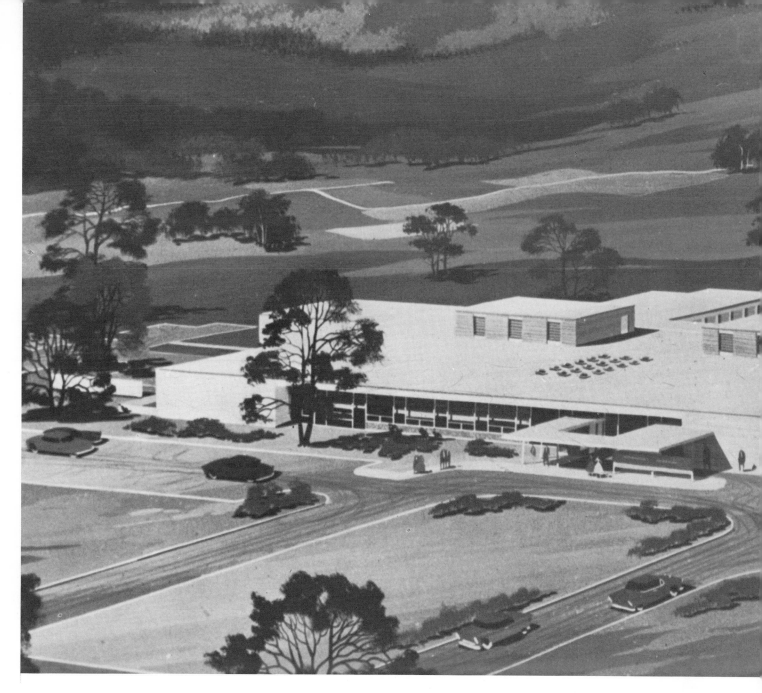

# Centralized Supply System Permits Logical Plan

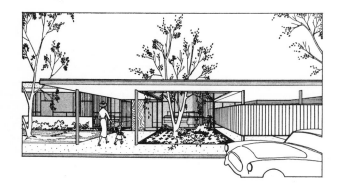

*Proposed Berwick Hospital, Berwick, Pa. Architects: Noakes & Neubauer; Associate Architect: Edmund George Good, Jr.; Medical Consultants: Gordon A. Friesen Associates; Consulting Engineers: Shefferman and Bigelson*

AN "AUTOMAT" SYSTEM of organizing and dispatching hospital supplies, developed by Consultant Gordon Friesen, has permitted Architect Edward Noakes to arrange a very interesting plan. A 92-bed hospital on one floor is a considerable expanse of complicated departmental dispositions, and the supply system of any hospital is an important determinant of the plan arrangements.

Friesen's supply scheme, developed from similar systems he used in the United Mine Workers hospitals, puts a dispatch center in the center of the building, where are grouped central sterilizing department, laundry, bulk and processed stores, laboratory, pharmacy

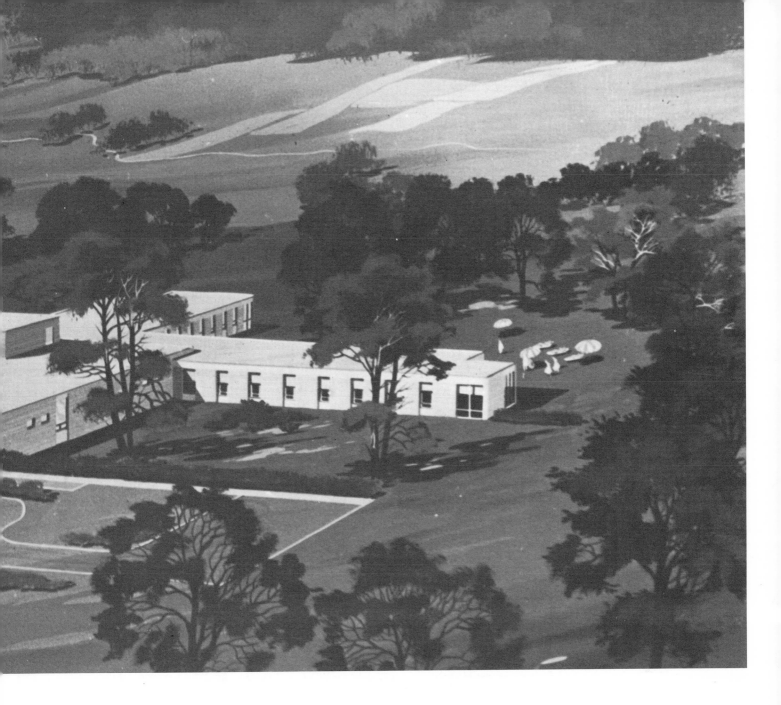

and linen rooms. From here, by special carts, supplies of everything needed in normal routines go out to every location in the hospital. The scheme is calculated to cut drastically a nurse's daily travel. Naturally the above listed grouping is a radical departure in hospital organization.

It doesn't require much study of the plan to see how logically various departments group themselves around the central supply department. The operating suite is perhaps most important; it is strategically placed with respect to supplies, laboratory, pharmacy, also x-ray and emergency. Incidentally, notice the unconventional arrangement of operating rooms with two-corridor approach — clean supplies separated from dirty, separate access for surgeons, and so on.

The delivery suite is well isolated, well separated from operating, but again close to the source of supplies. The maternity nursing unit takes off in its own wing from

the corner near the delivery group; it can expand toward the center of the building as required.

The nursing units cluster close around the central supply, coming to a focus in two nursing stations, well removed from traffic and noise.

The emergency suite is close to the main entrance, an idea Friesen rather insists upon. Notice that the receptionist can see into the emergency corridor, but waiting room guests are shielded from possibly unpleasant sights. This control from main desk would be very important in the wee small hours. So many people, in an emergency, naturally drive to the front of the hospital, points out Friesen, and how are they to know they should go around to the back, and then perhaps find only a locked door?

An especially good feature of this plan is the service entrance and short delivery corridor. The important departments to be served — boiler room, kitchen, stores,

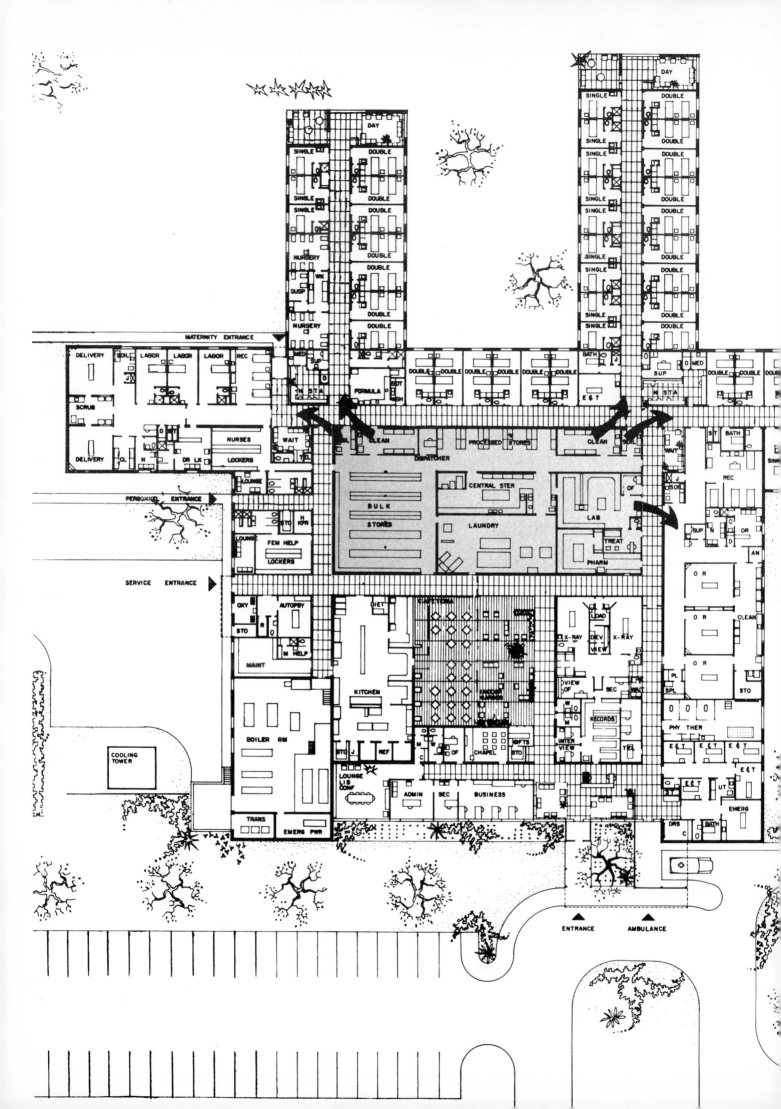

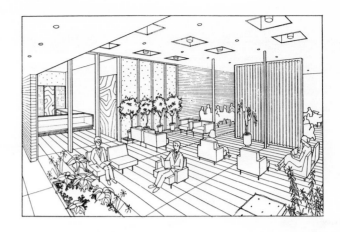

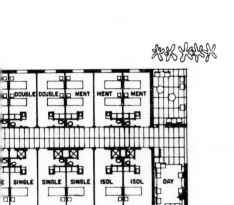

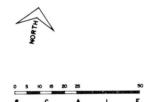

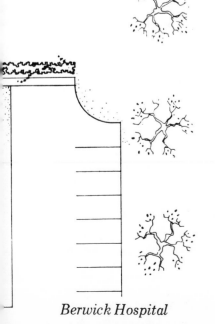

and so on, cluster neatly around this corridor.

The whole plan is worthy of study, representing an almost complete rearrangement of traditional groupings.

The architects express themselves as being quite happy about the cost data. The building itself came out quite reasonably — some 50 per cent of the total cost is represented by mechanical and electrical, allowing for future air conditioning of the whole plant. Total cost of the project, on the basis of bids, runs to $1,284,600, or $13,960 per bed for a capacity of 92 beds. The general construction contract puts this per bed cost at $12,174, or $18.24 per square foot, $1.53 per cube. (This is going up to $18.73 per square foot in a proposed change order involving air conditioning, the earlier figures representing air conditioning completely installed for only operating, delivery and nursery suites.) The total project cost included $75,600 for Group I equipment. Group II equipment, not included, is estimated at $88,800, though much Group II and Group III is being re-used, from their existing hospital.

Construction is masonry bearing walls, bar joist and poured gypsum roof construction, concrete slab on ground, concrete block partitions plastered.

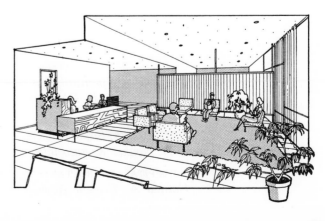

*Berwick Hospital*

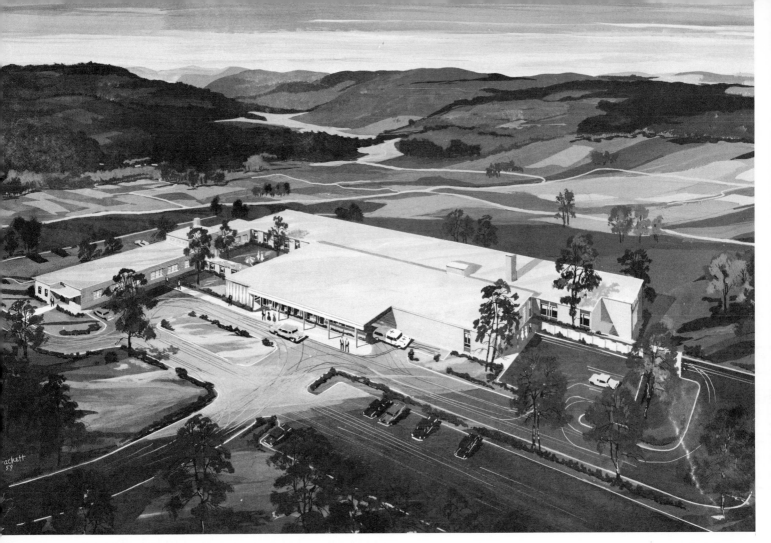

# Hospital Plan Based on Supply System Organization

CARROLL COUNTY
GENERAL HOSPITAL,
WESTMINSTER,
MARYLAND

ARCHITECT:
*(Working Drawings, Specifications)*
*B. E. Starr*

ASSOCIATE ARCHITECTS:
*(Design, Supervision)*
*Edward H. Noakes & Associates*

HOSPITAL CONSULTANTS:
*Gordon A. Friesen Assoc.*

The basic guiding principle behind the planning of this 64-bed general hospital was the idea that better nursing care is possible in a hospital if the nurses are freed from responsibility for supplies. In order to achieve this, the architects and hospital consultants worked out a design based on a highly organized and efficient supply system. In the hospital, clean supplies will be handled and distributed and soiled supplies collected and processed, by the supply crew. Control will be the responsibility of a dispatcher. Routine supply handling will be done automatically by the crew. An intercom station in each patient room will permit nurses to call for extra or special supplies, without leaving the room. These will be delivered by the supply crew.

All of the 32 patient rooms in the hospital are planned for double occupancy. Facilities were sized for eventual expansion of capacity to approximately 110 beds. The emergency entrance is controlled from the switchboard location and connects directly with the emergency suite, radiology, laboratory, and other patient facilities. A separate entrance is provided for maternity patients and doctors. This leads directly to the delivery suite and maternity nursing unit. Administrative elements are located in (and shared with) an existing health center adjoining the hospital.

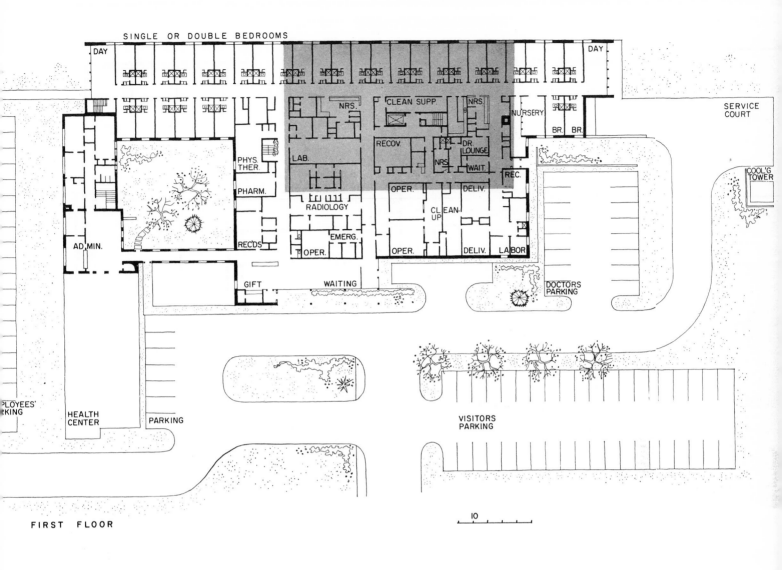

FIRST FLOOR

10

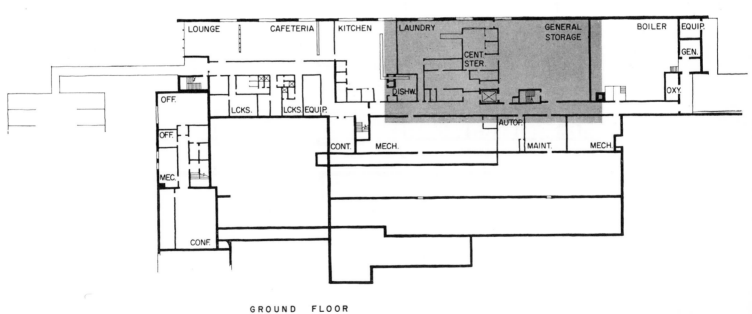

GROUND FLOOR

Utilizing the 10 per cent grade of the site, the architects placed all service elements in the basement, all patient facilities on the main floor. The core of the main floor plan is the central supply area. New supplies are received at special entrance on ground level. These and soiled supplies are processed on this level and distributed on special carts. Clean patient supplies are delivered to patient supply cabinets located near the entrance to each room where they are available to nurses within the rooms. Soiled supplies are placed by nurses in the soiled compartments of the cabinets. From here, they are picked up in the corridor and returned to central supply on carts. Total area: 52,000 sq ft. Total beds: 64. Estimated cost including site work and Group I equipment: $1,156,000. Estimated cost Group II and III equipment $150,000. Cost per bed: $20,400

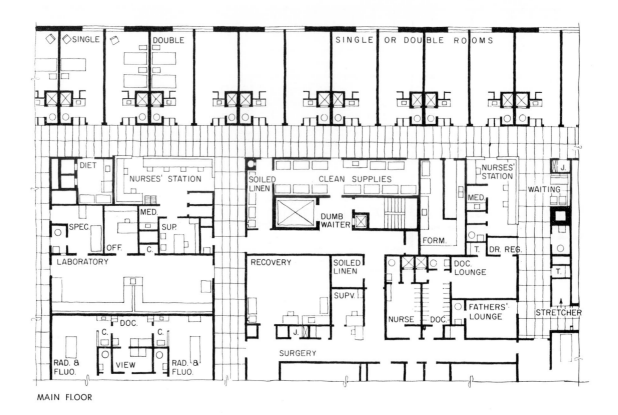

MAIN FLOOR

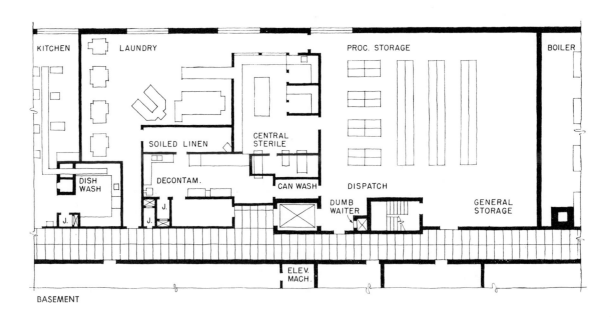

BASEMENT

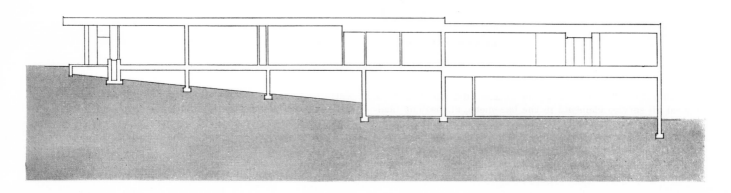

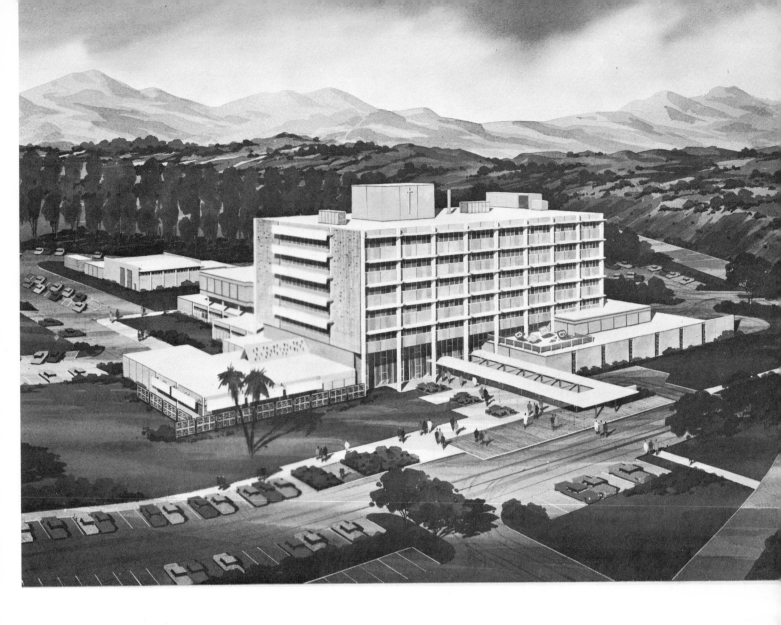

# Improved Supply System for Better Patient Care

*Holy Cross Hospital (Sisters of the Holy Cross), San Fernando, Calif.; Gene Verge and R. N. Clatworthy, Architects; Gordon Friesen and Associates, Consultants; Steed Brothers Construction Co., Contractors*

The central guiding principle for the design of this hospital was the provision of intensive personal nursing care for each patient when and if he needs it. This sounds easy, but as every hospital architect knows, it isn't. The costs of good nursing care together with the extreme shortage of trained personnel combine to prevent—usually—a workable solution to this problem. In addition, the high costs of construction today often prevent some of the best planning principles from being applied. In this hospital, the architects, the consultant, and the Sisters of the Holy Cross have given their best efforts to the provision of topflight nursing care, at minimum cost in nursing time (and therefore, money). In order to accomplish these objectives, the plan utilizes an extension of the automated supply systems employed in the United Mine Workers hospitals and a few other institutions. In the main, the systems involve the prepackaging of sterile supplies, and their distribution through a flow system similar in many respects to those in industry. Through the use of this system and careful planning, it is expected that the patients of this hospital can be cared for in private rooms, at reasonable costs, and, in addition, that construction costs can be held down.

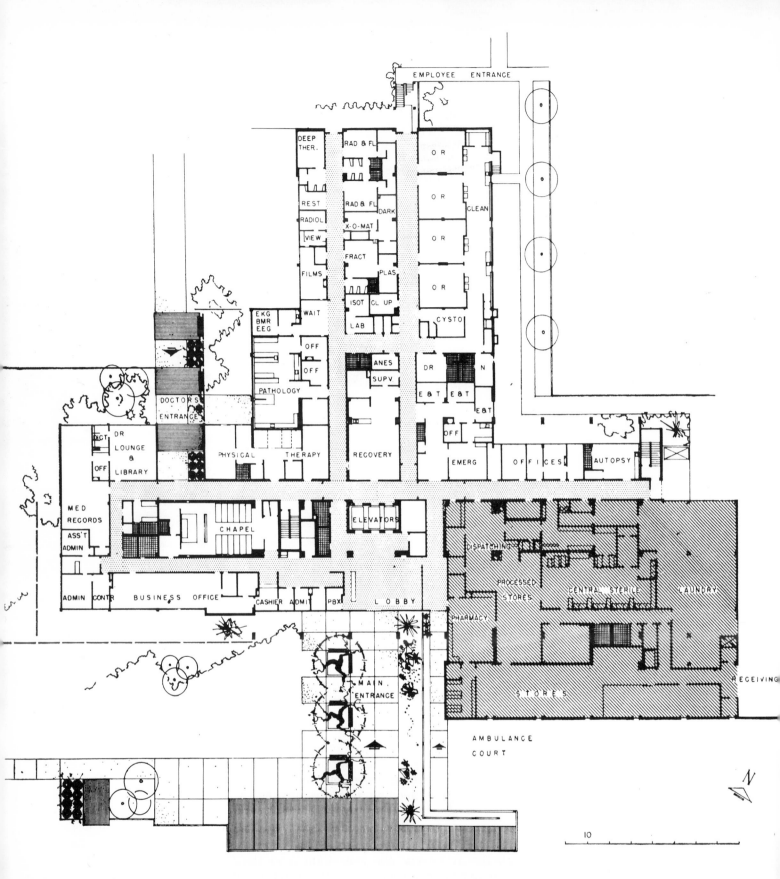

## MAIN FLOOR

The hub of the supply system is the central area shown above and right. Incoming supplies are received and transferred to their respective storage areas; from here, the supplies are sent to the preparation area, and sterilized or otherwise processed, and then sent to the dispatcher. Soiled supplies arrive in their receiving area via chutes or conveyors. Waste and refuse go to the incinerator; linen and dry goods go to the laundry. Utensils and similar items are cleaned and sterilized. All clean supplies pass through the preparation area, and if not sterilized previously, pass on to the sterilizing area. From here, they go to processed stores, where the dispatcher sends them to their destinations via mechanized tray conveyors with ejector systems for automatic unloading

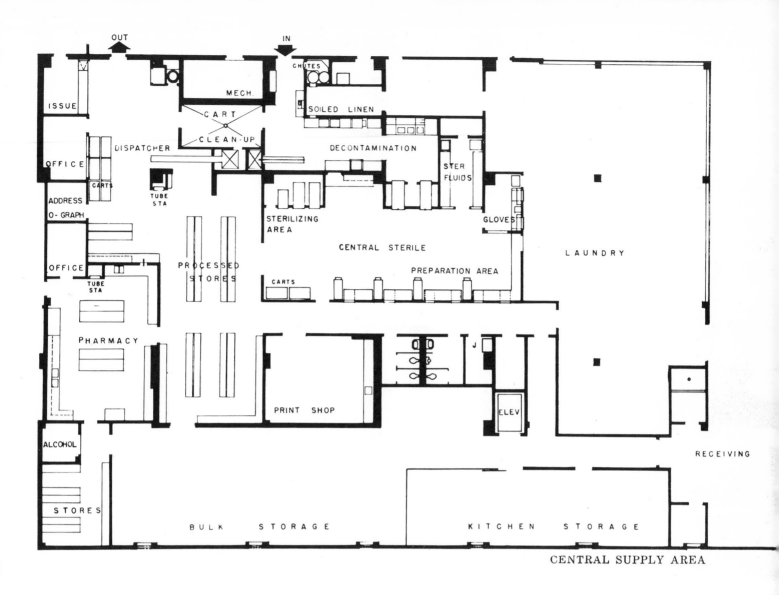

CENTRAL SUPPLY AREA

Of utmost importance in reducing bacterial count and reducing the spread of infection are the techniques and equipment to be used in this hospital for processing soiled supplies and other items. Cleaning equipment to be provided in the soiled supply area of central supply will include a clinical hopper sink, a pair of manual washing sinks, an automatic mechanical utensil washer, an automatic mechanical laboratory glass washer, a needle cleaner, a large combination action ultrasonic cleaner and two large double door sterilizers. Items such as bedpans will be cleaned with brushes and germicide in the clinical hopper sink. Items that require more precise cleaning will be thoroughly processed in the ultrasonic cleaner. In this machine, sound waves of a proper type will be introduced into a germicidal detergent solution, causing great pressure differentials to build up (the process is called cavitation). The energy released as these pressures move toward equilibrium tears the soil from the items being cleaned, and breaks up bacterial clumps. In this way, the germicide can more effectively attack the bacteria, resulting in more efficient than usual germicidal action. The bacterial count is appreciably reduced. The mechanical washers are operated in the usual manner. The two large sterilizers (autoclaves) are both of the high-speed type, and are equipped with high pressure steam. In addition, one is provided with equipment for ethylene oxide gas sterilization. After all of the cleaning and sterilization processes have been completed, each item will be enclosed in a sterile plastic bag to insure that it is not contaminated with bacteria enroute to the place where it will be used. Handling of supplies after sterilization will be kept to a minimum, for the same reasons and for efficiency. After final cleaning, sterilization, and packaging, they will be checked and dispatched to patient floors on the tray conveyors.

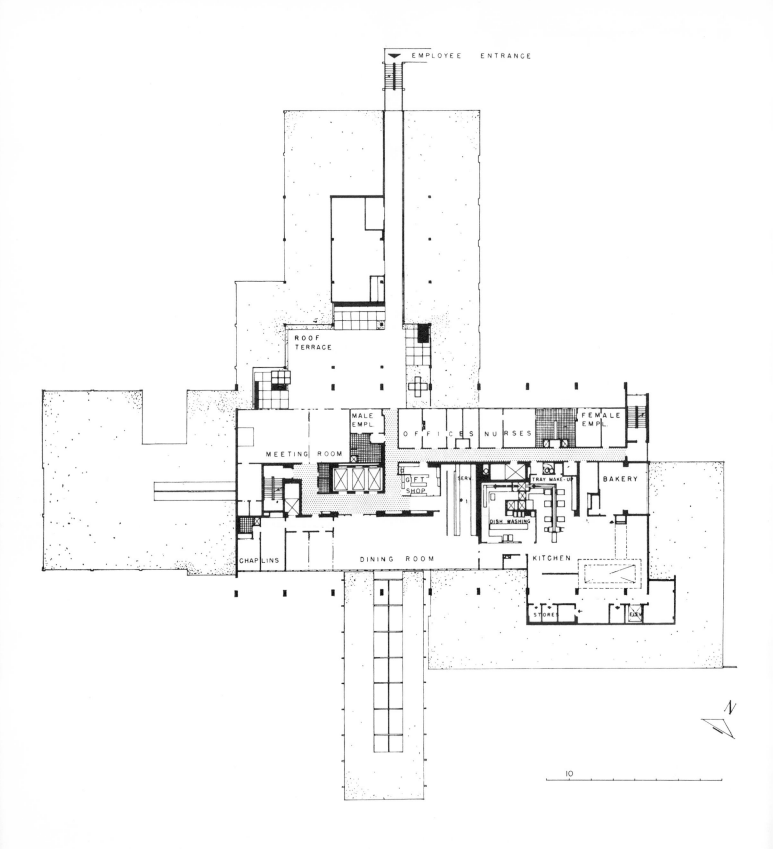

EMPLOYEE ENTRANCE

ROOF
TERRACE

MALE
EMPL.

OFFICES NURSES

FEMALE
EMPL.

MEETING ROOM

GIFT
SHOP

SERV.

TRAY MAKE-UP

BAKERY

DISH WASHING

CHAPLINS

DINING ROOM

KITCHEN

STORES

ELEV.

N

10

## SECOND FLOOR

Shown in the plan is the second floor, which acts as a buffer between the main hospital
floor below and the nursing floors above. Only non-medical facilities are located on this
floor. These include offices for nurses and administration, the chaplains' offices, a large
meeting room with adjacent roof terrace, a gift shop, and the dining-kitchen facilities.
By concentrating these non-medical functions on one floor of the building, it has been
possible to physically remove them from any direct interference with the major work
of the hospital. The kitchen, in addition to servicing the dining area on this floor,
prepares the food for patients in the rooms above. Prepared food is dispatched from
the kitchen to nursing floors via automatic tray conveyors and several dumbwaiters

## TYPICAL NURSING FLOOR

Clean supplies from the central supply area below arrive in the core areas on the patient floors via automatic subveyors. Included in the system are facilities for handling food as well as other supplies. From this area, items are sent directly to patient rooms or other places where they are needed. Soiled supplies collected will be brought to the soiled receiving area on the patient floors and dispatched via the chutes or conveyor to the main soiled supply area directly below.

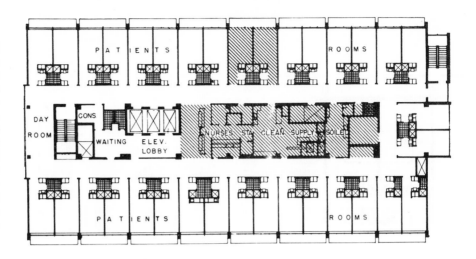

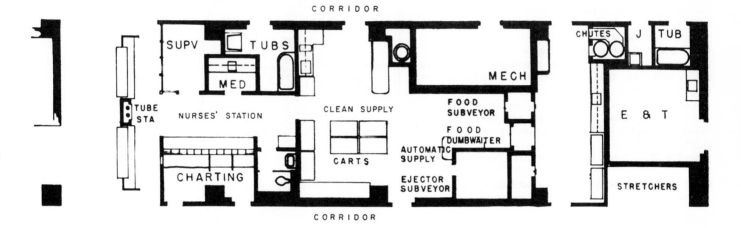

The installation of the very advanced supply system in this hospital is expected to bring about many other benefits in addition to increased efficiency, and its corollary, better nursing care for the patients. Obviously, an important advance has been made if it is possible, as projected here, to give each patient a private room and complete bath, without increasing the budget to astronomical proportions. The amenities in this are most apparent. Additionally, patients are expected to benefit from a sharp decrease in cross-infection. This will be partially due to their isolation from each other brought about by the private rooms. Of equal importance in the reduction of infection will be the extremely good control of sterilization and handling of supplies throughout the entire system. The installation of the individual supply cabinets to be used in each patient room represents a long-cherished dream of the consultant, Mr. Friesen, who has felt that the supplies must be put where the nurses are. It is his conviction that the place of the nurse is at the bedside of the patient. The best way to keep her there is to give her what she needs, where and when she needs it. In this way, the nurses may spend their time profitably looking after the patients, rather than looking for supplies. Nurses may go from one patient to the next, giving care without ever doubling back to the supply area. If some item is missing, the nurse may have it dispatched immediately from the central supply area, by simply calling the floor dispatching center to deliver it. All of this, of course, adds up to increased performance in meaningful activities for the nurses, leading to increased benefits for the patients and, undoubtedly, speeded up healing processes.

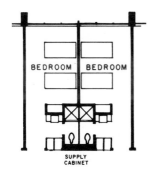

BEDROOM | BEDROOM

SUPPLY CABINET

Each patient room is provided with a utility section which contains a complete bathroom with shower stall and a supply cabinet especially designed to become an integral part of the overall supply system. The supply cabinet is built into the wall, next to the entrance door. It is divided vertically in the center. One side is used for clean supplies, the other for soiled. Double doors are provided on both the hall and the patient room sides. Clean supplies (in plastic bags) are placed in the cabinet by an attendant. They may be removed from the opposite side when needed. Soiled supplies are handled in a similar manner with the flow reversed

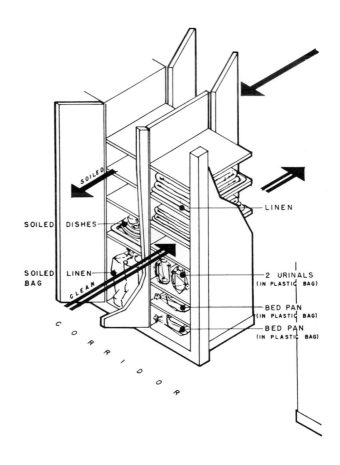

The general treasurer of the Sisters of the Holy Cross, Sister Mary Gerald, says of the hospital, "the sisters of the Holy Cross are dedicated to caring for the physical, mental, social, spiritual, and financial needs of their patients. Their dedication recognizes the moral obligation to discharge with economy and efficiency the responsibility of spending the millions entrusted to them for the care of the sick to whom they are privileged to minister. Countless hours of valuable time are lost in hospitals because nurses, aides, and orderlies must obtain essential supplies from dozens of sources, generally remote from the surgery, delivery, or patients' rooms. Transporting supplies through busy corridors and elevators by day results in confusion and waste of time. Holy Cross Hospital will have a revolutionary system of supply that will save, it is estimated, about 30 per cent of the nurses' time. The basic principle for the system is the placement of all supplies on a production line. Much of the supply handling will be done at night. Early ambulation has decreased the need for bed baths. Therefore, each patient room is equipped with a shower. The private shower room enables the nurse to make the bed while the patient bathes, and makes unnecessary the need to walk with the patient to and from a general shower room. Since nursing service is the largest item of expense in any hospital's budget, the cost of individual showers will be amortized within a short time through the saving of nursing time. The entrance to the emergency department will be adjacent to the main entrance, enabling the night attendant to see that emergency cases receive immediate attention. The chapel, located off the lobby, will be convenient for patients, personnel, and visitors. All patients' rooms will provide excellent views of the towering mountains of the San Fernando Valley."

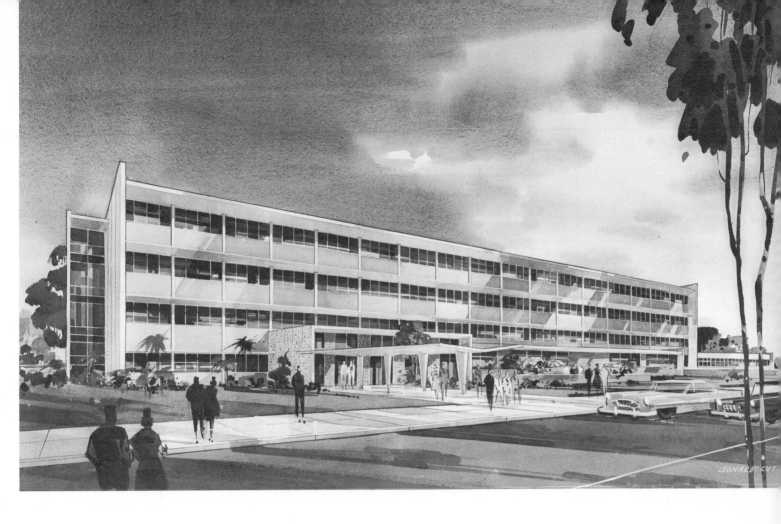

# General Hospital Planned for Expansion

*South Bay Hospital, Redondo Beach, California; Walker, Kalionzes, and Klingerman, Architects; August W. Koenig, Hospital Consultant*

This hospital is a good example of a solution to a problem which often faces the architect. The need for an institution in this location having been established, its size was determined by a projection of future requirements, and then pared down to a size which would be feasible at the present time. Thus, all decisions made during the design and planning stages had to take into consideration not one, but actually two projects— the hospital to be built now, and the one into which it must grow later.

The hospital was designed for 250 beds. Only 149 of these will be provided for in the first stage of construction, the remainder to be included in a four-story nursing wing to be constructed later on the south side of the building. Most of the medical, surgical, and auxiliary facilities which will be needed for the complete hospital will be included in the first phase. In this way, all general hospital services will be available from the time the first phase is completed. The hospital is to be located on a ten-acre site, overlooking the Pacific Ocean. The decision to build it here grew out of a survey and study of this area made by the consultant, in 1955. The complete institution will serve a hospital district of approximately 40 square miles, which includes the cities of Manhattan Beach, Hermosa Beach, and Redondo Beach. The approximately 12 square miles these cities occupy is one of the most densely populated areas of California. The site is near the geographical and population center of the hospital district.

Close attention to expansion, the site, and other problems has resulted in a multi-story structure which is quite simple and compact. It is expected to be economical to build and operate, because of the importance given in the planning to details of traffic flow, general services, and vertical transportation.

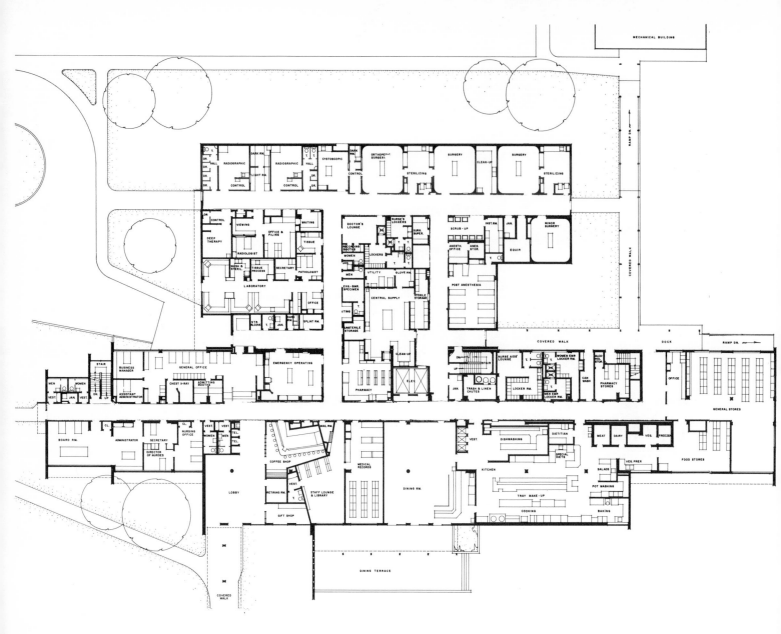

FIRST FLOOR

The over-all scheme for this hospital includes four floors and a partial basement. A separate building houses the boilers and other equipment. Future additions will include an additional 100 beds in a new nursing wing, and an extension of the boiler room to provide the additional capacity that will be required. The basement will contain equipment rooms, laundry, morgue, and physical therapy spaces. Approximately one-half of its area will be unassigned at present, but earmarked for future expansion of these facilities.

The first floor is devoted to admission facilities, administration areas, dining and kitchen, central supply, and complete surgical facilities with all necessary auxiliary spaces. As may be seen in the plan, these areas are zoned away from each other when possible. However, related facilities are conveniently placed near each other; all areas are connected by a system of interlocking halls. The second floor contains complete obstetrical facilities, including delivery suites, nurseries, nursing wings, and all auxiliary spaces required. The third and fourth floors are complete nursing units. They are quite similar in plan, except that a portion of the fourth floor is to be used for a separate pediatric nursing unit with a minimum of ten beds and its own nurses' station. A special post anesthesia room near the surgical suite has been provided for recovery of patients who have undergone surgery.

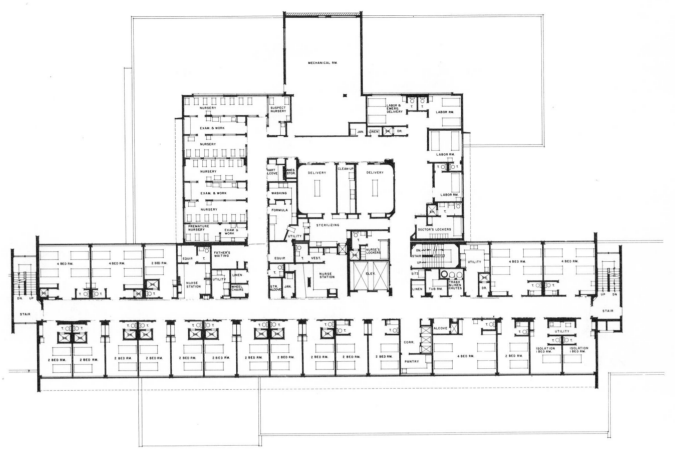

SECOND FLOOR

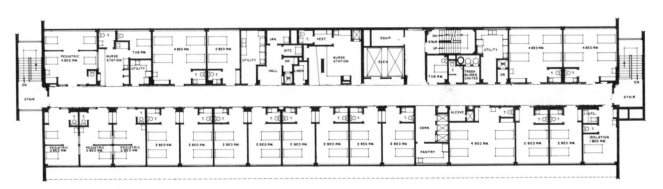

TYPICAL NURSING FLOOR

The supply system of this hospital revolves around the central supply area, located near the geographical center of the first floor. In this area, all of the necessary medical and surgical supplies are prepared and sent to surgery, emergency, and delivery departments, and to other areas of the hospital where patients are cared for. Complete sterilizing facilities are provided here. From central supply and the pharmacy located nearby, supplies are dispatched via dumbwaiters to the floors above, and are received in the delivery suite or nurses' stations on the patient floors. Another design feature of interest is the placement of the emergency near the admitting office rather than adjacent to surgery. It seems logical, in many respects, for emergency to be located in this position. It is intended that all surgery for emergency cases will be handled in the regular surgical suite, although cleaning up and preparation will be performed in the emergency room. In this way, it will be possible for emergency cases to receive the same high standard of surgical care available to any other patient, in the regular surgical suites away from the crowds which often gather in the emergency rooms during crises

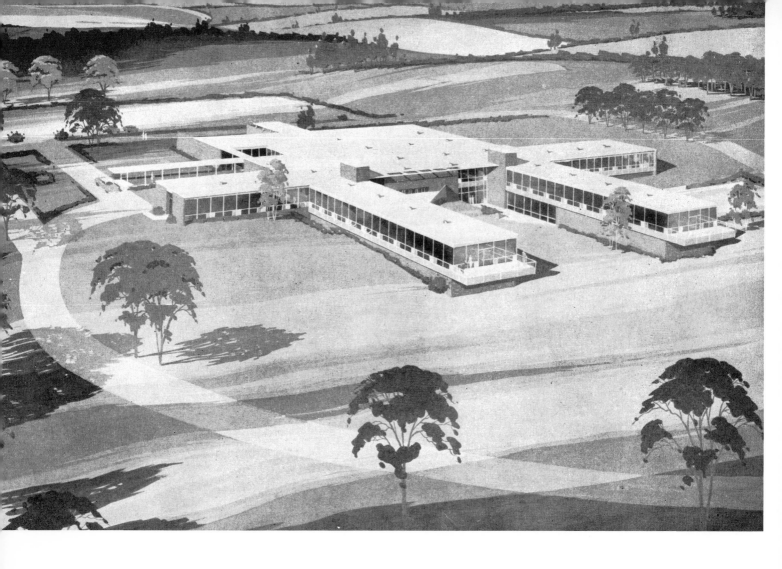

# Hospital Planned for Unusual Emergency Requirements in Industrial Area

NORTH KANSAS CITY
MEMORIAL HOSPITAL,
NORTH KANSAS CITY,
MISSOURI

ARCHITECTS & ENGINEERS:
*Hewitt and Royer;*
*Harry L. Wagner, Associate;*
*F. Wm. Shuler,*
*Supervising Architect*

CONTRACTOR:
*Bennett Construction Company*

A major problem which was solved in the design of this 100-bed general hospital was the abnormally large number of accident cases to be treated. The number of emergency cases of this type is due largely to the industrial nature of the surrounding area and the frequency of auto accidents occurring on the nearby highways. To facilitate the efficient handling of accident cases, the emergency entrance is prominently located, and easily identified. The area allotted to this section is larger than might otherwise have been provided. For purposes of control, it is located in a position adjacent to the central business office. Although the number of outpatients is relatively small, facilities for them were also located near the business office, thus facilitating treatment. Double-loaded corridors are used throughout the surgery, delivery, and outpatient areas in order to minimize patient circulation between these and other areas in the hospital. Plans include provisions for eventual expansion to 250 beds if required.

A steel frame structure, with concrete floor and steel roof deck, is used in the building. Exterior walls are brick with a curtain wall of porcelain enamel panels and glass in aluminum frames. Ceilings throughout are finished with acoustical plaster. Interior partitions throughout the entire building are metal studs with plaster.

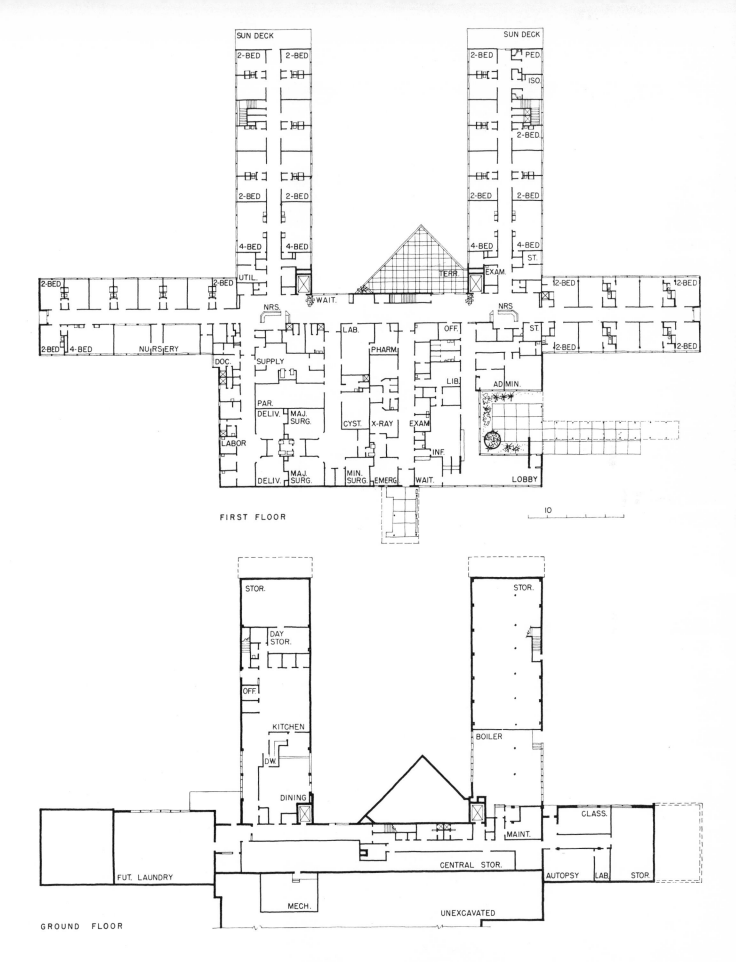

**FIRST FLOOR**

SUN DECK

2-BED 2-BED

2-BED 2-BED

4-BED 4-BED

2-BED 2-BED UTIL. WAIT. TERR. EXAM.

NRS NRS

2-BED 4-BED NURSERY LAB. OFF. ST.

DOC. SUPPLY PHARM.

LIB. ADMIN.

PAR. DELIV. MAJ. SURG.

LABOR CYST. X-RAY EXAM.

INF.

DELIV. MAJ. SURG. MIN. SURG. EMERG. WAIT. LOBBY

10

SUN DECK

2-BED PED.

ISO.

2-BED

2-BED 2-BED

4-BED 4-BED ST.

2-BED 2-BED

ST.

2-BED 2-BED

**GROUND FLOOR**

STOR. STOR.

DAY STOR.

OFF.

KITCHEN BOILER

D.W.

DINING

MAINT. CLASS.

FUT. LAUNDRY CENTRAL STOR. AUTOPSY LAB. STOR.

MECH. UNEXCAVATED

As may be seen in the plans, the scheme for this hospital involves a one-story building with a basement, part of which is unexcavated. All patient facilities are located on the main floor. Nursing wings are arranged for segregation of different types of patients. The two nurses' stations are placed so that each has control over two of the four nursing areas. In this way, approximately one-half (50) of the patients are handled from each station. Four-bed wards and semi-private rooms only are provided. The only private accommodations are the isolation and psychiatric rooms required under the Hill-Burton program. Because of the slope of the site, the basement is partially above grade. In it are located various service areas

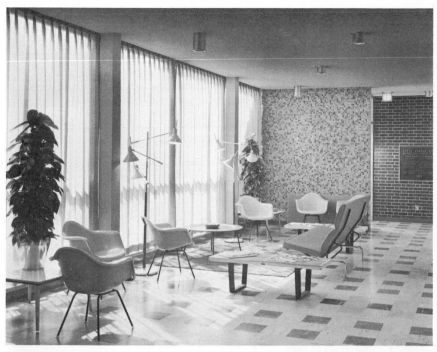

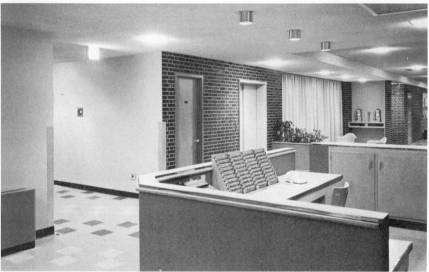

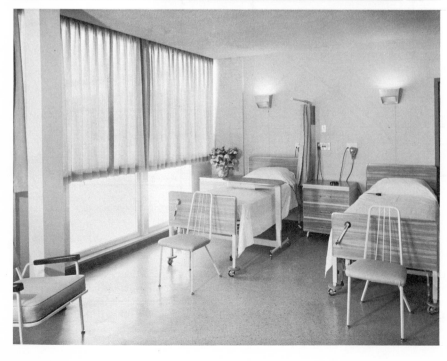

Left, top: view of waiting room toward the entrance vestibule. Left, center: each nurses' station is located at the intersection of two nursing wings. Stations are larger than normal, because of greater than usual number of nurses needed for handling of 50 patients from each station. Left, bottom: typical rooms have two patient beds. The large glass area permits unrestricted view of the river and provides patients with maximum amount of light and sun. Heavy glass fiber curtains are used for sun control. Space economy was achieved in the patient rooms by the decision not to build any private rooms. However, all rooms are air conditioned and have individual controls. Each room is equipped with radio and television with individual pillow speakers, nurse call, telephone, and piped oxygen

HOSPITAL BUILDINGS

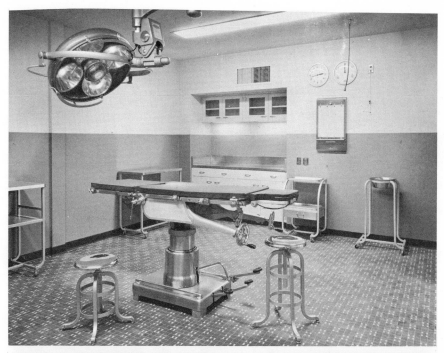

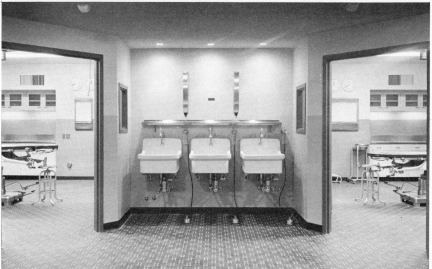

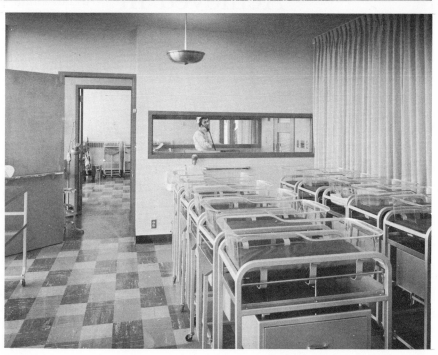

Right, top: view of one of two major surgeries. The surgeries are connected to each other by a scrub-up room (right, center). Right bottom: view of a nursery toward the workroom which connects it with the second nursery. Double-loaded corridors are provided for these areas and throughout other hospital areas in order to minimize patient and staff travel between various facilities.

COST TABULATION:

| | |
|---|---|
| Total Area (sq ft) | 50,480 |
| Total Usable Beds | 100 |
| Basic Construction Cost | $1,116,731 |
| Group I, II, III Equip., Fees, other equipment | 253,269 |
| **TOTAL PROJECT COST** | **$1,370,000** |
| **TOTAL COST PER BED** | **$13,700** |

Hospital constructed with assistance of Hill-Burton funds, administered by Division of Health, State of Missouri

*North Kansas City Memorial Hospital*

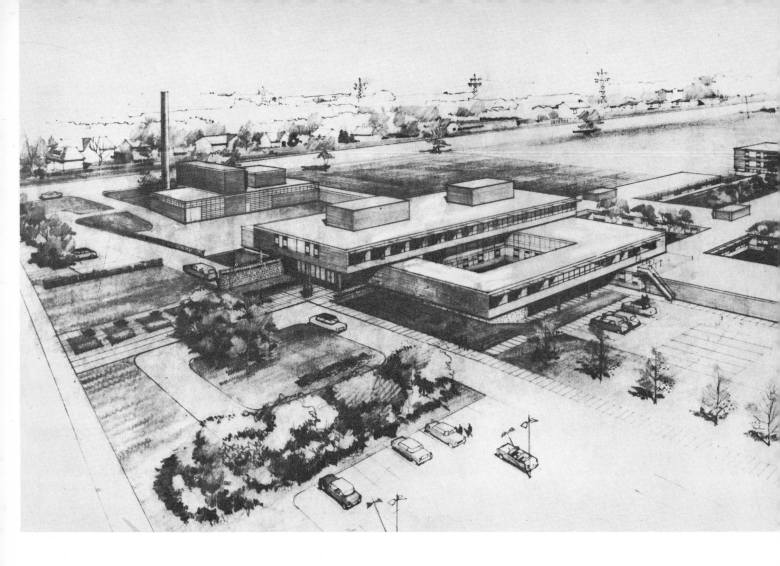

# High Efficiency, Lower Costs Achieved in Low-Rise Hospital

THE GREATER NIAGARA
GENERAL HOSPITAL
NIAGARA FALLS,
ONTARIO

ARCHITECTS & ENGINEERS:
*John B. Parkin Associates*

HOSPITAL CONSULTANTS:
*Agnew, Peckham & Associates*

CONTRACTORS:
*Smith Brothers Construction, Ltd.*

The scheme for this hospital was based on studies made by Dr. MacKinnon Phillips, former Provincial Minister of Health. These studies showed that a large percentage of the beds in a general hospital are occupied by non-acute cases. These patients require a minimum of care. Using this information, the architects placed nursing units for intensive care patients near the core of the building where diagnostic and treatment facilities are located; patients requiring a minimum of care are housed in a series of one-story nursing wings connected to the central core. The three-story central core contains all diagnostic and active treatment facilities on the main floor. Below this are the service departments. The natural slope of the site allowed both floors to have grade level entrances. On the third floor, over the center of the core, the acute medical and surgical unit is located.

The structure of the main (core) building consists of fire-proofed steel columns supporting reinforced concrete flat slab floors. For the wings, structural clay tile bearing walls are used with poured-on-grade floor slab and a precast concrete roof. Exterior walls are brick with double glazed aluminum sash. Interior partitions are structural clay tile-glazed in halls, operating and delivery rooms, pantries, and utility rooms, plastered elsewhere.

Panda photos

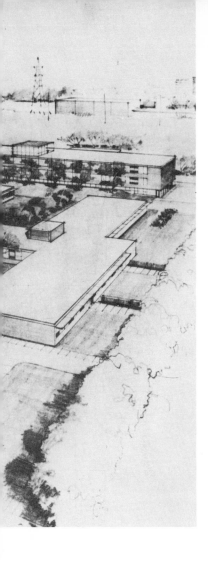

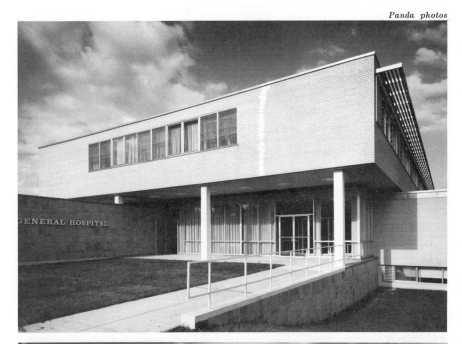

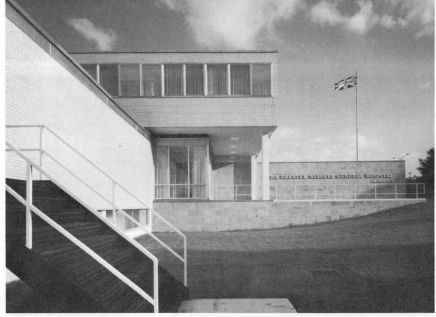

Above: in the rendering may be seen the three-story central core, with the boiler and laundry room at the extreme left, the sub-acute nursing wings to the right, and the nurses' residence in the background. Right and below: views of the core building. The projecting wall separates the emergency entrance from the main entrance. The grade slopes from this side down to the rear, permitting a grade level entrance to the basement on the rear

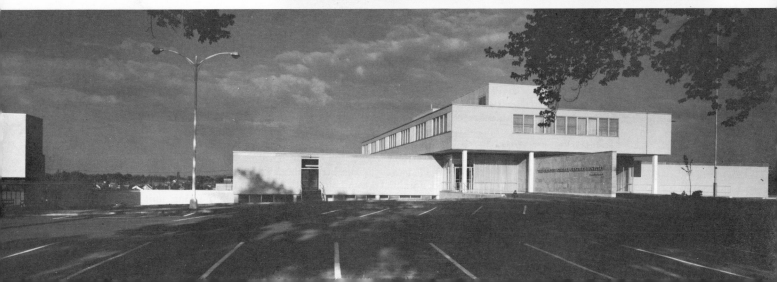

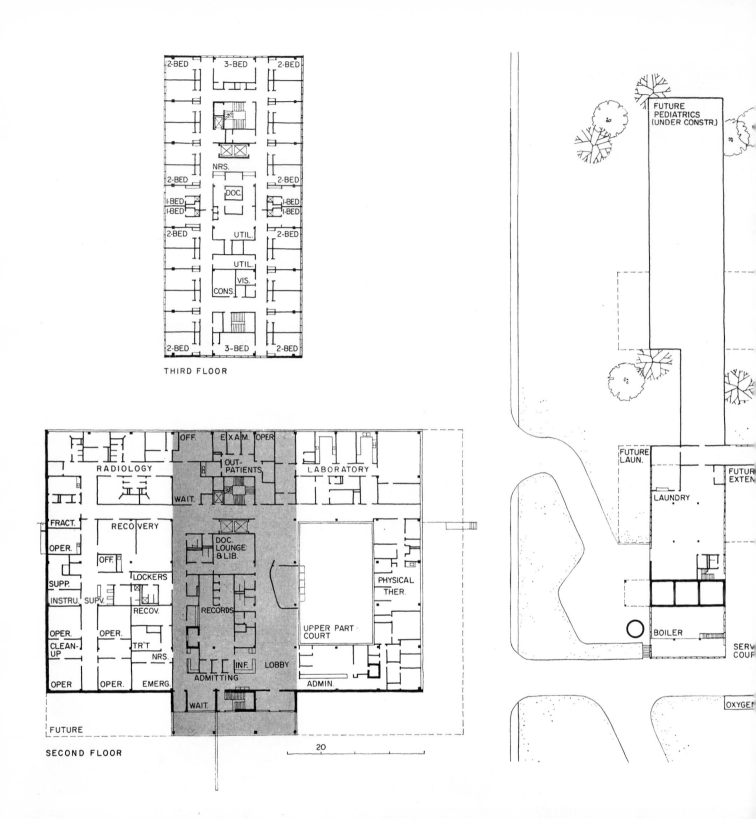

THIRD FLOOR

SECOND FLOOR

The ground level of the central core (shaded in main floor plan) contains areas for supply, kitchen and cafeteria, storage, and related facilities. On the same level, the delivery suite is connected to the maternity nursing wing by the nursery. Wings are provided for medical, surgical, and pediatric patients. As indicated, future wings have been planned and a separate pediatric nursing unit is now under construction. In the view of the hospital (opposite page, bottom), the various levels of the buildings and their relationships with finished grades may be seen. A separate entrance for maternity patients is provided, located on the extreme right side of the building. The second floor of the core is located over the shaded area of the large plan. This floor (immediately above) contains zoned areas for administration, physical therapy, laboratories, outpatients, radiology, surgery, and emergency. The third floor contains a nursing unit for intensive care

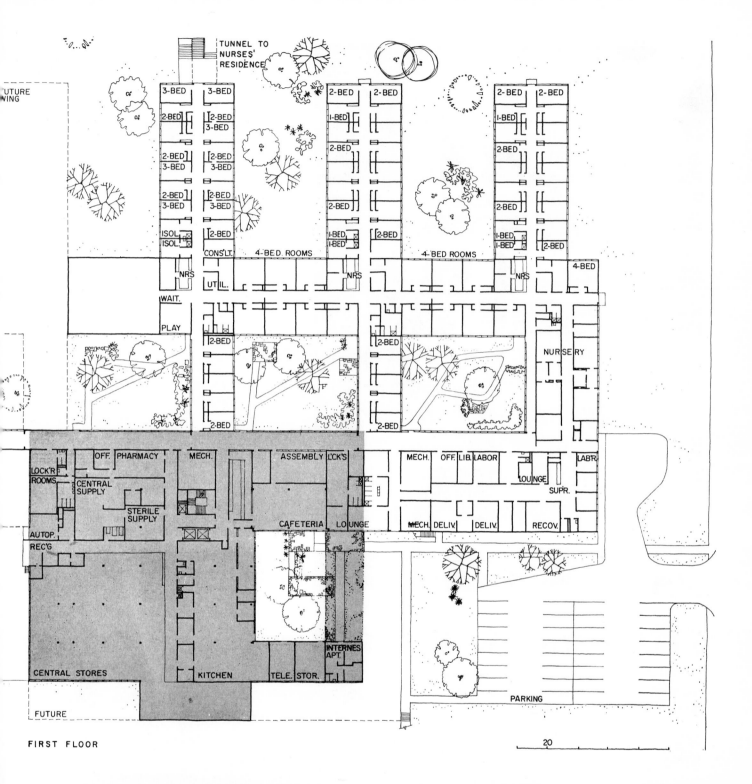

TUNNEL TO NURSES' RESIDENCE

FUTURE WING

3-BED 3-BED 2-BED 2-BED 2-BED 2-BED
2-BED 2-BED 1-BED 1-BED
3-BED
2-BED 2-BED 2-BED
3-BED 3-BED 2-BED 2-BED
2-BED 2-BED 2-BED
3-BED 3-BED 2-BED 2-BED
ISOL 2-BED 1-BED 1-BED 1-BED
ISOL 1-BED 1-BED 2-BED
CONS'LT. 4-BED ROOMS 4-BED ROOMS 4-BED
NRS UTIL. NRS NRS
WAIT.
PLAY 2-BED NURSERY
2-BED 2-BED

2-BED 2-BED

LOCK'R ROOMS OFF. PHARMACY MECH. ASSEMBLY L'CK'S MECH. OFF. LIB. LABOR. LABR.
CENTRAL SUPPLY LOUNGE SUPR.
STERILE SUPPLY CAFETERIA LOUNGE
AUTOP. MECH. DELIV. DELIV. RECOV.
REC'G

INTERNES APT.
CENTRAL STORES KITCHEN TELE. STOR.

PARKING

FUTURE

FIRST FLOOR                                    20

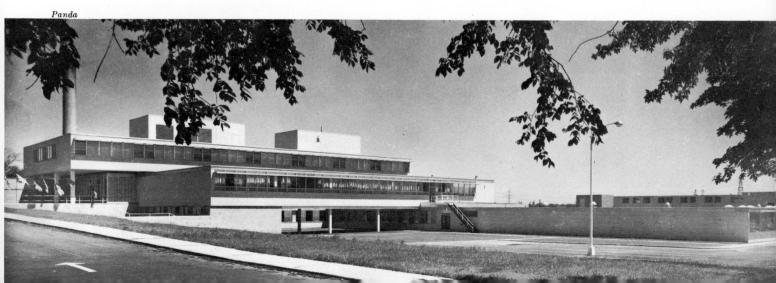

Panda

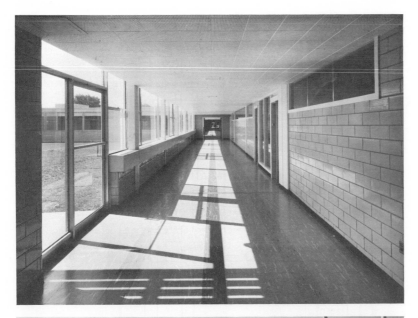

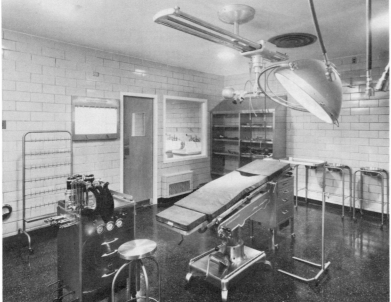

*Panda photos*

Left, top: view of a typical corridor. Nursing unit corridors are no longer than is usual in hospitals of this size. Less frequently used corridors are quite long, but are pleasant and open. Left, center: view of one of the four major operating rooms. In addition, there is a surgery for minor operations. All are closely related. Below: view of the lobby, toward the reception desk. In the background may be seen the meditation room. To the left are located the information desk, administrative offices, the medical records room

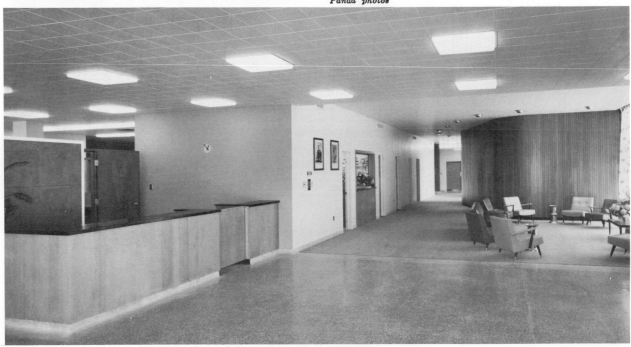

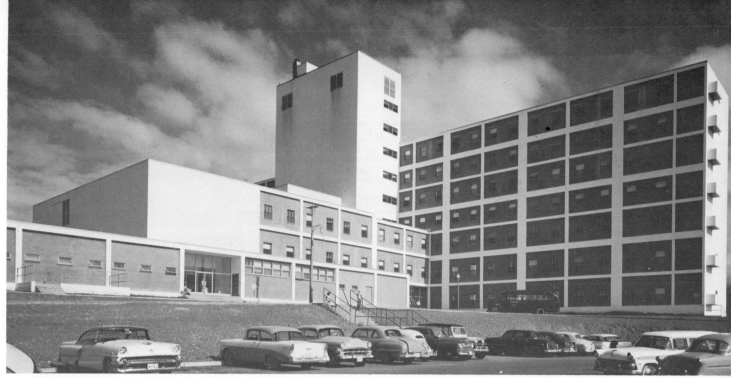

# Large Hospital for Military and Civilian Use in Alaska

*Elmendorf Hospital*
*Elmendorf Air Force Base*
*Anchorage, Alaska*

*Architects: Skidmore Owings & Merrill*

*Structural Engineer: Isadore Thompson*
*Mechanical Engineers: Keller & Gannon*
*Contractor: J. C. Boespflug*
*Construction Company*

*Construction Supervision by:*
*Alaska District Office*
*Corps of Engineers, U. S. Army*

As if the circulation problems of a large hospital were not complicated enough normally, here they are especially intricate because of the multiple purposes of this hospital. It is a combined military and civilian institution, to serve a large area in the developing territory (pardon, state) of Alaska. Strictly speaking, it is an Air Force hospital, serving the Elmendorf Air Force Base and administered as such. It serves also the adjacent civilian population, not only as a hospital but also as a sort of health center. Thus it has an exceptionally large outpatient department, large nursery and obstetrical suite. It is, moreover, a large hospital, around 400 beds, in an area where health facilities have to be self-sufficient.

So its problems of programming were taken seriously. The plan makes clean separations of diverse departments and functions; typical nursing unit floors take the narrow slab form, but lower stories have an essentially three-wing scheme to provide those separations. A large square-shaped wing on the first floor gives a clinic and outpatient department as virtually a separate building, though it does connect to the main portion at the elevator bank, so that hospital patients have convenient access to the clinic departments. Most importantly, outpatients are kept entirely out of the main hospital traffic lanes. This plan, with this feature, has been approved for the military for use in others of its hospital installations.

Above the first floor this same wing narrows down to suitable dimensions of the surgical suite (third floor) and the obstetrical suite (second floor). Above the third floor the wing becomes merely an elevator and stair tower, this transport core being nicely placed with respect to main traffic routes. Also it keeps individual floors free of the interruption of elevators and elevator lobbies.

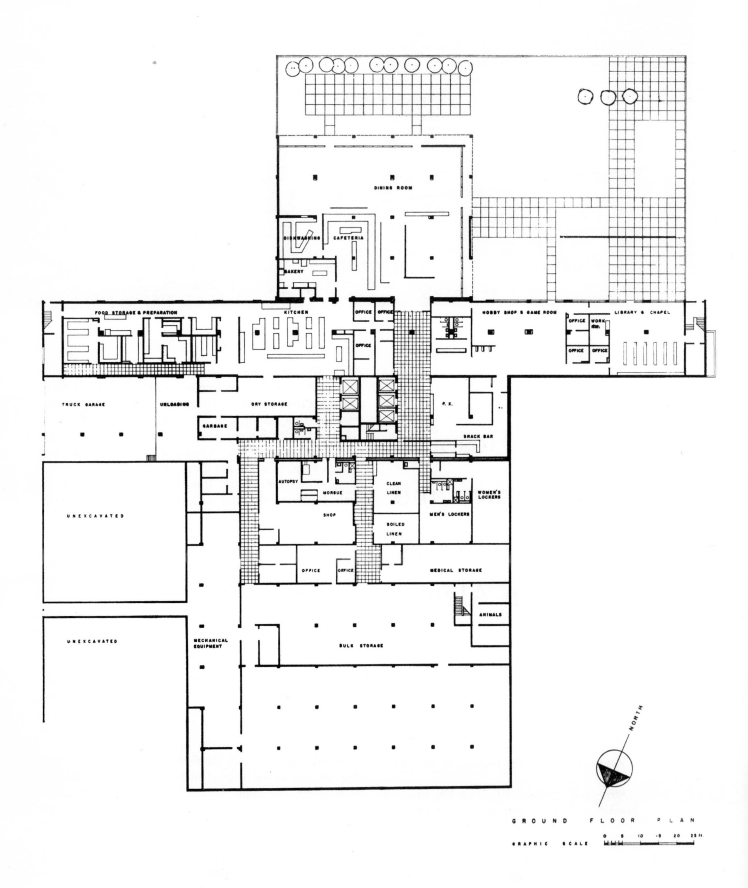

Ground floor (mostly a basement level) takes advantage of grade to make a gesture
toward outdoor living in cold Alaska; the dining room, PX, library and chapel open to
the outdoors. Truck garage and loading dock are also at this level. The large first floor
coverage gives ample room for storage at the ground floor

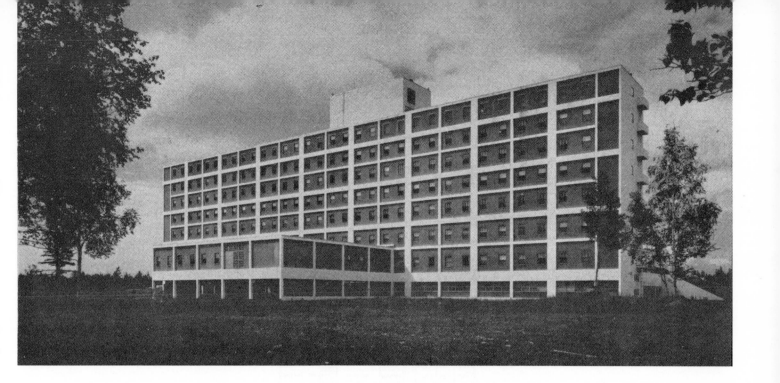

The building is oriented with the nursing unit wing facing south, with the majority of the bedrooms and wards facing south where there is an excellent view of the mountains. The sloping site presented the opportunity of providing two levels of access for ambulant traffic, also for truck and ambulance entrances. Access to ground floor has been provided at dining room, recreation rooms, library and the chapel, and by stairs at ends of nursing units. Recreation, dining and PX areas have been grouped to join outside areas for whatever outdoor activities the climate permits.

The four typical nursing floors consist of two nursing units each of either 28 or 34 beds, with a centrally located floor-serving kitchen. The majority of the patients' rooms are oriented to the southeast with the nurse's stations, utility rooms and offices to the north. Fenestration and sun control presented a problem due to the extreme north latitude of the Anchorage area. The low angle of winter sun made impractical any "eyebrow" solution to sun control and the extremely low design temperature of -30°F made strip windows costly due to the necessity of providing insulating sash. The solution provides 5- by 5-ft windows at 10 ft-9 in. centers with a low sill height to enable bedridden patients to take advantage of the view of the mountains in the distance. The typical window consists essentially of two superimposed double hung windows providing the greatest insulating effect and flexibility of ventilation at minimum cost. Light-proof shades and venetian blinds are provided as a method of controlling sunlight and to provide darkness during the summer nights. A Women's and Pediatric nursing unit is located on the sixth floor and a neuropsychiatric ward and treatment and consultation facilities on the seventh floor.

The structural system for the building is rein-forced concrete, with flat slab construction for floors and roof. The flat slab was chosen for economy of construction, in addition to keeping floor-to-floor heights at a minimum and providing plain surfaces for application of insulation to the slab at the walls. Climatic conditions required insulating all exterior walls, and insulating floor slabs, top and bottom, for a distance of four feet from the exterior walls to prevent freezing of water in pipes in these areas. Tile floors in bathrooms and other locations are installed with adhesive to avoid complicating the floor structure with depressions for mortar setting beds.

Exterior walls are of concrete block installed within the structural panels. Window area is used judiciously due to the climatic conditions.

The main lobby, and waiting areas in clinic and outpatient department have terrazzo floors, and acoustical ceilings with perforated cement asbestos finish. Wall finish in the main lobby is terrazzo and hardwood. The clinic and outpatient waiting areas have vinyl wall finish.

Typical finishes in nursing units and other areas above the first floor are asphalt tile flooring, acoustical ceilings with perforated cement asbestos finish in corridors, plaster ceilings in bedrooms, and ceramic tile in toilets, utility rooms, operating rooms, etc. Operating rooms have conductive terrazzo floors and base.

An underground tunnel provides access for piping to the power plant which supplies hot water and steam for heating, sterilizing, etc.

The heating system consists of radiators, convectors, and extended-surface steel tube type radiators, thermostatically controlled. Tempered outside air is distributed to rooms from corridor ceiling ducts and exhausted by fans. Operating rooms, recovery areas, outpatient therapy department and similar areas are fully air conditioned, including dust removal.

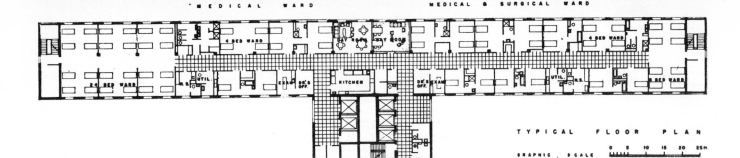

TYPICAL FLOOR PLAN

GRAPHIC SCALE

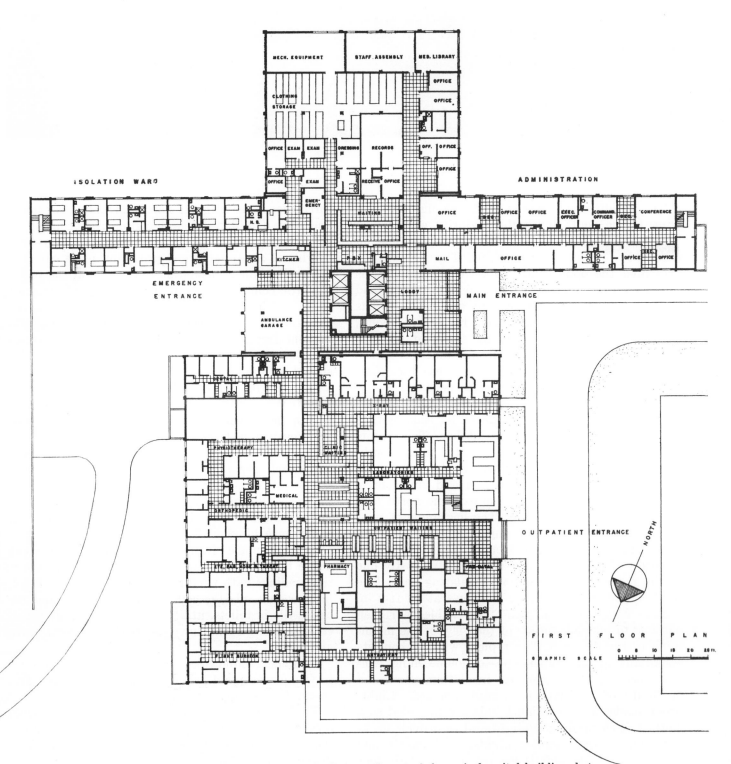

FIRST FLOOR PLAN

GRAPHIC SCALE

First floor outpatient wing keeps all clinic traffic out of the main hospital building, but is easily accessible to inpatients. Ambulance entrance is at this level, above the truck garage and loading dock. Typical floor has only nursing units, with vertical transportation in a core outside the wall dimension. Most beds are in two- or four-bed wards

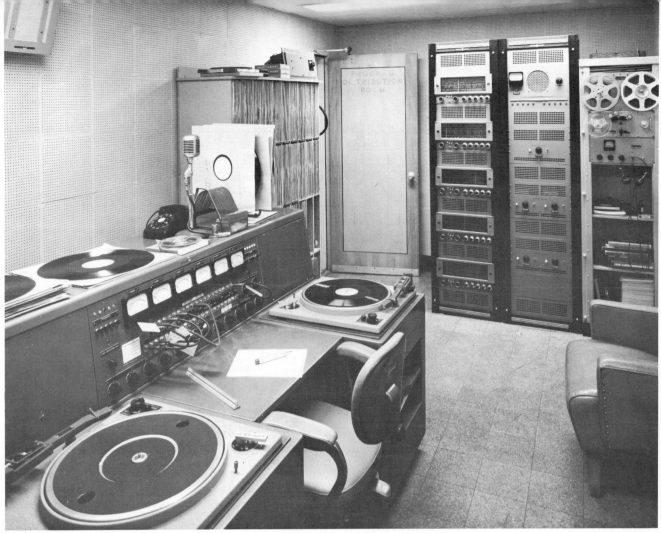

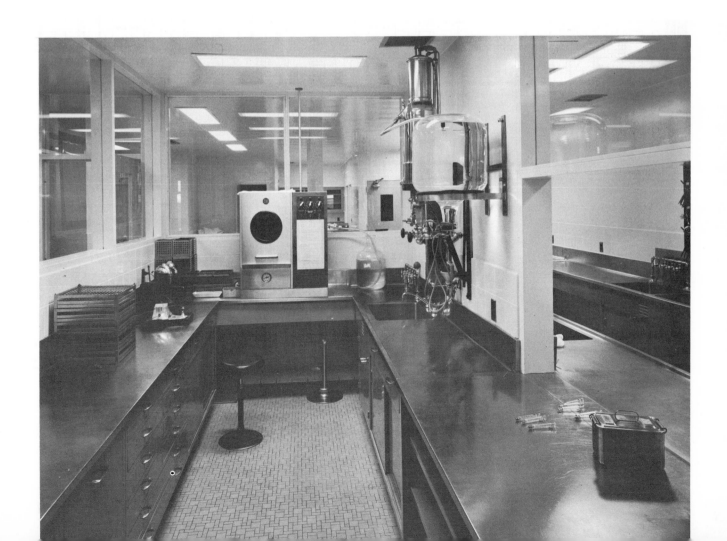

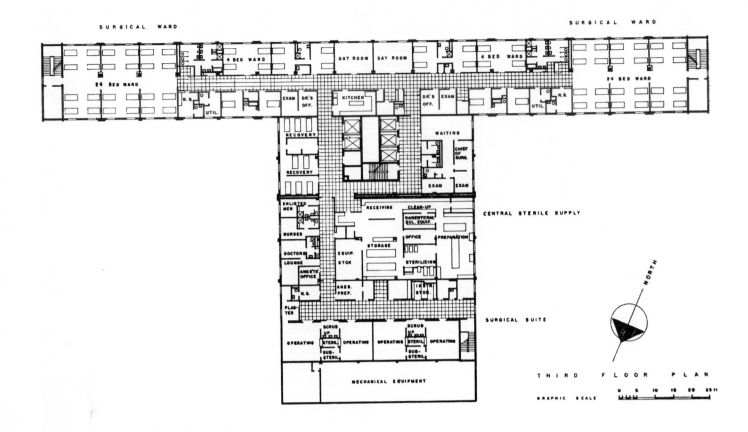

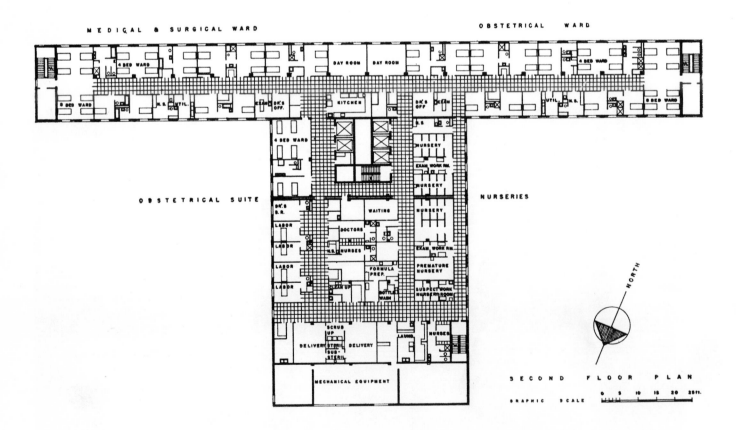

The obstetrical suite, nurseries and o.b. nursing unit are on the second floor, because of the high traffic generated by this department. Labor and delivery rooms and so on have their own cul de sac locations, as do operating rooms on the floor above. The elevator cores separate these departments from the corresponding nursing units

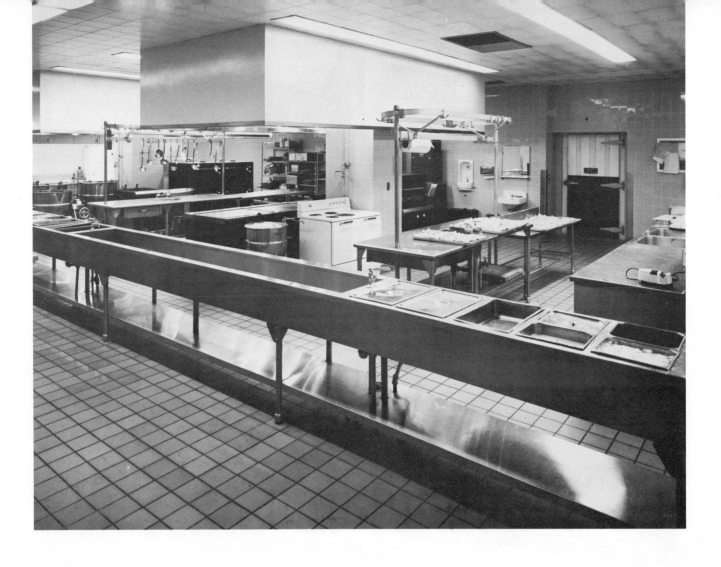

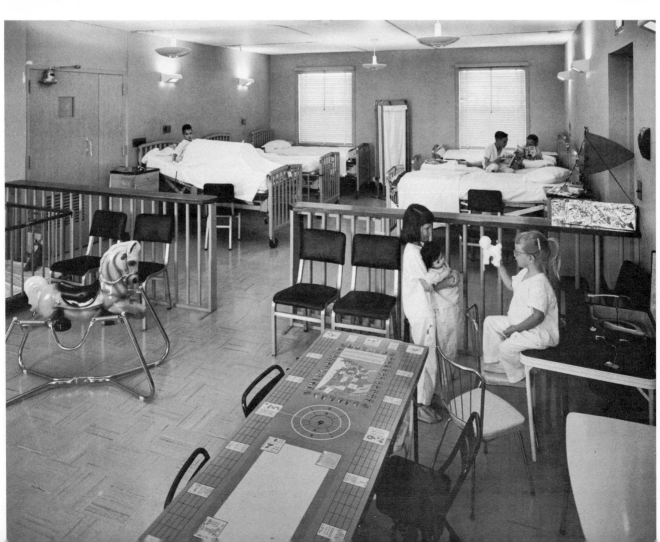

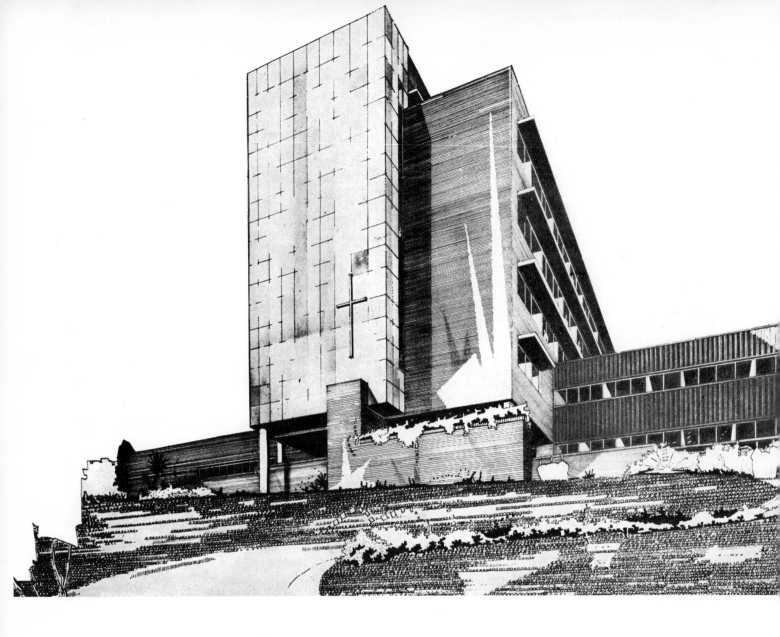

# Large Hospital with Imaginative Plan

A LARGE HOSPITAL with a basically L-shaped plan, this building shows careful development of the principles of hospital planning. Each major department has its own cul de sac location where it can go about its own business without any confusion from cross traffic. If the L form of the lower floors is unusual it is, here, quite effective.

The surgical suite has the far end of the first floor with maximum isolation and protection from the rest of the hospital. Of itself the surgical suite is not unconventional, though it does have a larger than usual sterile storage room, complete with autoclave. And the recovery room has an unusual layout, with two private rooms for critical cases and the nurses' work space right between for effective control. It is unusual to have the emergency suite open into the surgical corridor, and the merits of this could be debated both ways. Normally it is considered that the surgical corridor should be protected against possible "dirty" cases in the emergency

room, but a firm closing of the door should be effective. In case of a community disaster with a sudden load of injury cases, the operating suite could become an adjunct of the emergency room.

Also on the first floor, the out-patient department is quite effectively placed for both good control from the main lobby and for isolation of outpatients from the rest of the hospital.

On the second floor, the L form works out well for the isolation of the delivery suite, and the nursery corridor adjoins the delivery suite but has its own cul de sac location. If the nurses have to walk a long way to take the babies to the mothers' rooms, the nursery is exceptionally well protected against unauthorized entry and the possibility of contamination.

On the upper floors, where the building takes the simple slab form, there is still an extra spur beyond the elevators, where special units can enjoy isolation.

## MERCY HOSPITAL

*Laredo, Texas*

*Wade · Gibson · Martin, Architects*

*Tom A. Vernor, Electrical Engineer*
*Martin Staley, Mechanical Engineer*
*Frank T. Drought, Structural Engineer*

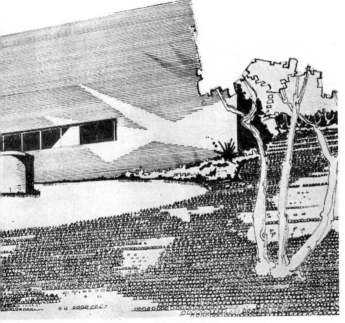

*Site is a high plot at the edge of town, overlooking the Rio Grande River. The hospital, replacing an outdated one in a downtown location, will serve an area of 150-mile radius, taking some patients from Mexico. H. H. Moeller was recently awarded the general contract, in the amount of $2,264,000*

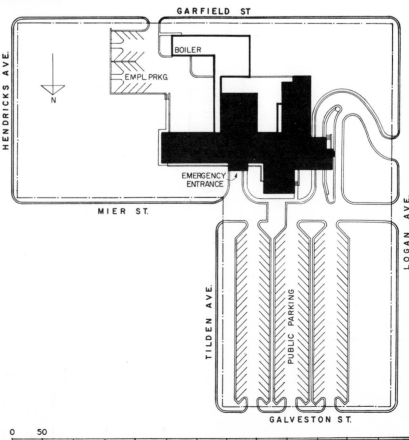

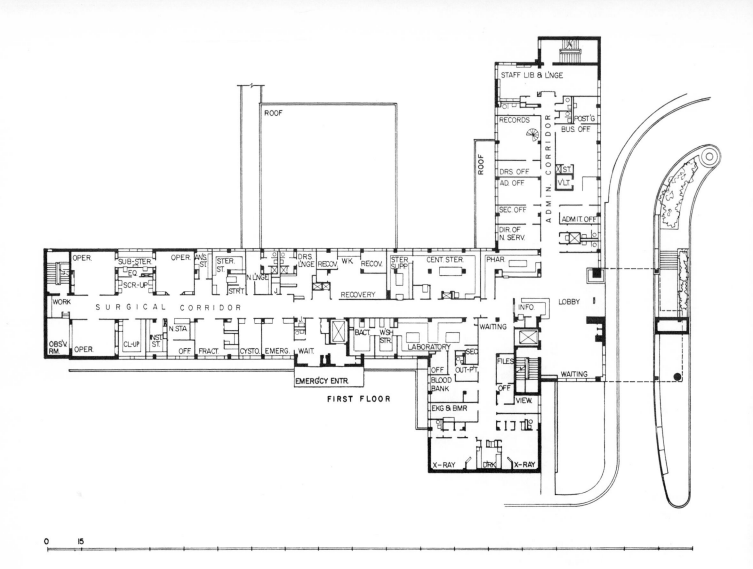

ROOF

STAFF LIB & L'NGE

RECORDS · BUS. OFF · POST'G

DRS. OFF · AD. OFF · ST · VLT

SEC. OFF · ADMIT. OFF

DIR. OF N. SERV.

ROOF

ADMIN. CORRIDOR

OPER. · SUB-STER. · OPER. · ANS. ST · STER. ST. · DRS. L'NGE · RECOV · WK · RECOV. · STER. SUPP. · CENT. STER. · PHAR.

SCR-UP · EQ · N L'NGE · STRT · J

WORK

SURGICAL CORRIDOR

RECOVERY

OBS'V. RM. · OPER. · CL-UP · INST. ST. · N.STA. · OFF. · FRACT. · CYSTO. · EMERG. · WAIT.

LOBBY

INFO.

WAITING

BACT. · WSH STR · LABORATORY

SEC.

FILES

OFF

VIEW.

WAITING

EMERG'CY ENTR.

OFF. · OUT-PT.

BLOOD BANK

EKG & BMR

X-RAY · DRK · X-RAY

**FIRST FLOOR**

0    15

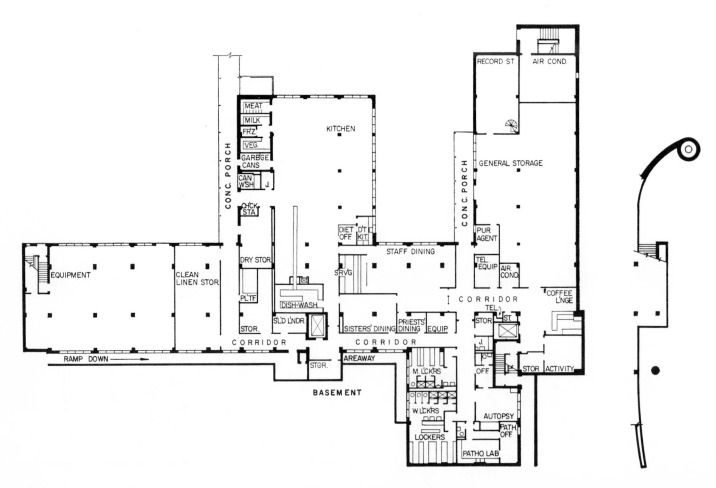

RECORD ST. · AIR COND.

MEAT
MILK
FR'Z.
VEG.

KITCHEN

CONC. PORCH

GARBAGE CANS

CAN WSH · J

CH'CK STA

GENERAL STORAGE

CONC. PORCH

DIET OFF · DT KIT.

PUR. AGENT

STAFF DINING

EQUIPMENT

CLEAN LINEN STOR.

DRY STOR.

SRVG

TEL. EQUIP · AIR. COND.

COFFEE L'NGE

PL'TF

DISH-WASH

CORRIDOR

TEL.

STOR.

ST.

SL'D L'NDR.

SISTERS' DINING · PRIESTS' DINING · EQUIP

J.

STOR.

RAMP DOWN ⟶

CORRIDOR

CORRIDOR

OFF. · STOR · ACTIVITY

STOR. · AREAWAY

M. L'CKRS

W. L'CKRS

LOCKERS

AUTOPSY

PATH OFF

PATHO. LAB

**BASEMENT**

HOSPITAL BUILDINGS

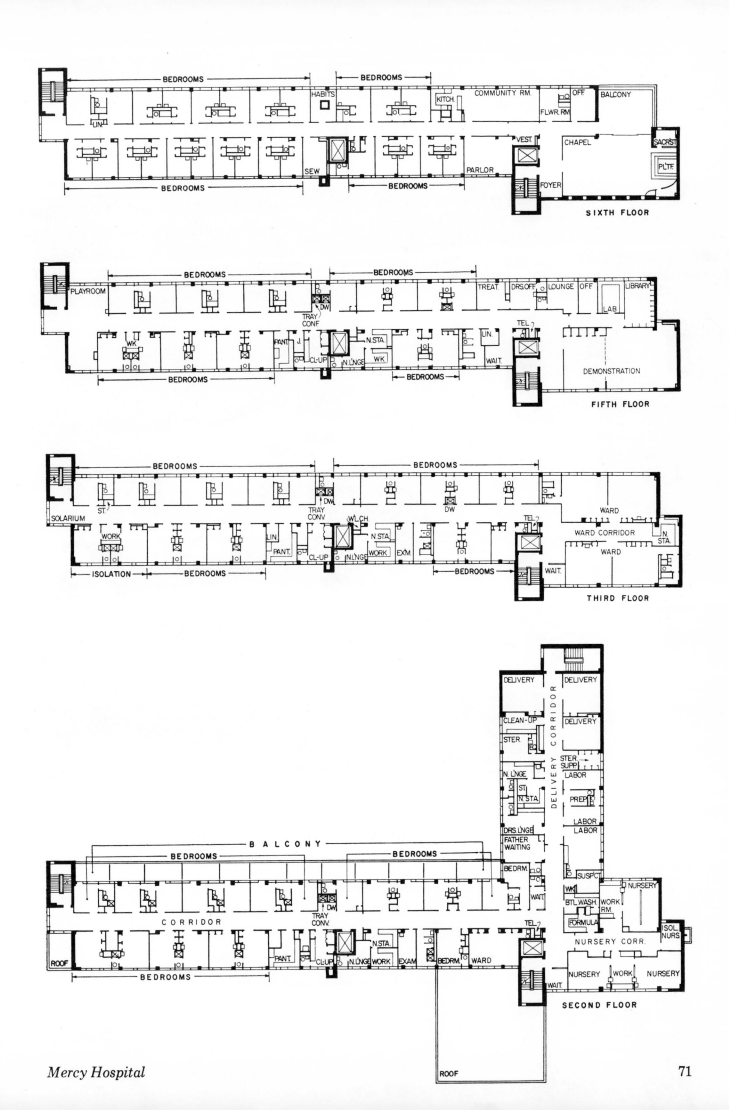

*Mercy Hospital*

# Hospital Based on Research

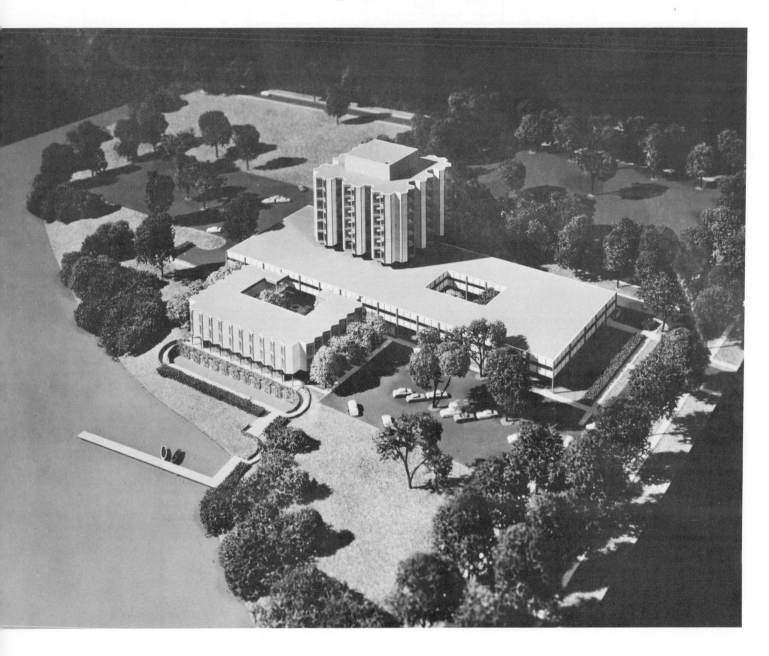

DAVIS MEDICAL FOUNDATION, MARION, INDIANA

ARCHITECTS: Harry Weese, Bruce Adams, John van der Meulen

ASSOCIATE: John Dinkeloo

PLANNING CONSULTANT: Carl W. Walter, M.D.

ADMINISTRATION CONSULTANT: A. C. O'Connor

STRUCTURAL ENGINEER: Frank J. Kornacker

MECHANICAL ENGINEER: Samuel R. Lewis

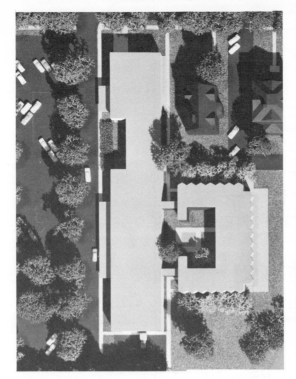 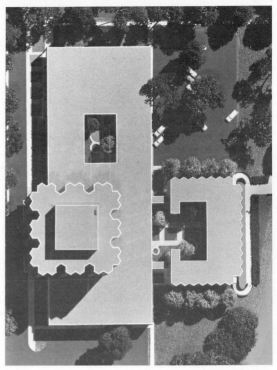

Orderly growth of the hospital is made possible by the scheme for 80 beds, shown at the left, with provisions for eventual expansion to 300 beds with additional medical and surgical facilities at a later time. The final layout is shown at the right. Separation of the 80 bed wing and the future nursing tower will permit the additions to be made with minimum disturbance to the patients and staff using the 80 bed complex

## THE PROBLEM:

The research and design for the hospital were sponsored by Davis Medical Foundation, Marion, Ind. Its president, Merrill S. Davis, M.D., says: "Remarkable advances have been made in medicine and its related sciences in the past fifteen years. As a result of the great strides, virtually every community in this country can have the very best medical care.

"The most apparent defect in this picture of medical progress is the failure to provide physical facilities which are economically feasible. The efficiency with which physicians and their assistants can function has been greatly handicapped by obsolete design. Patient comfort and provisions for expansion have often been overlooked. The need for an entirely new concept for the design, construction, maintenance, and operation of hospitals is apparent.

"The Davis Medical Foundation has sponsored a study of these problems. The work has been going on for five years. To confirm the opinions developed through the research, consultants were employed. This hospital design is the result of the translation of their studies into a concrete proposal."

## THE CRITERIA:

The Planning Consultant, Carl W. Walter, M.D., says: "Planning a general hospital for wage earners in a community has increased in complexity as medical care has improved due to the increase in medical knowledge and to appreciation of the role that personality plays in disease. Care of the patients as a whole can only be accomplished in an integrated unit where a patient's physician, his consultant specialists and laboratory technicians have the opportunity to study the patient under optimum circumstances and where all the diagnostic facilities are readily at hand. With fatigued, anxious patients who are not properly prepared for medical examinations, the medical staff is handicapped.

"The hospital care of the patient has undergone an enormous change in emphasis. Early ambulation, control of infection, the role of the psychiatric factors in well-being, and the maintenance of homeostasis introduce new concepts in hospital design. The elaboration of medical technology and the development of team nursing all bring changes to the design of a nursing unit.

"The ill patient is apprehensive and anxious. The stress stimulates defense mechanisms. Personalities change. Patients become irritable, suspicious, and defensive. They long for security; in most people's minds this means the seclusion of a private room. Here the patient can find protection from annoyances. The sick patient in our culture appreciates privacy because he is as loath to inflict unpleasantness on his fellow as he is unwilling to share others' miseries. Patients like to have their own needs determine the degree of privacy they wish. It is their need for their rest or sleep which is most important to them. In modern society, the physician-patient relationship can only blossom in privacy. The days of sharing confidences in a noisy ward with a blustering doctor have disappeared.

"Habits among patients are deeply ingrained. They like fresh, running water to drink; they want to wash their hands. Many have a deep revulsion against the use of the public toilet; they have learned to wash their hands after attending to their sanitary needs. A hospital that does not provide water at the bedside and individual toilets offends most patients.

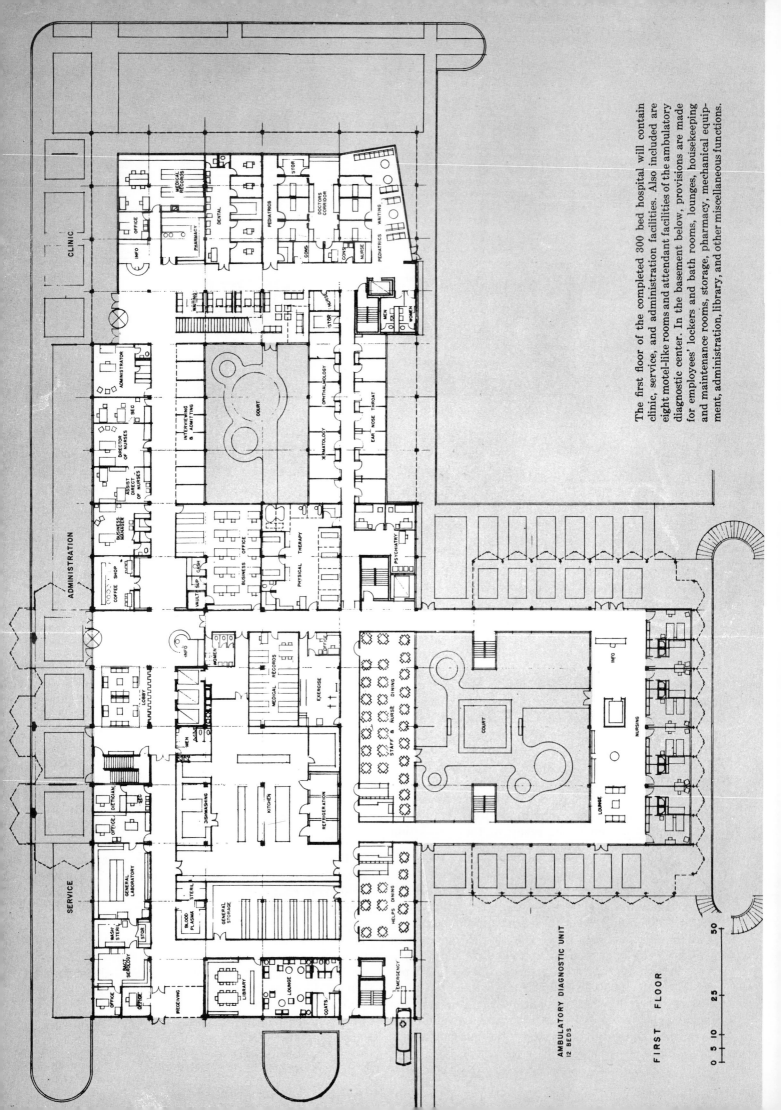

The first floor of the completed 300 bed hospital will contain clinic, service, and administration facilities. Also included are eight motel-like rooms and attendant facilities of the ambulatory diagnostic center. In the basement below, provisions are made for employees' lockers and bath rooms, lounges, housekeeping and maintenance rooms, storage, pharmacy, mechanical equipment, administration, library, and other miscellaneous functions.

AMBULATORY DIAGNOSTIC UNIT
12 BEDS

FIRST FLOOR

0 5 10    25    50

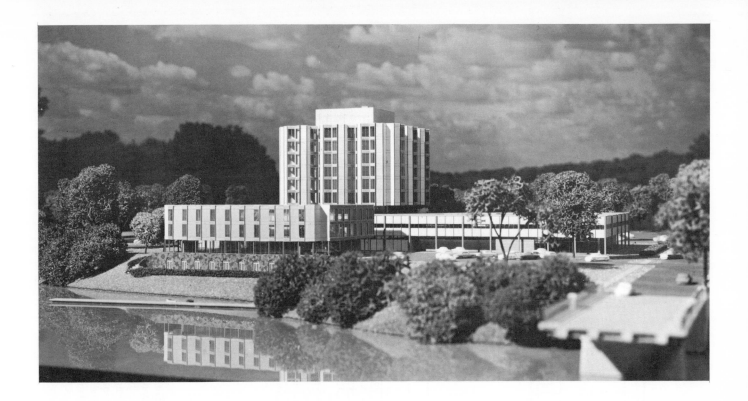

"As patients get better they like to roam. Exercise aids in bodily functions. Most convalescent patients are gregarious. They like to exchange experiences with their fellows; they like to eat together. Ultimately, they develop the urge to help others. This means that hospitals must provide Commons Rooms where these activities can occur under supervision."

The architects, Harry Weese, Bruce Adams, and John van der Meulen and associate, John Dinkeloo, say: "The Davis Medical Foundation wanted to achieve a hospital design based on their long research, one which would solve the Marion, Ind., community medical problems in a manner consistent with advances in medicine, hospital organization and design, and long-range community planning. The Foundation's research indicated that there would soon be a need in the community for a general hospital of 300 beds to supplement the already overcrowded city hospital.

"The new hospital, planned to be located at the site of the existing Foundation clinic, is the answer to the needs set forth in the program developed by the planning team. The advanced ideas in hospital organization and planning of Dr. Carl Walter of the Harvard Medical School staff are responsible for many of the differences in this scheme.

"The hospital scheme assumes that the Foundation acquire more land at their present attractive site (as they have already begun to do) and that they maintain their practice in the existing facilities while the new hospital is under construction. The site is located on the north bank of a river a few blocks away from the center of the town. The only unusual site planning problem is the danger of flood which limits the lower level of the building to non-critical uses."

The eighty rooms of the original construction, shown below, will be converted to the use of ambulatory or convalescent patients after construction of the nursing tower. These rooms are like motel or hotel rooms, each with a private bath, parking nearby and a view of the river. Patients here will ordinarily walk to the dining rooms, recreation areas and medical facility spaces. Many patients will be able to come and go at will when not being treated or examined.

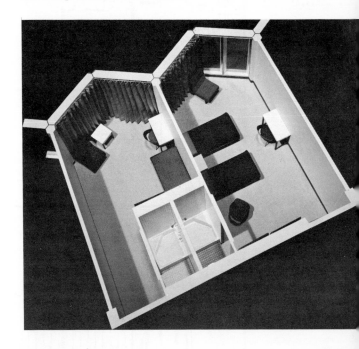

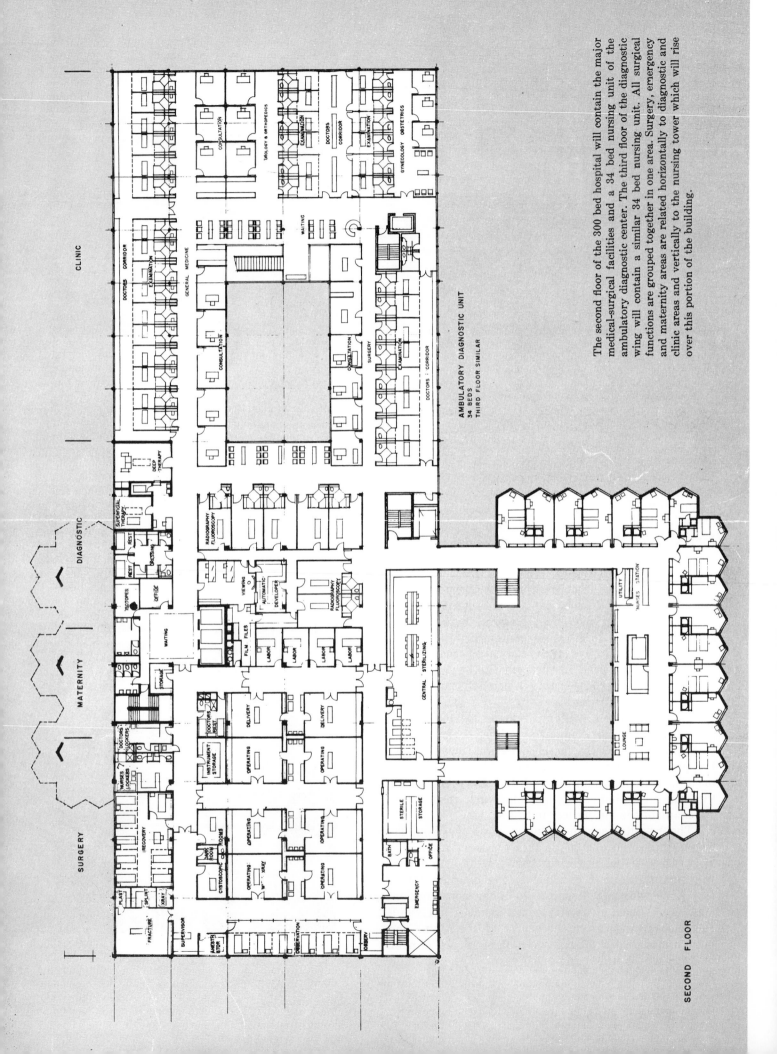

The second floor of the 300 bed hospital will contain the major medical-surgical facilities and a 34 bed nursing unit of the ambulatory diagnostic center. The third floor of the diagnostic wing will contain a similar 34 bed nursing unit. All surgical functions are grouped together in one area. Surgery, emergency and maternity areas are related horizontally to diagnostic and clinic areas and vertically to the nursing tower which will rise over this portion of the building.

AMBULATORY DIAGNOSTIC UNIT
34 BEDS
THIRD FLOOR SIMILAR

SECOND FLOOR

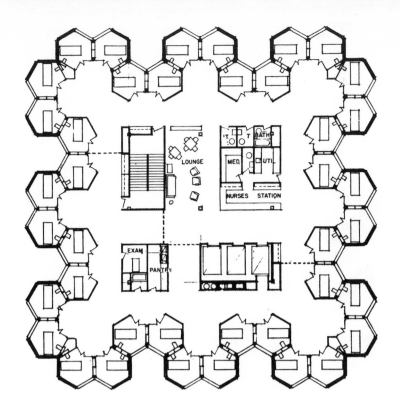

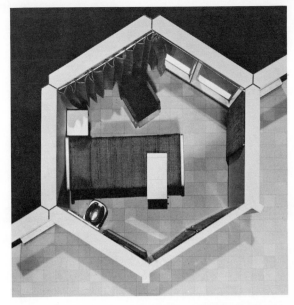

Each floor of the tower contains 40 beds in private rooms. The planning team felt that this was the optimum size for a nursing unit. Each room is equipped with a built-in toilet-lavatory at the bedside. These fold into the wall when not actually in use

## THE SOLUTION:

The planning consultant, Dr. Walter, says: "The design joins a group practice clinic with diagnostic and consultation facilities, a motel-like ambulatory diagnostic unit, and a hospital to provide the facilities for the physician to care for his patients under ideal circumstances. Ample parking space assures an unharrassed arrival, the ambulatory diagnostic unit gives opportunity for overnight preparation and collection of laboratory samples in the resting state, and private consultation rooms are an enormous aid in arriving at a proper diagnosis. Well-equipped examining rooms, where consultation with specialists is easy and where diagnostic procedures can be carried out quickly by the interested physician, save the patient time and inconvenience and add to the ease of caring for patients by supplying the necessary information while the physician's interest in that particular patient is at its height.

"The ambulatory diagnostic unit accommodations also provide minimal care facilities for patients who are recovering from a procedure, those who are being rehabilitated in the physiotherapy department, or chronic care patients who return periodically for observation.

"The design gives expression to patient needs by providing well-equipped, small, private rooms. The hexagonal-shaped rooms have working spaces at the sides of the beds, provide running water within easy reach of every patient, and enable him to use the toilet, adequately screened by a sturdy partition. Odor and noise are eliminated by proper ventilation and acoustic treatment. The maximum of privacy is afforded by the location of the bed. The properly placed window permits the patient to see the landscape without being exposed mercilessly to the sun or light.

"Nursing care is facilitated by shortening the path between patients and the source of supply by grouping the hexagonal-shaped rooms about a short working corridor. The doors to each room are located so that the nurse can readily inspect each patient without disturbing him. In this way many patients can be checked by nurses while en route to another destination. Isolation of the nursing floors from the remainder of the hospital insures quiet and permits exploitation of mechanical services in providing food and care for dishes.

"Functional grouping of the high traffic areas, such as X-ray, physiotherapy, kitchen-dining areas, laboratories, operating and delivery rooms, and clinics on two floors, permit concentration of hospital activities in a manageable unit where expansion or change, wrought by progress, can be accomplished without disturbing the nursing areas."

The architects say: "Noteworthy qualities of this hospital include integration of the various functions of a complete medical center, separation of seriously ill patients from convalescent or ambulatory patients, consolidation of surgical functions in one area, nursing units of 40 beds each grouped around nursing service cores, the motel-like ambulatory patients' rooms, and provision for orderly expansion.

"The clinic areas relate to diagnostic facilities which in turn relate to surgical and nursing areas in a close and direct way. Administration areas are grouped at the entrance between the clinic and nursing elements. Service areas are related directly to their uses.

"The nursing floors contain the most apparent changes from existing standards. All seriously ill patients will be provided with single rooms grouped together to allow maximum supervision with minimum travel by the nurses."

*Davis Medical Foundation*

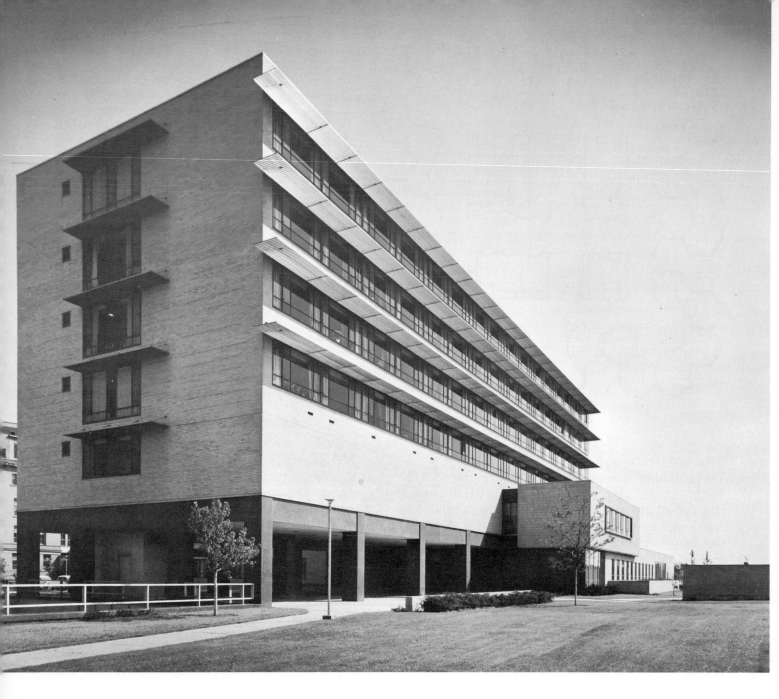

# Pavilion for a Large Hospital

*M. S. Kaplan Pavilion, Michael Reese Hospital, Chicago. Architects: Loebl, Schlossman & Bennett; Consultants: The Architects Collaborative; Medical Consultants: Dr. Jacob Golub; Mechanical Engineer, Robert E. Hattis; Structural Engineer: Alfred Benesch and Associates; Landscape Architects: Sasaki & Novak; Furnishings and Interior Colors: Watson and Boaler, Inc.*

A FAMOUS OLD INSTITUTION on Chicago's South Side, Michael Reese Hospital, is registering advances to match those of its neighborhood. This is the great area along the lake front that is being completely redeveloped with huge apartments. To match this activity, Michael Reese has projected a complete rebuilding program that will replace all its old buildings and will increase bed capacity from 700 to 1200. The Kaplan Pavilion forms the nucleus of the new campus scheme.

The architectural solution strives to combine the many hospital activities, facilities and equipment into convenient functional relationships; and by the use of simple easily maintained materials, cheerful colors, pleasant, sunny exposures, and carefully proportioned spaces to create a pleasant non-institutional environment. To this end the interiors have been kept small in scale where possible. Most patient rooms face south, and windows extend from wall to wall and sill to ceiling, in order to provide a large expanse of glass and an open feeling; light and view are controllable by the patient, as suits season, lighting conditions or moods.

In this present building all food service comes from the kitchen of another building on the campus, by food truck through a tunnel. A later addition to this pavilion will house a new kitchen for the whole hospital.

This building is completely air conditioned. Minimal

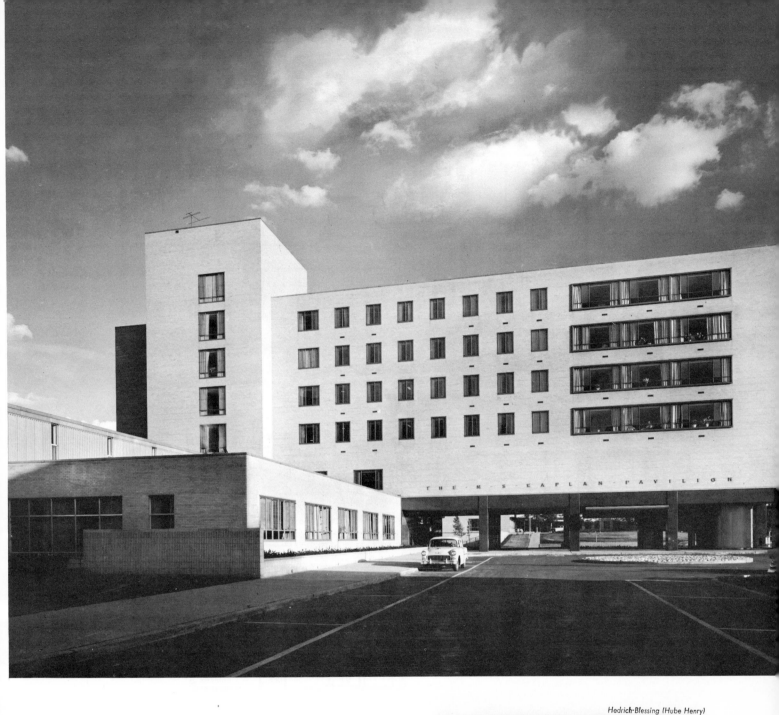

cost was achieved by using individual cooling and ventilating units in each room of patient areas. Each patient thus has been given individual control of his room conditioning. The same piping circulates chilled water in summer and hot water in winter.

A single-conduit type send-and-return automatic switch pneumatic type system interconnects the pavilion and all other buildings. The central doctor's call and message center also integrates all campus buildings and is so arranged that any doctor can register his arrival and departure from any point on the campus.

Expansion of this unit will be vertical; six added floors of nursing units are provided for in mechanical installations. The scheme also calls for a two-story wing to house central facilities for the whole campus, such as central record room (a present office wing is omitted in the plans here shown), main kitchen, new operating department, out-patient facilities and doctors' offices.

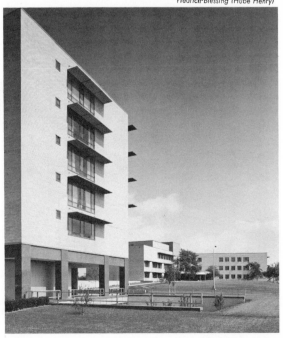

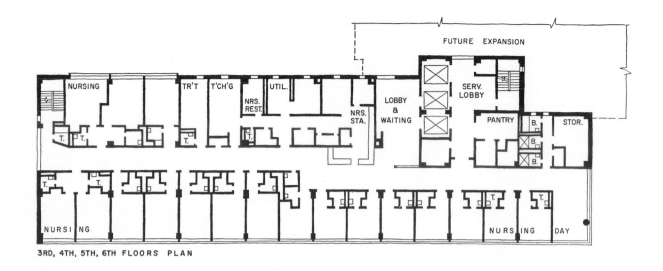

### 3RD, 4TH, 5TH, 6TH FLOORS PLAN

Labels visible: NURSING · TR'T · T'CH'G · UTIL. · NRS. REST. · NRS. STA. · LOBBY & WAITING · FUTURE EXPANSION · SERV. LOBBY · PANTRY · B. · STOR. · T. · NURSING · NURSING · DAY

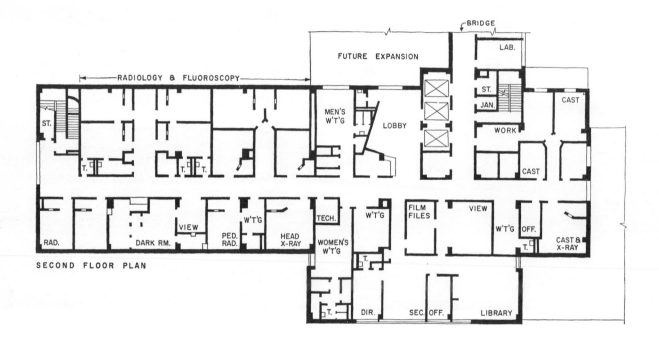

### SECOND FLOOR PLAN

Labels visible: RADIOLOGY & FLUOROSCOPY · FUTURE EXPANSION · BRIDGE · LAB. · ST. · JAN. · CAST · WORK · CAST · MEN'S W'T'G · LOBBY · ST. · T. · RAD. · DARK RM. · VIEW · PED. RAD. · HEAD X-RAY · TECH. · WOMEN'S W'T'G · W'T'G · FILM FILES · VIEW · W'T'G · OFF. · CAST & X-RAY · T. · DIR. · SEC. OFF. · LIBRARY

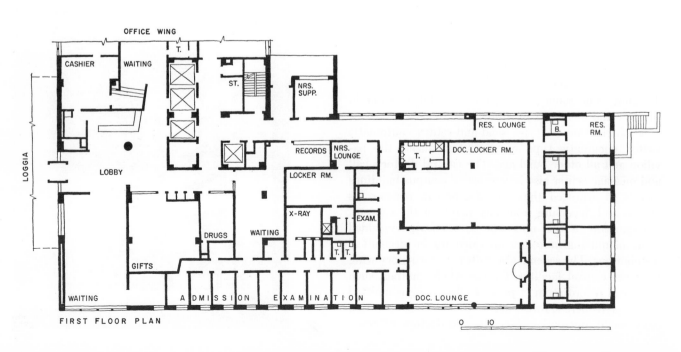

### FIRST FLOOR PLAN

Labels visible: OFFICE WING · CASHIER · WAITING · T. · ST. · NRS. SUPP. · RES. LOUNGE · B. · RES. RM. · LOGGIA · LOBBY · RECORDS · NRS. LOUNGE · T. · DOC. LOCKER RM. · LOCKER RM. · X-RAY · EXAM. · DRUGS · WAITING · T. · T. · GIFTS · WAITING · ADMISSION EXAMINATION · DOC. LOUNGE

0    10

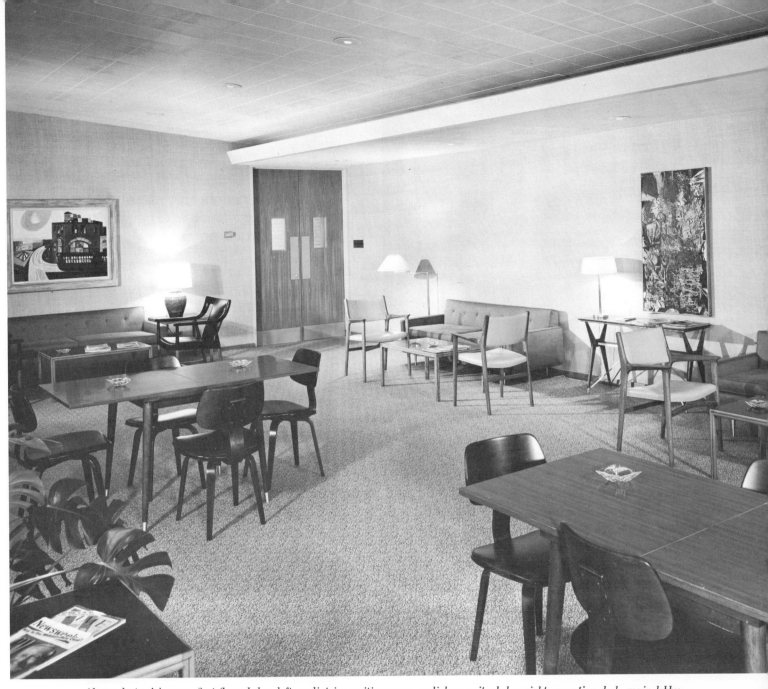

*Above: doctors' lounge, first floor; below left: pediatrics waiting room, radiology suite; below right: reception desk, main lobby*

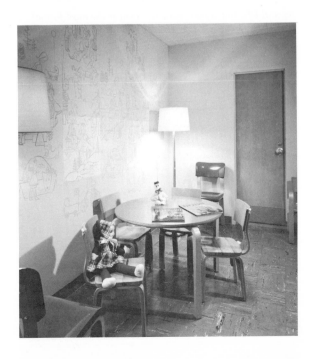

Hedrich-Blessing (Bill Engdahl & Hube Henry)

*M. S. Kaplan Pavilion*

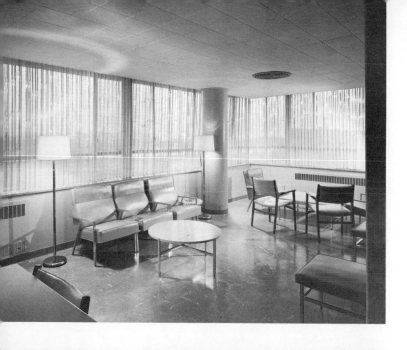

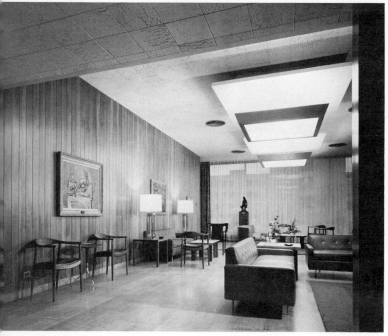

*Left: each nursing room floor has a large, bright day room*

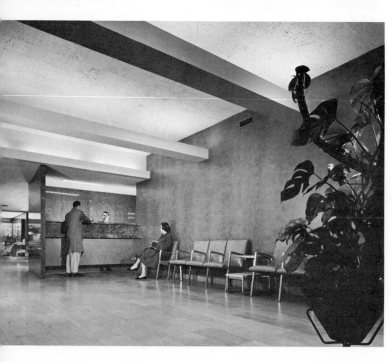

Hedrich-Blessing (Bill Engdahl & Hube Henry)

*Above and left: main floor waiting room is the most formal*

*Left: office wing has smaller waiting room, cashier counter*

HOSPITAL BUILDINGS

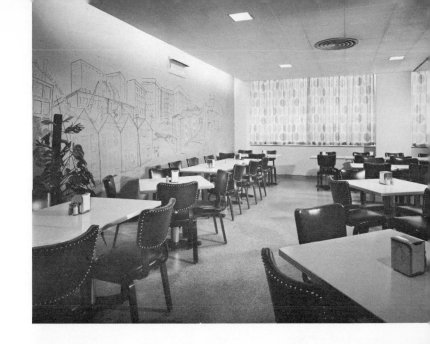

*Right: staff dining room, basement floor, plan not shown*

*Right: administrator's office is large enough for meetings*

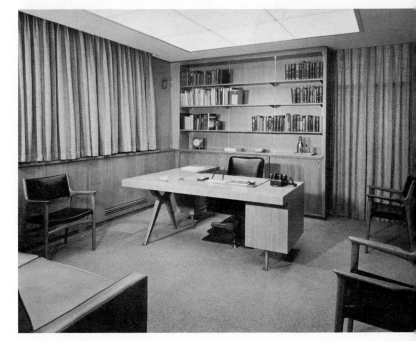

*Below and right: gift shop and pharmacy off main lobby*

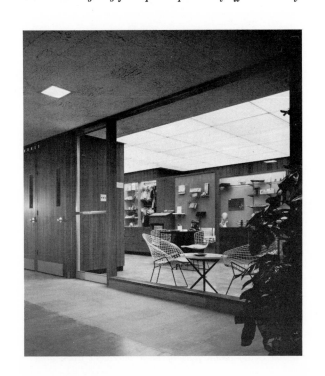

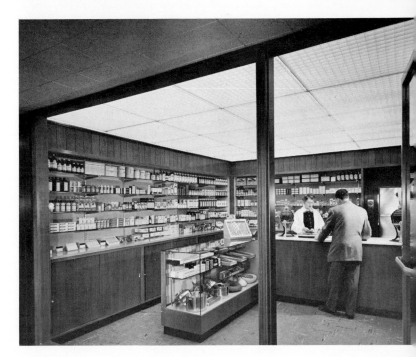

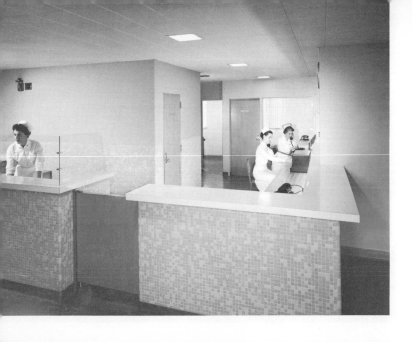

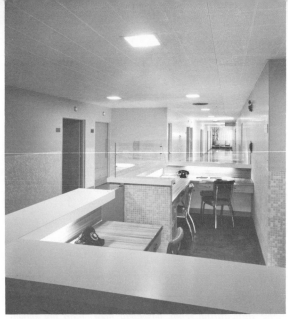

Hedrich-Blessing (Bill Engdahl & Hube Henry)

*Above and left: nurses' station is roomy, has full view*

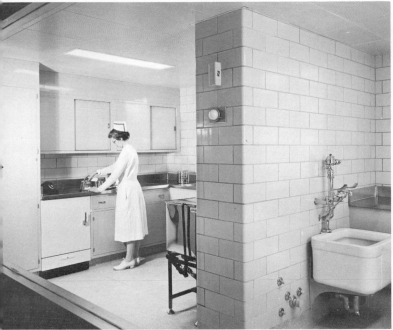

*Left: utility rooms, part of nurses' station grouping*

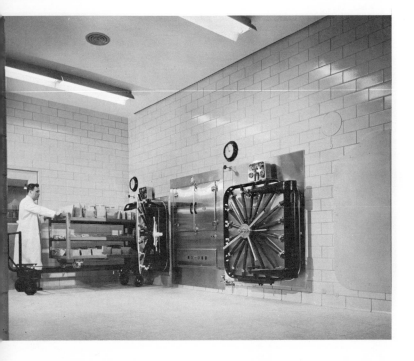

*Left: sterilizing room, part of large basement work area*

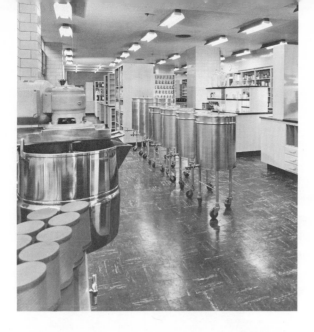

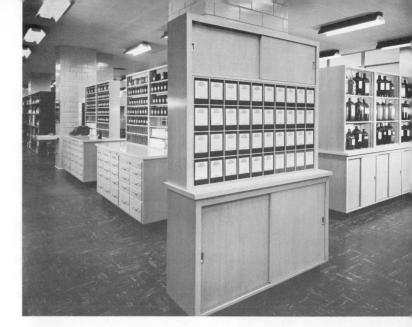

*Above and right: large manufacturing pharmacy, basement*

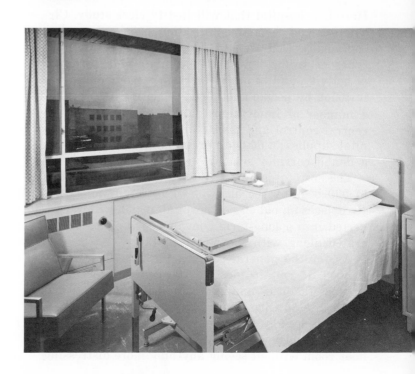

*Right: typical two-bed room, beds aligned on one wall*

*Right: single bed room illustrates window arrangement*

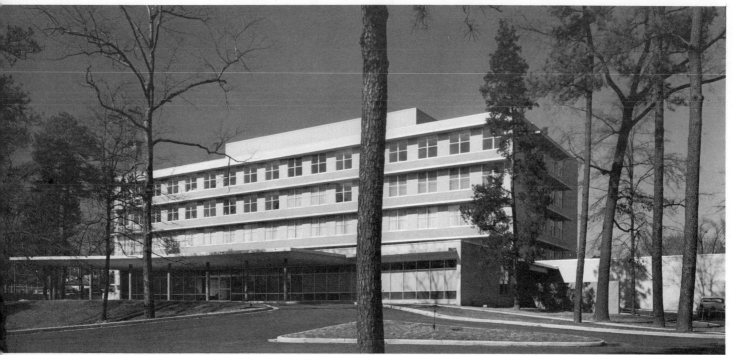

*Dewey G. Mears photos*

# Large General Hospital with Several Innovations

*Wadley Hospital, Texarkana, Texas. Page, Southerland & Page; Reinheimer & Cox, Associated Architects; Gordon A. Friesen Associates, Hospital Consultants; B. Segal, Mechanical Engineer; Frank B. Johnson, Mechanical Engineer; Montgomery & Williams, Civil Engineers; Boner and Lane, Acoustical Consultants*

Here is a hospital that will justify close study. Circulation and departmentalization problems are exceptionally well worked out, to separate different types of traffic, to isolate hospital units by types of activity, and to protect certain departments from invasion by people and germs. Also the hospital has a number of innovations: a psychiatric section; a central control and dispatching system for all hospital supplies; a 50-bed nursing unit arrangement in a double-corridor scheme.

The hospital is now a 180-bed facility, expandable to 300 beds by the addition of new nursing floors. It replaces an old 50-bed hospital, which will be converted into a long-term convalescent unit to be operated along with the new hospital.

As for the general scheme, the first floor is expanded to contain most of the heavy-traffic areas, adjunct facilities and operating suite. These disparate types of areas are well separated and grouped. Notice especially the separation of public and staff elevators and corridors. A visitor can get to an upper floor room without seeing anything more distressing than a few offices, gift shop or "cafetorium" and staff personnel are free to go their own ways without interference from wandering visitors. Upper floor corridors are also arranged (with the help of the double-corridor plan) to keep working areas bunched together and isolated. First floor plan divides roughly in half, with kitchen, stores, laundry and such at one end, medical facilities at the other. Laundry and boiler room are nicely banished in a rear projection. Above the first floor the building reduces to the dimensions of a 50-bed nursing unit, plus some special department on each floor: delivery suite, nursery, pediatric unit (on third floor, plan not shown), and psychiatric nursing unit. Elevators are so placed that one end of each floor can be cut off for these special facilities, reachable by staff elevators but not by public ones.

On the first floor plan, between pharmacy and stores, is a dispatcher's office, central focus of a supply control system developed by the hospital consultant. This office is staffed round the clock, and the dispatcher is responsible for all supplies for all areas. Deliveries are by tube system, dumbwaiter or cart, normal deliveries being made in light-traffic hours.

The psychiatric section represents a forward step, particularly in this community. There is no mental facility within 75 miles, and only after inclusion of this section in the plans was it possible to induce a psychiatrist to locate in the community.

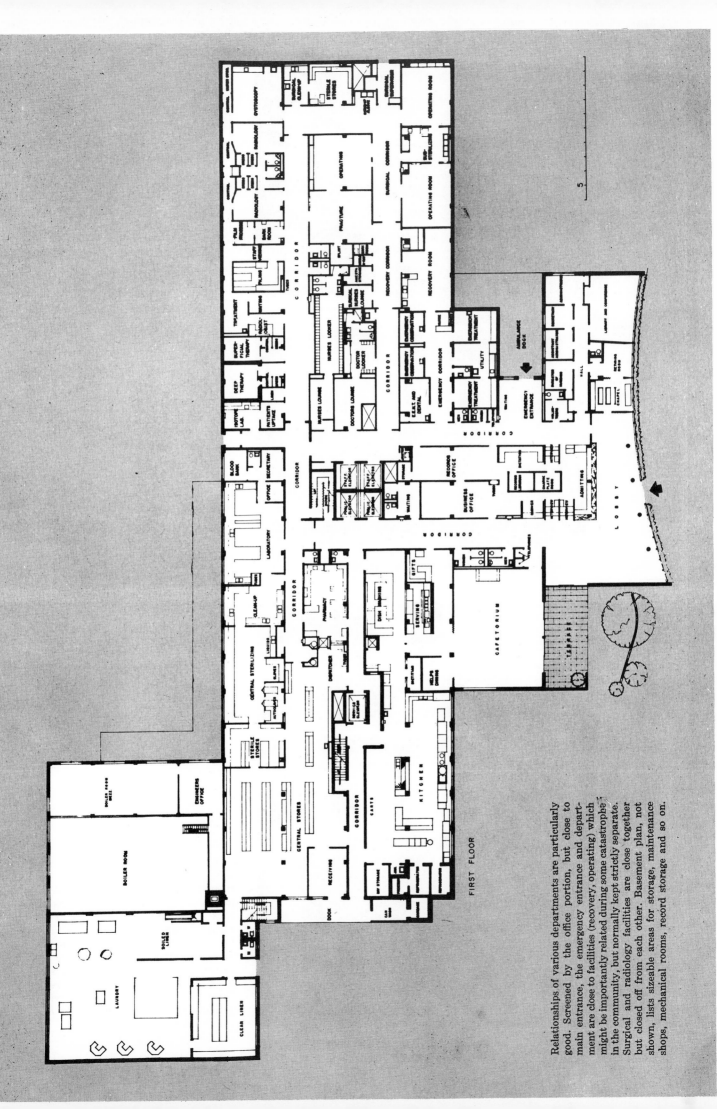

Relationships of various departments are particularly good. Screened by the office portion, but close to main entrance, the emergency entrance and department are close to facilities (recovery, operating) which might be importantly related during some catastrophe in the community, but normally kept strictly separate. Surgical and radiology facilities are close together but closed off from each other. Basement plan, not shown, lists sizeable areas for storage, maintenance shops, mechanical rooms, record storage and so on.

FIRST FLOOR

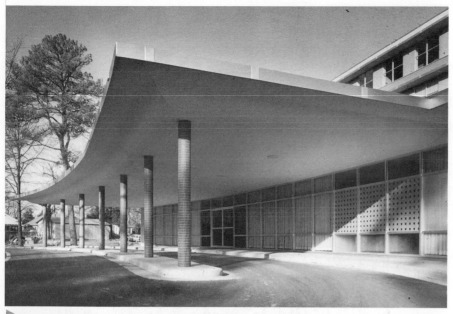

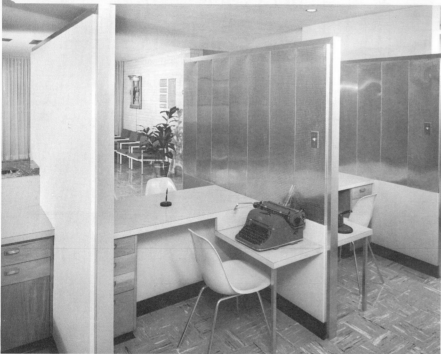

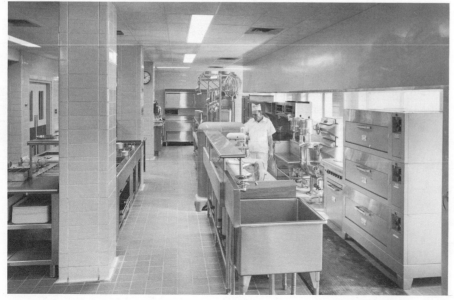

*Dewey G. Mears photos*

Hospital presents a commodious and pleasant main entrance to visitors; backed by nothing more sinister than offices. Large turnaround leads to visitor parking; there are separate parking areas for staff and for employe cars. Center photograph at the left shows interview booths, acoustically treated. From the main kitchen food service to patients' rooms is by heated food carts, via elevators

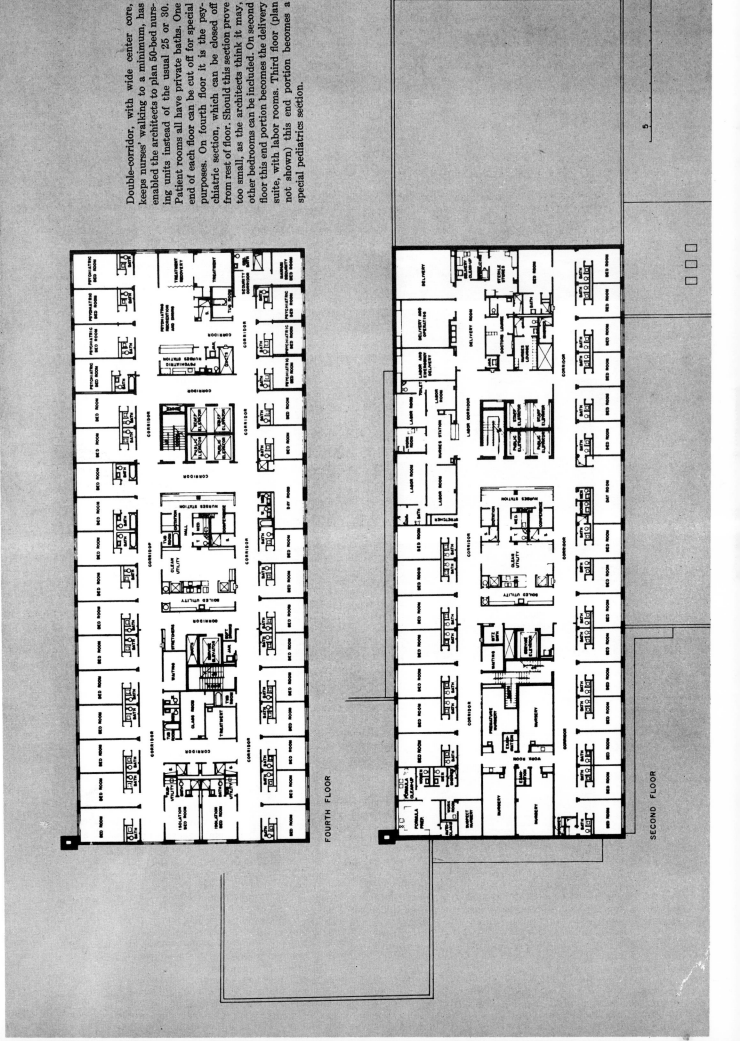

Double-corridor, with wide center core, keeps nurses' walking to a minimum, has enabled the architects to plan 50-bed nursing units instead of the usual 25 or 30. Patient rooms all have private baths. One end of each floor can be cut off for special purposes. On fourth floor it is the psychiatric section, which can be closed off from rest of floor. Should this section prove too small, as the architects think it may, other bedrooms can be included. On second floor this end portion becomes the delivery suite, with labor rooms. Third floor (plan not shown) this end portion becomes a special pediatrics section.

FOURTH FLOOR

SECOND FLOOR

5

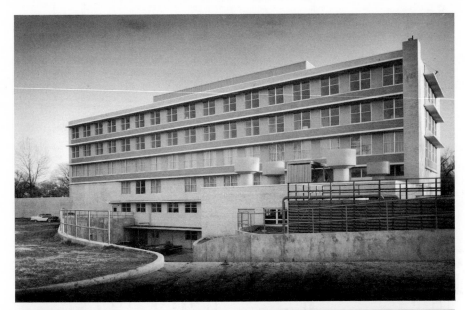

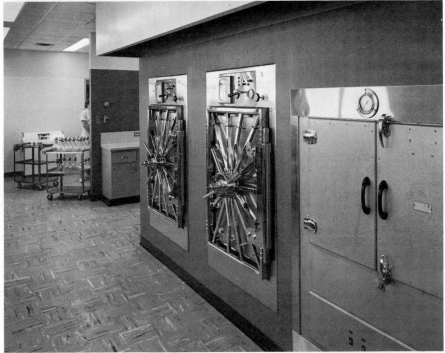

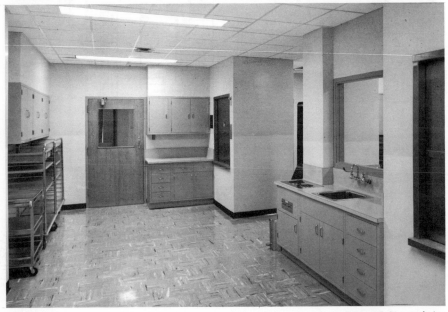

*Dewey G. Mears photos*

At the rear of the building a ramped service drive leads to basement, though main service entrance is at ground level, to the right in the upper photograph. Center photograph shows autoclaves in central sterilizing room. Sterile supplies, like all other materials, are controlled by a central dispatcher, with a cubby-hole office near central sterilizing room on first floor. Lower view at left shows one of the large utility rooms between double corridors on nursing floors

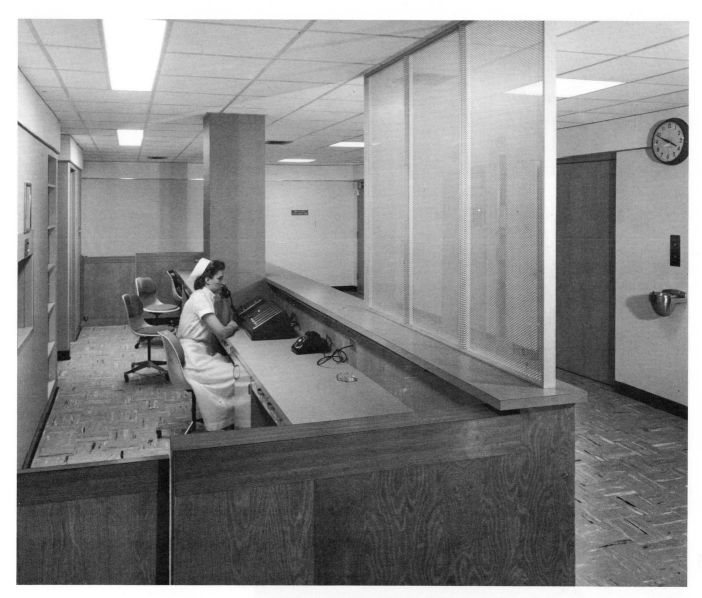

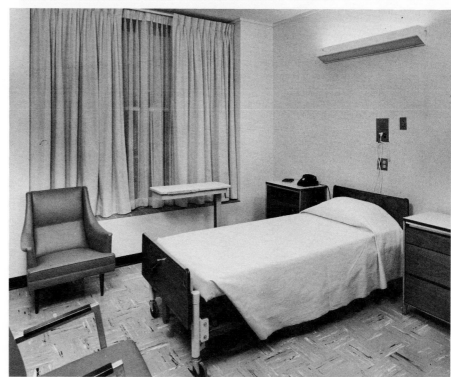

Nurses' station occupies full length of space between two corridors, facing the public elevators. Immediately behind nurses' station is a panel of pneumatic tubes. Opening off the station are two small rooms, one for private conference with doctors, another for doctors to dictate the records. Patient rooms are decorated to have as little institutional atmosphere as possible in a hospital

*Wadley Hospital*

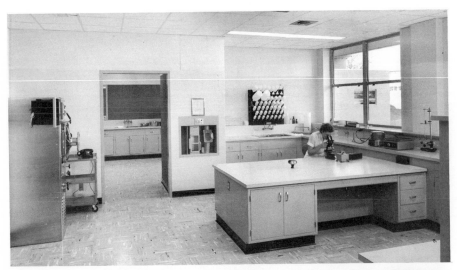

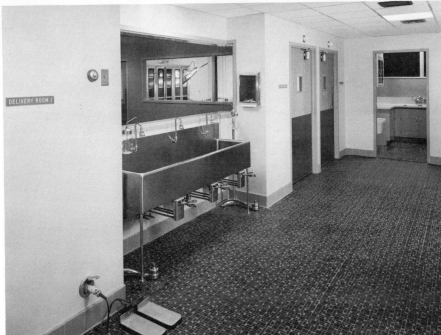

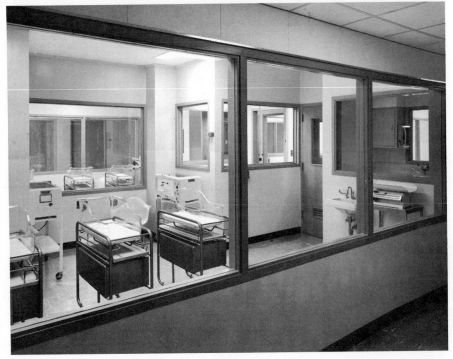

*Dewey G. Mears photos*

*Upper left:* the hospital has an exceptionally large laboratory, which is well located with respect to its traffic—close to radiology corridor and surgical suite. View looks through laboratory into cleanup room. *Center left:* the scrubup sink in the delivery corridor. *Lower left:* view into one of the nurseries, located between the two corridors on the second floor

*Opposite page:* Above, one of the delivery rooms; and, *below*, one of the major operating rooms

*Wadley Hospital*

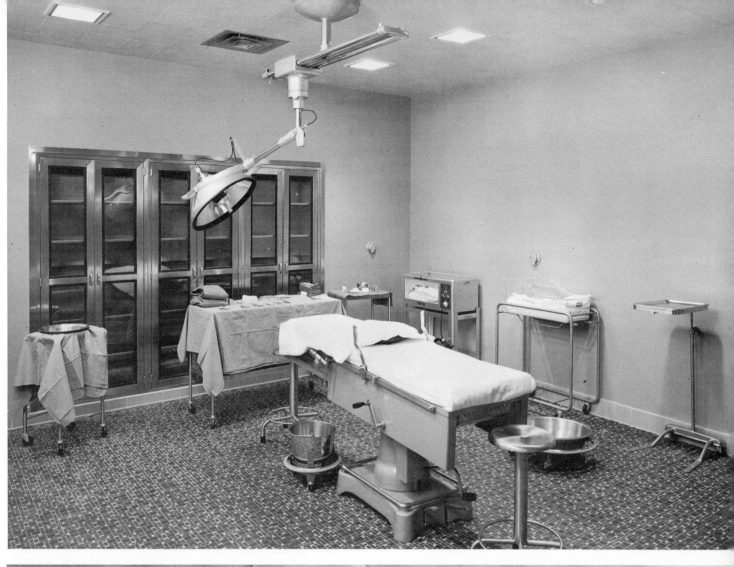

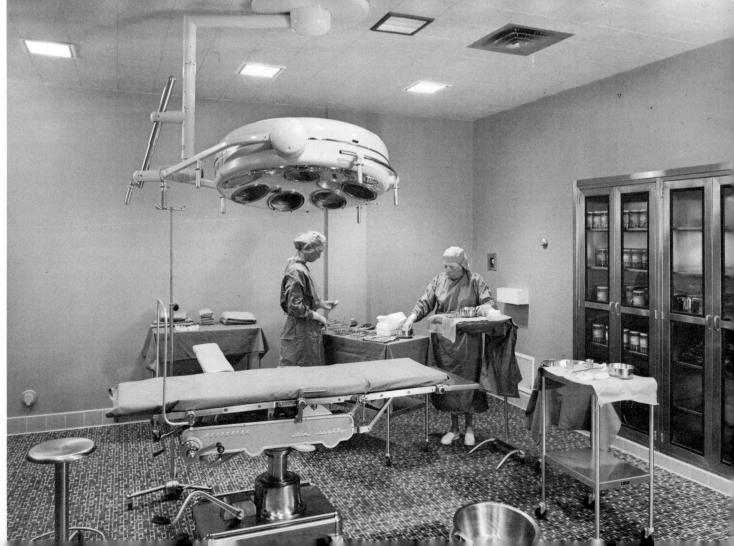

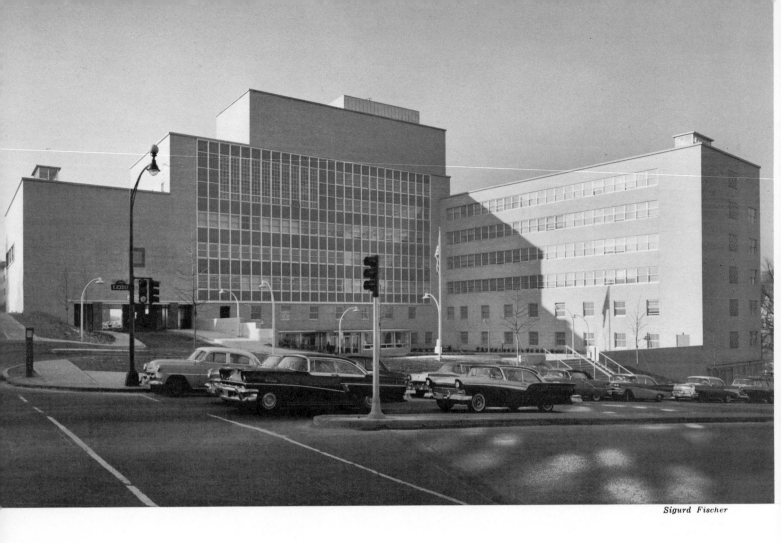

# Limited Site Size, Extreme Grade Helped Determine Hospital Plan

MISERICORDIA HOSPITAL, BRONX, NEW YORK

ARCHITECTS:
*Kiff, Colean, Voss & Souder,*
*The Office of York & Sawyer*

STRUCTURAL ENGINEERS:
*Di Stasio & Van Buren*

MECHANICAL &
ELECTRICAL ENGINEERS:
*Meyer, Strong & Jones*

FOOD SERVICE CONSULTANT:
*Howard L. Post*

CONTRACTOR:
*Vermilya-Brown Company, Inc.*

This is a complicated hospital. In addition to the usual medical and surgical requirements for a 210-bed general hospital, there is a nursing school with 150 student nurses, a home for 32 unwed mothers, and a convent for the Sisters of Misericorde who operate the hospital. An extensive research program is carried on; a large number of emergency cases is cared for.

In order to achieve the best solutions to the many intricate and interrelated problems inherent in the functions of the hospital, in the limited size of the 4-acre site, and in the steep grade, the architects designed a scheme with three buildings: main hospital (seven floors and basement), nursing school, and unwed mothers home. These are interconnected with covered walkways. The extremely steep grade made it possible to provide major entrances on three floors: service entrances on the ground floor, main hospital entrance on the first, outpatient and emergency entrances on the second floor. Because of the grade, the two-level parking system was feasible. Thus, various types of circulation to and from the hospital have been separated, making increased efficiency possible.

Building structure is concrete frame with flat plate floor arches. Exterior walls are aluminum framed porcelain enamel curtain walls and brick with limestone trim. Interior walls are plastered concrete block; ceilings are plastered.

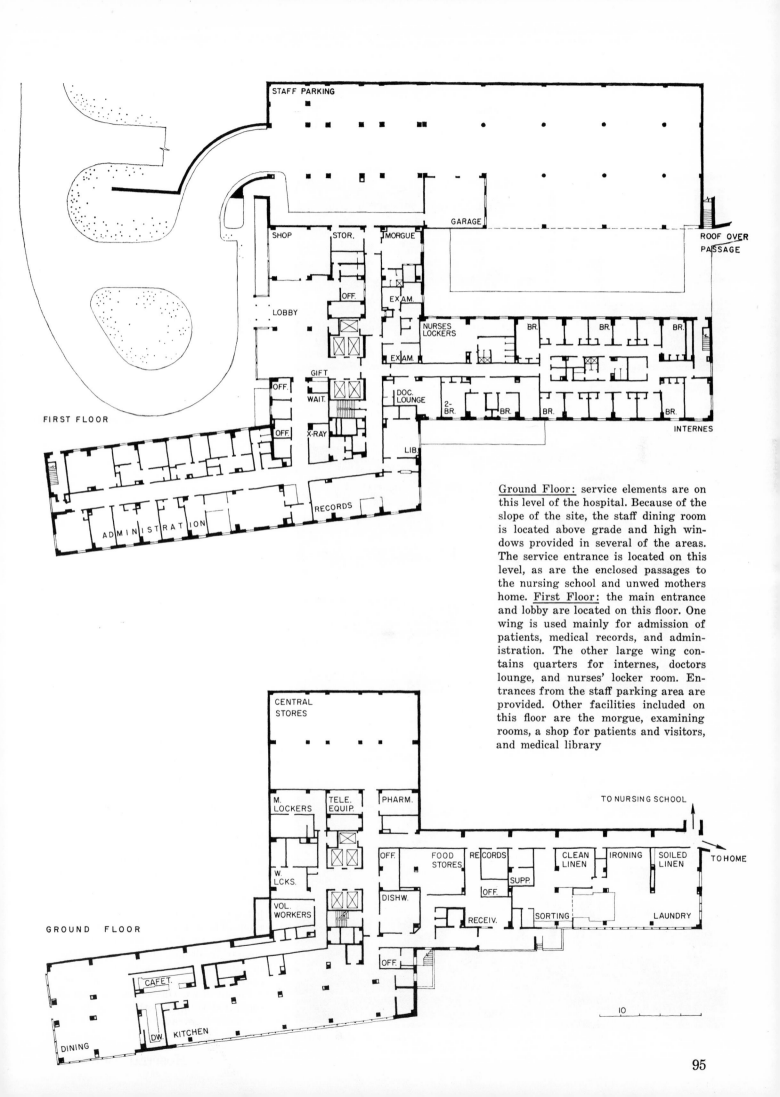

**STAFF PARKING**

SHOP

STOR.

MORGUE

GARAGE

ROOF OVER PASSAGE

LOBBY

OFF.

EXAM.

NURSES LOCKERS

BR.

BR.

BR.

EXAM.

OFF.

GIFT

WAIT.

DOC. LOUNGE

2- BR.

BR.

BR.

BR.

OFF.

X-RAY

LIB.

INTERNES

**FIRST FLOOR**

ADMINISTRATION

RECORDS

Ground Floor: service elements are on this level of the hospital. Because of the slope of the site, the staff dining room is located above grade and high windows provided in several of the areas. The service entrance is located on this level, as are the enclosed passages to the nursing school and unwed mothers home. First Floor: the main entrance and lobby are located on this floor. One wing is used mainly for admission of patients, medical records, and administration. The other large wing contains quarters for internes, doctors lounge, and nurses' locker room. Entrances from the staff parking area are provided. Other facilities included on this floor are the morgue, examining rooms, a shop for patients and visitors, and medical library

**CENTRAL STORES**

M. LOCKERS

TELE. EQUIP.

PHARM.

TO NURSING SCHOOL

TO HOME

W. LCKS.

OFF.

FOOD STORES

RECORDS

SUPP.

CLEAN LINEN

IRONING

SOILED LINEN

VOL. WORKERS

DISHW.

OFF.

RECEIV.

SORTING

LAUNDRY

**GROUND FLOOR**

OFF.

CAFET.

DINING

DW.

KITCHEN

10

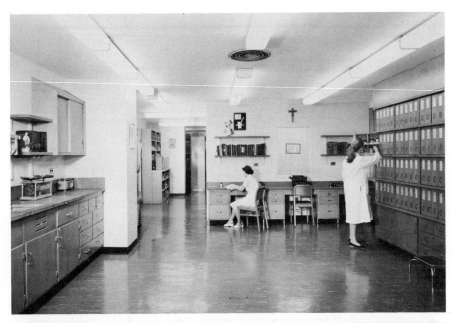

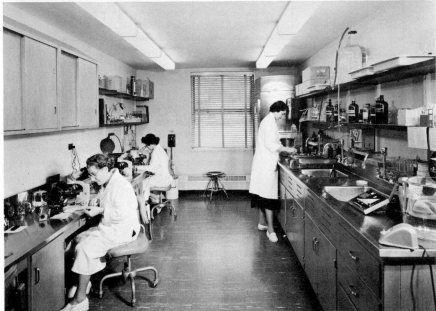

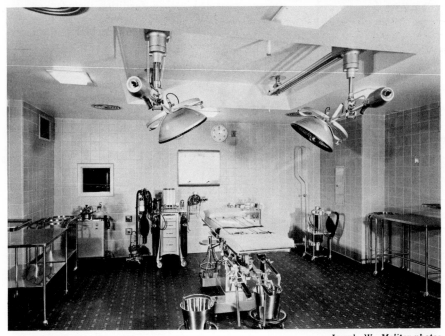

Left, top: view of medical records room which is located on the first floor. Adjoining this area are a small room for dictation and the medical library. Left, center: view of a laboratory. All labs are located on the second floor, as are the pharmacy, radiographic and fluoroscopy suite and similar facilities. Thus all facilities required for examination and treatment of outpatients are on the floor where the outpatient clinic is located. Efficiency is improved and the load on elevators is decreased. Left, bottom: view of a typical operating room. There are five of these rooms, located on the third floor. All are quite similar in design. They are arranged in surgical suites, each having two operating rooms connected by a shared scrub-up room. One operating room is separated from the others and is used for special operations

*Joseph W. Molitor photos*

HOSPITAL BUILDINGS

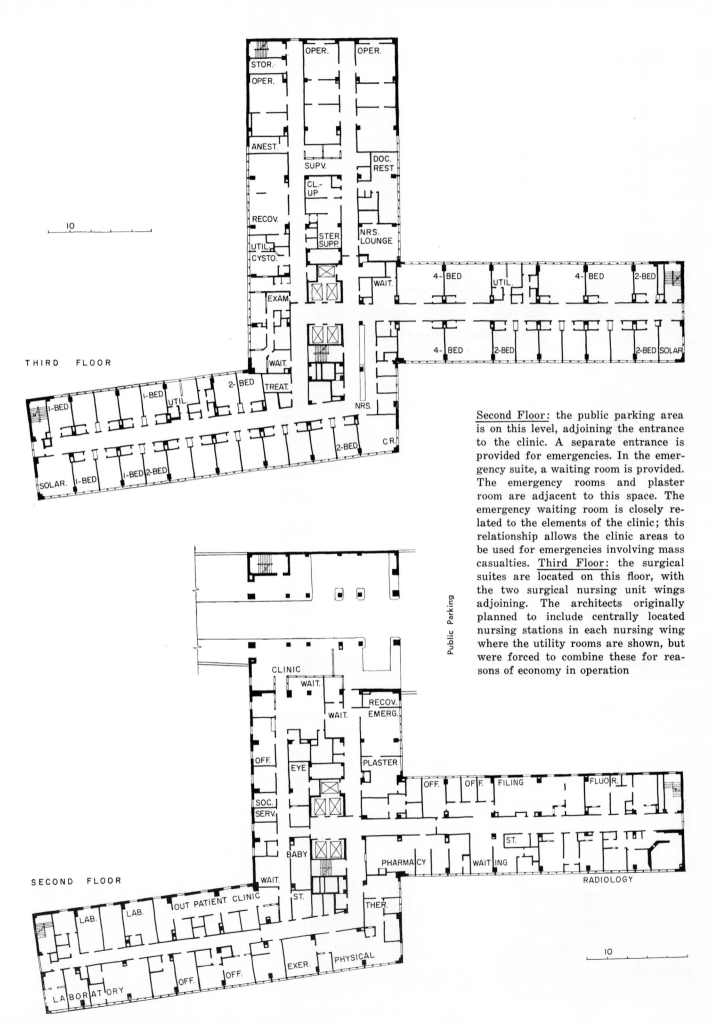

THIRD FLOOR

STOR.
OPER.
OPER.
OPER.
ANEST.
SUPV.
DOC. REST
CL.-UP
RECOV.
STER. SUPP
NRS. LOUNGE
UTIL.
CYSTO.
WAIT.
4-BED
UTIL.
4-BED
2-BED
EXAM
WAIT.
4-BED
2-BED
2-BED SOLAR
2-BED
TREAT.
1-BED
UTIL.
1-BED
NRS.
2-BED
1-BED
2-BED
C.R.
SOLAR.
1-BED
1-BED 2-BED

Second Floor: the public parking area is on this level, adjoining the entrance to the clinic. A separate entrance is provided for emergencies. In the emergency suite, a waiting room is provided. The emergency rooms and plaster room are adjacent to this space. The emergency waiting room is closely related to the elements of the clinic; this relationship allows the clinic areas to be used for emergencies involving mass casualties. Third Floor: the surgical suites are located on this floor, with the two surgical nursing unit wings adjoining. The architects originally planned to include centrally located nursing stations in each nursing wing where the utility rooms are shown, but were forced to combine these for reasons of economy in operation

Public Parking

CLINIC
WAIT.
RECOV.
WAIT.
EMERG.
OFF.
EYE
PLASTER
OFF.
OFF.
FILING
FLUOR.
SOC. SERV.
ST.
BABY
SECOND FLOOR
PHARMACY
WAITING
WAIT.
RADIOLOGY
OUT PATIENT CLINIC
ST.
LAB.
LAB.
THER.
EXER.
PHYSICAL
OFF.
OFF.
LABORATORY

10

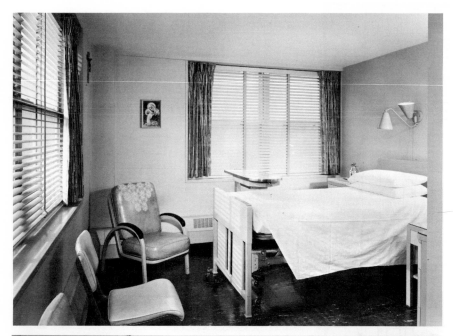

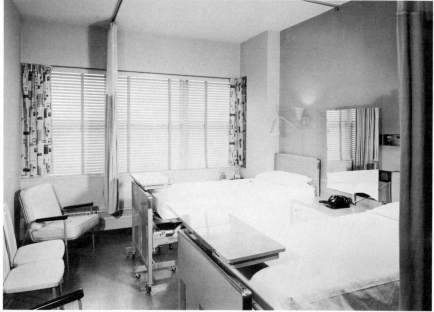

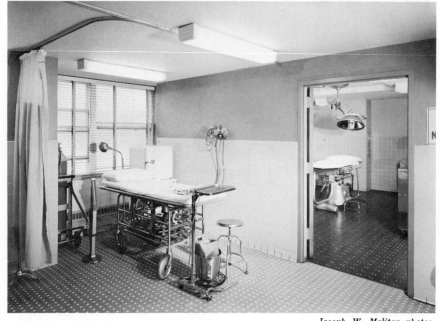

*Joseph W. Molitor photos*

Left, top: view of a typical private patient room. Nearly all of these rooms are exactly the same size as semi-private rooms. They were planned for use as either private or semi-private rooms as required. All patient rooms have at least two large windows; most have three, but a few corner rooms have more as shown. Left, center: view of a typical semi-private room showing the interior arrangements, curtains hung from the ceiling, and furnishings. In addition to rooms of this size, several four-bed wards are provided in the hospital nursing wings. Left, bottom: view of the emergency suite, located on the second floor. As shown, the emergency room is directly connected with the plaster room. Ceiling-hung curtains are provided for division of the rooms into several areas when required

HOSPITAL BUILDINGS

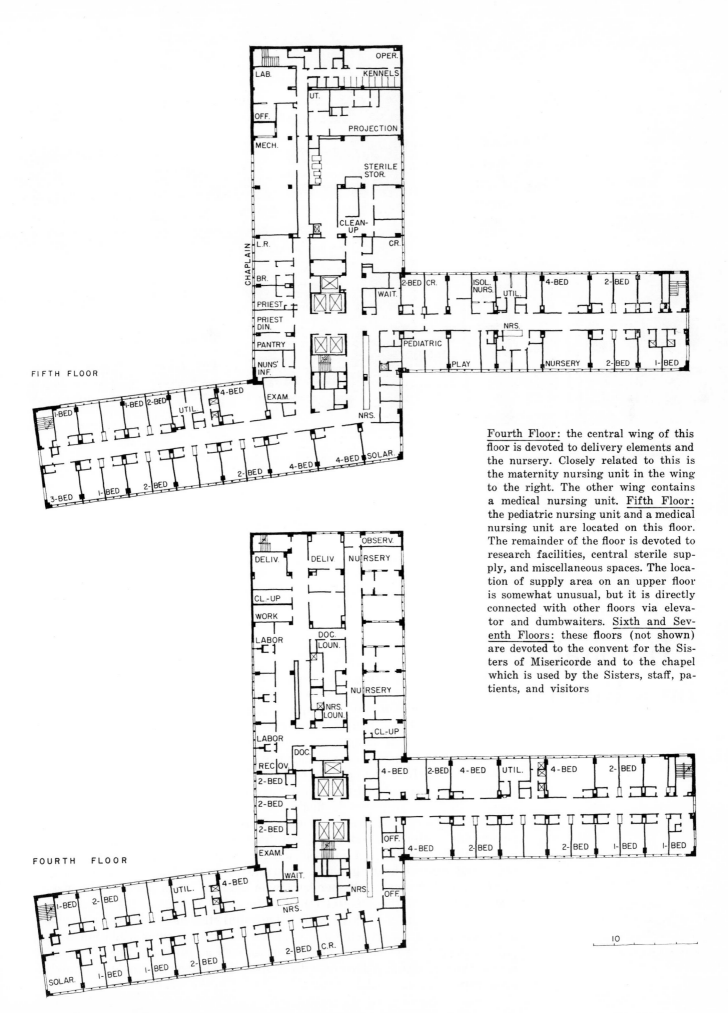

**FIFTH FLOOR**

**FOURTH FLOOR**

Fourth Floor: the central wing of this floor is devoted to delivery elements and the nursery. Closely related to this is the maternity nursing unit in the wing to the right. The other wing contains a medical nursing unit. Fifth Floor: the pediatric nursing unit and a medical nursing unit are located on this floor. The remainder of the floor is devoted to research facilities, central sterile supply, and miscellaneous spaces. The location of supply area on an upper floor is somewhat unusual, but it is directly connected with other floors via elevator and dumbwaiters. Sixth and Seventh Floors: these floors (not shown) are devoted to the convent for the Sisters of Misericorde and to the chapel which is used by the Sisters, staff, patients, and visitors

*Misericordia Hospital*

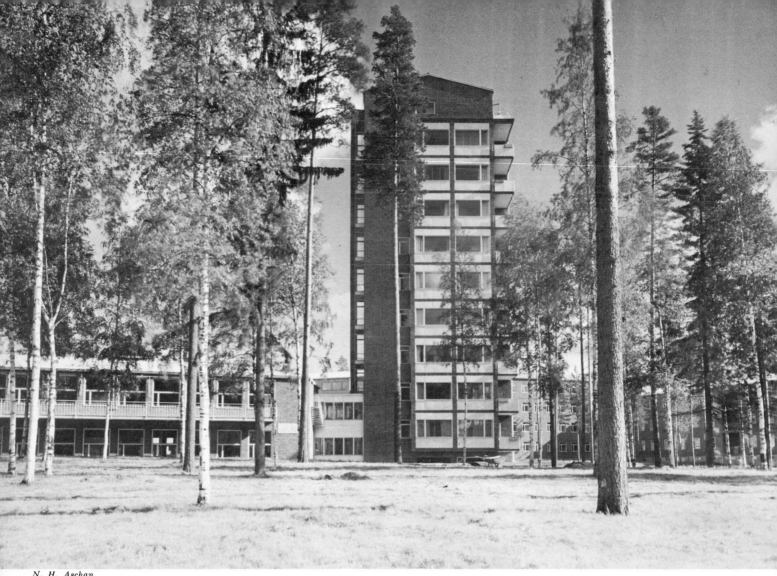

N. H. Aschan

# An Efficient Hospital, on a Rural Site

*Central Hospital for Middle Finland, Jyväskylylä, Finland; Jonas Cedercreutz and Helge Railo, Architects; Esko Päivärinne, Lighting Engineer; Lasse Ollinkari, Interior Designer*

While practices and procedures used in European hospitals differ in many respects from those in this country, there are a number of universal ideas and viewpoints which may, perhaps, be seen at their best in Scandinavian institutions. In the creation of an atmosphere for healing, efficient yet scaled to the human being (especially the one who is sick), the Scandinavian architects often seem to achieve successes in situations in which other designers fail. The hospital contains 375 beds. Contrary to American practice, these are placed in six-bed wards. Its site is rural, and partially because of this, provision is made for every conceivable function of a hospital. Included here are complete facilities for surgery, medicine, gynecology and obstetrics, pediatrics, ophthalmology, and otolaryngology. To service these medical functions efficiently, the hospital has its own power plant and central heating plant. Quarters are provided for the doctors, nurses, and technical staff members who operate it. In spite of the size and complexity of the hospital (the site includes 55 acres), the architects and their consultants working with the hospital staff have achieved a pleasant environment for patients and staff members. Particular attention was paid to the details of design for comfort as well as function. For example, a new type of lighting fixture with a special reflector to shield patients' eyes from glare was custom designed and used in the wards.

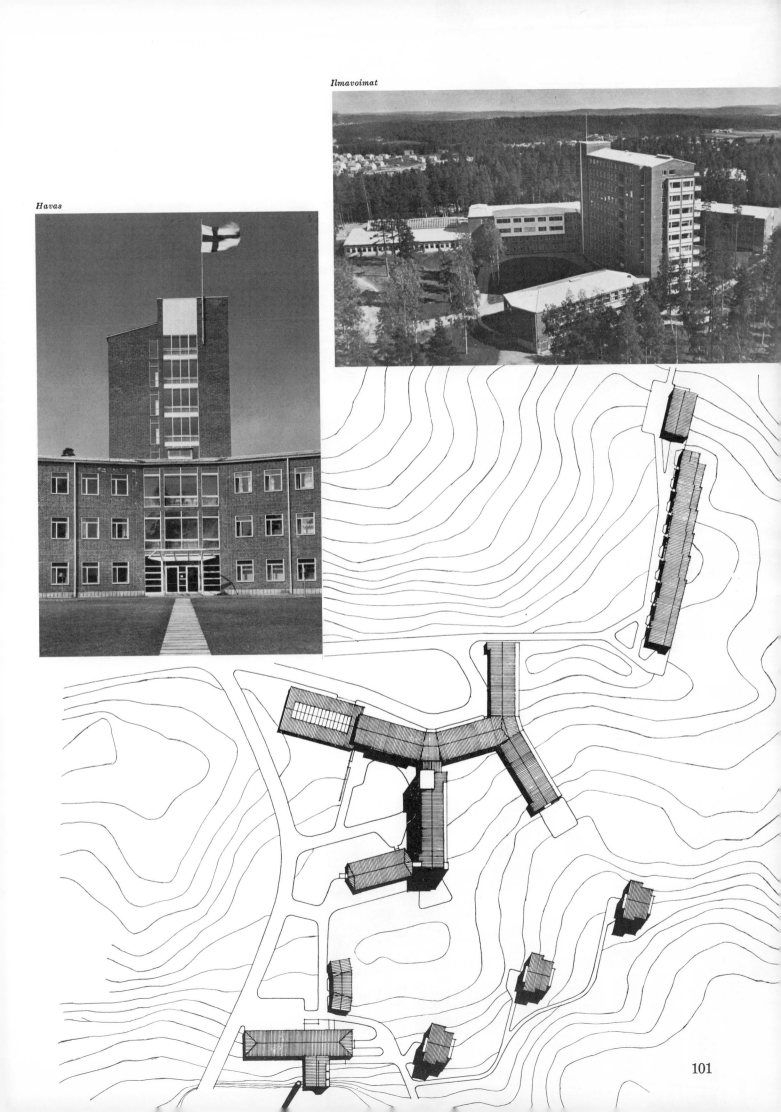

*Havas*

*Ilmavoimat*

101

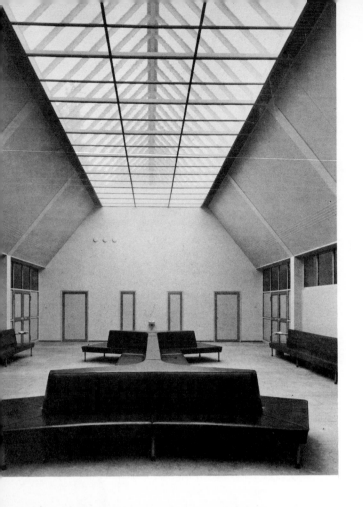

Left, above: waiting room-solarium in the outpatients' department. Left, center: view of an operating room from adjacent surgeons' scrub room. Left, bottom: entrance to outpatients' waiting room-solarium. Below: patients' dayroom (typical of facilities provided for each patient wing through the hospital) and staff dining room (also used for an assembly hall at times)

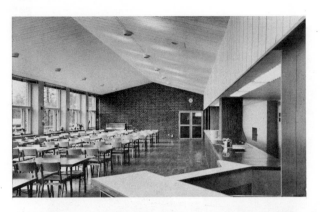

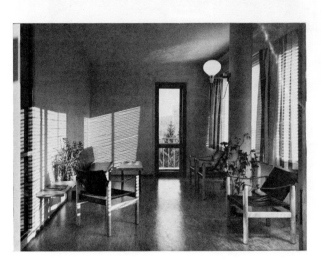

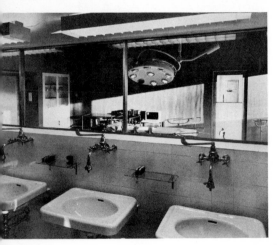

*photos: Havas*

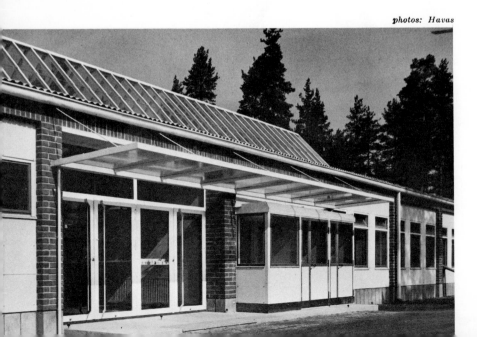

*Central Hospital*

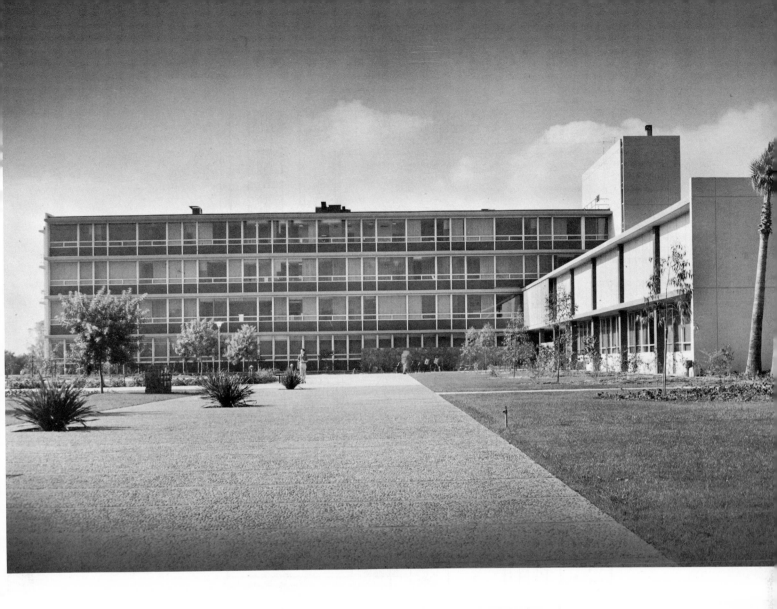

# Psychiatric Unit for a General Hospital

*Methodist Hospital of Southern California, Arcadia, Cal. Architects: Neptune and Thomas; Structural Engineer: John Minasian; Mechanical Engineers: Levine & McCann; Electrical Engineer: John R. Kocher; Landscape Architect: V. H. Pinckney*

ONE OF THE ADVANCES registered in this hospital is the inclusion of a 25-bed psychiatric nursing unit, first in a California general hospital. Another first is a ceramic veneer panel for a curtain wall exterior, conceived by the architects for this building.

The psychiatric unit is especially pleasant; it is on the first floor, and has two enclosed patios for use by patients; some of the patients' rooms open, through shatterproof glass, directly into the larger court. The unit is arranged for the isolation of a group of disturbed patients, with access to the smaller patio. A large day room occupies the space between the courts.

The hospital is planned in bi-nuclear fashion, with the nursing units stacked up in one section, surgical, administrative, in fact most non-bedroom spaces, grouped in a second portion. This scheme has the advantage, of course, of keeping, in at least the nursing

unit, all columns, mechanical systems, plumbing, and so on, in uniform stacks. It permits a great deal of prefabrication of plumbing assemblies on the ground. This placing of masses was also important to the economy of the structural system, since the building is done with lift-slab floors. Columns could be positioned for the floor system, and rooms uniformly designed around them, at least in nursing wings.

The architects, along with Walter R. Hoefflin, Jr., executive secretary of the hospital, worked out a non-conventional arrangement of delivery suite, operating department, recovery room and so on.

The proposed expansion is planned as horizontal, rather than vertical, with another nursing wing added end-to-end to the first one. The building will then take the form of the conventional T, with elevators at the juncture, nursing units on either side.

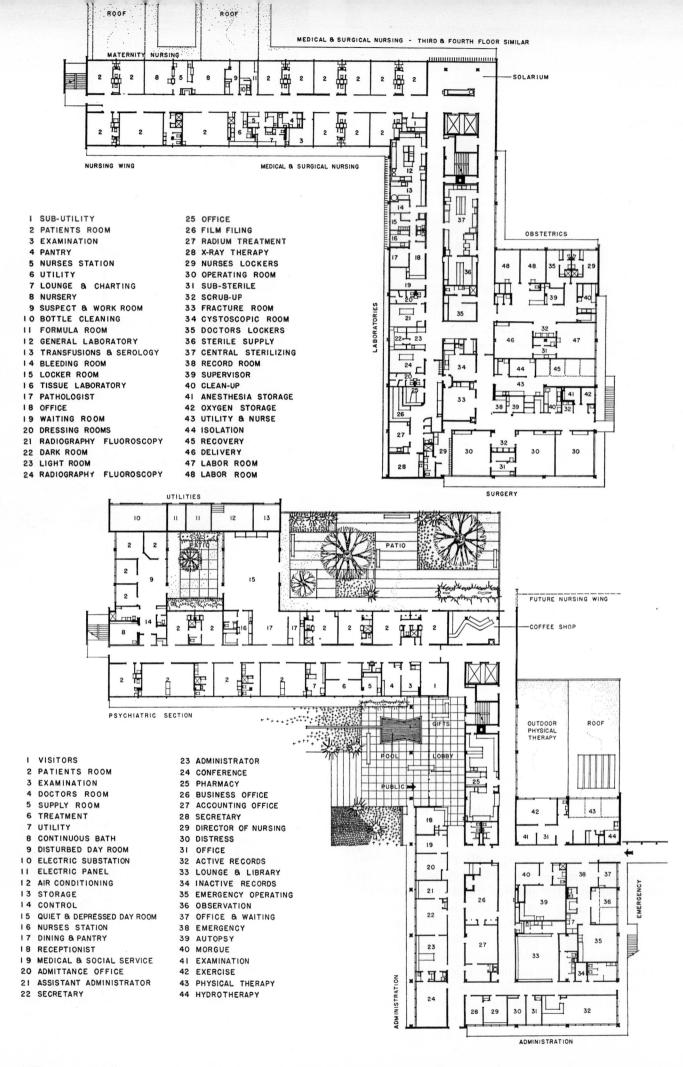

ROOF     ROOF

MEDICAL & SURGICAL NURSING - THIRD & FOURTH FLOOR SIMILAR

MATERNITY NURSING

SOLARIUM

NURSING WING     MEDICAL & SURGICAL NURSING

OBSTETRICS

LABORATORIES

| 1 | SUB-UTILITY | 25 | OFFICE |
|---|---|---|---|
| 2 | PATIENTS ROOM | 26 | FILM FILING |
| 3 | EXAMINATION | 27 | RADIUM TREATMENT |
| 4 | PANTRY | 28 | X-RAY THERAPY |
| 5 | NURSES STATION | 29 | NURSES LOCKERS |
| 6 | UTILITY | 30 | OPERATING ROOM |
| 7 | LOUNGE & CHARTING | 31 | SUB-STERILE |
| 8 | NURSERY | 32 | SCRUB-UP |
| 9 | SUSPECT & WORK ROOM | 33 | FRACTURE ROOM |
| 10 | BOTTLE CLEANING | 34 | CYSTOSCOPIC ROOM |
| 11 | FORMULA ROOM | 35 | DOCTORS LOCKERS |
| 12 | GENERAL LABORATORY | 36 | STERILE SUPPLY |
| 13 | TRANSFUSIONS & SEROLOGY | 37 | CENTRAL STERILIZING |
| 14 | BLEEDING ROOM | 38 | RECORD ROOM |
| 15 | LOCKER ROOM | 39 | SUPERVISOR |
| 16 | TISSUE LABORATORY | 40 | CLEAN-UP |
| 17 | PATHOLOGIST | 41 | ANESTHESIA STORAGE |
| 18 | OFFICE | 42 | OXYGEN STORAGE |
| 19 | WAITING ROOM | 43 | UTILITY & NURSE |
| 20 | DRESSING ROOMS | 44 | ISOLATION |
| 21 | RADIOGRAPHY FLUOROSCOPY | 45 | RECOVERY |
| 22 | DARK ROOM | 46 | DELIVERY |
| 23 | LIGHT ROOM | 47 | LABOR ROOM |
| 24 | RADIOGRAPHY FLUOROSCOPY | 48 | LABOR ROOM |

SURGERY

UTILITIES

PATIO     PATIO

FUTURE NURSING WING

COFFEE SHOP

PSYCHIATRIC SECTION

OUTDOOR PHYSICAL THERAPY     ROOF

GIFTS

POOL     LOBBY

PUBLIC

EMERGENCY

| 1 | VISITORS | 23 | ADMINISTRATOR |
|---|---|---|---|
| 2 | PATIENTS ROOM | 24 | CONFERENCE |
| 3 | EXAMINATION | 25 | PHARMACY |
| 4 | DOCTORS ROOM | 26 | BUSINESS OFFICE |
| 5 | SUPPLY ROOM | 27 | ACCOUNTING OFFICE |
| 6 | TREATMENT | 28 | SECRETARY |
| 7 | UTILITY | 29 | DIRECTOR OF NURSING |
| 8 | CONTINUOUS BATH | 30 | DISTRESS |
| 9 | DISTURBED DAY ROOM | 31 | OFFICE |
| 10 | ELECTRIC SUBSTATION | 32 | ACTIVE RECORDS |
| 11 | ELECTRIC PANEL | 33 | LOUNGE & LIBRARY |
| 12 | AIR CONDITIONING | 34 | INACTIVE RECORDS |
| 13 | STORAGE | 35 | EMERGENCY OPERATING |
| 14 | CONTROL | 36 | OBSERVATION |
| 15 | QUIET & DEPRESSED DAY ROOM | 37 | OFFICE & WAITING |
| 16 | NURSES STATION | 38 | EMERGENCY |
| 17 | DINING & PANTRY | 39 | AUTOPSY |
| 18 | RECEPTIONIST | 40 | MORGUE |
| 19 | MEDICAL & SOCIAL SERVICE | 41 | EXAMINATION |
| 20 | ADMITTANCE OFFICE | 42 | EXERCISE |
| 21 | ASSISTANT ADMINISTRATOR | 43 | PHYSICAL THERAPY |
| 22 | SECRETARY | 44 | HYDROTHERAPY |

ADMINISTRATION

ADMINISTRATION

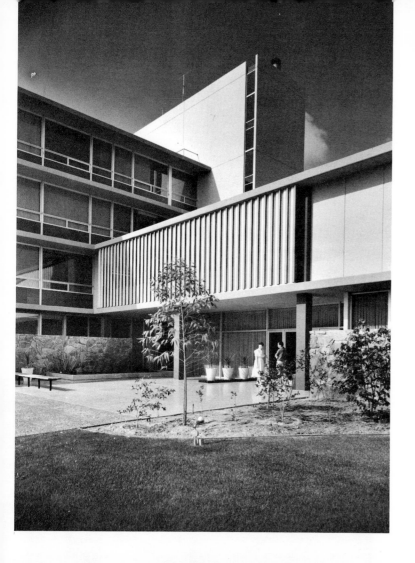
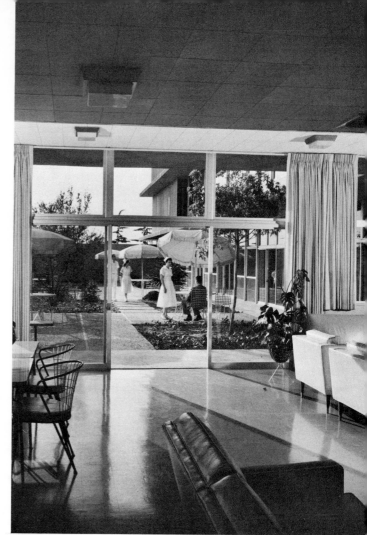
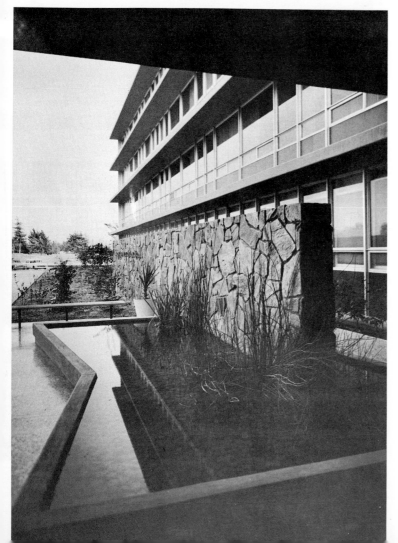
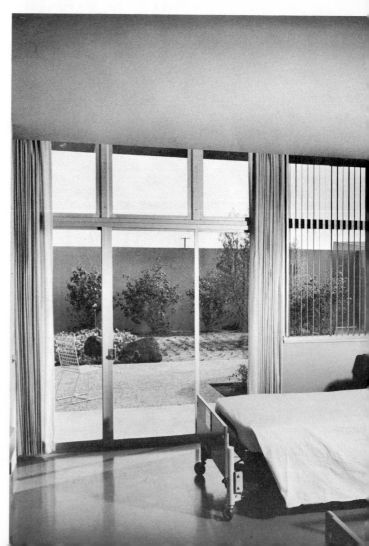

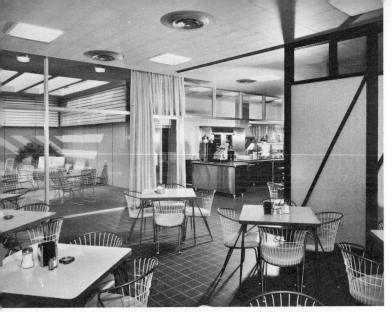

*Above: staff dining room*

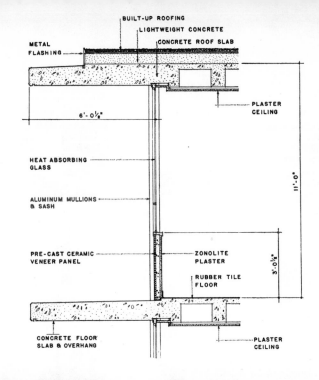

BUILT-UP ROOFING
LIGHTWEIGHT CONCRETE
CONCRETE ROOF SLAB
METAL FLASHING
PLASTER CEILING
6'-0½"
HEAT ABSORBING GLASS
11'-0"
ALUMINUM MULLIONS & SASH
PRE-CAST CERAMIC VENEER PANEL
ZONOLITE PLASTER
RUBBER TILE FLOOR
3'-0"
CONCRETE FLOOR SLAB & OVERHANG
PLASTER CEILING

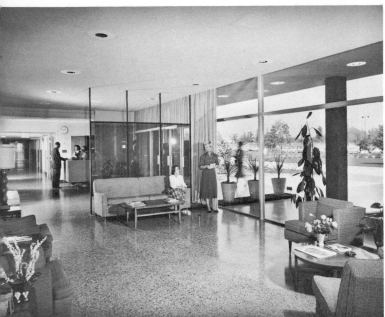

*Above: main waiting room; main entrance is behind*

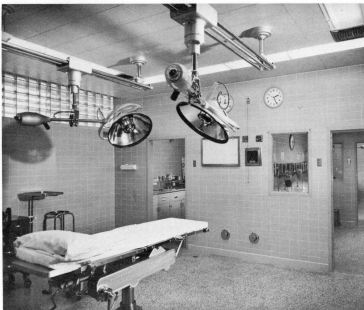

*Above: operating room has conductive terrazzo floors*

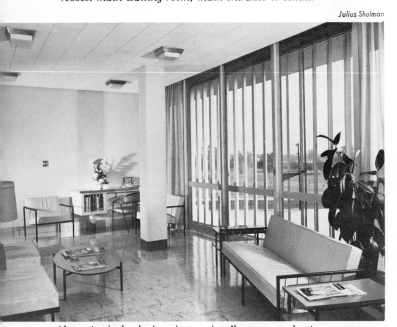

*Above: typical solarium in nursing floors, near elevators*

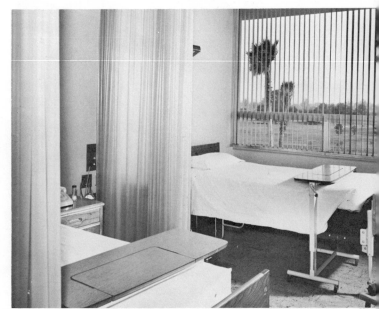

*Above: typical patient's bedroom*

*Methodist Hospital of Southern California*

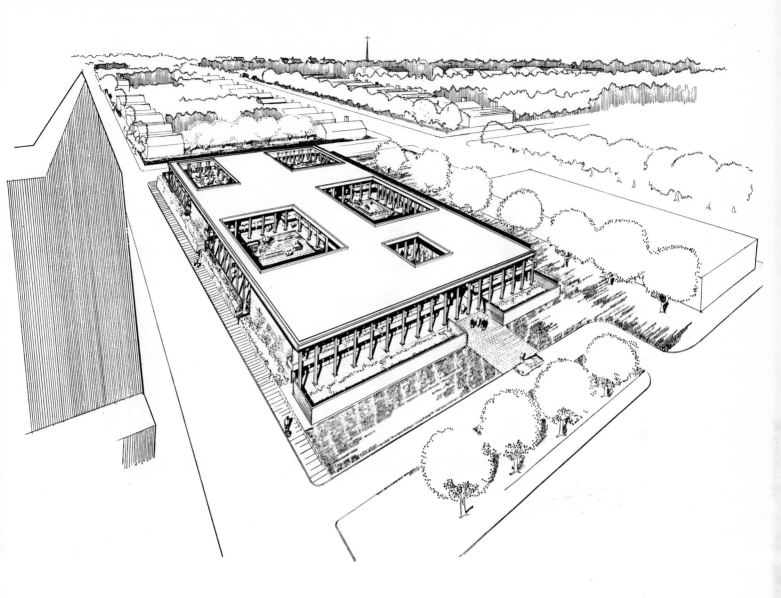

# Pleasant and Open Plan for Psychiatric Patients

*David Wohl Health Institute of St. Louis University, St. Louis, Mo.; Hellmuth, Obata, and Kassabaum, Inc., Architects & Engineers; Eason, Thompson and Associates, Structural Engineers*

This psychiatric hospital has almost nothing in common with most other institutions of its type, except the specific illnesses of the patients to be cared for. Most psychiatric hospitals of the past have more closely resembled the maximum security prisons of the past. In them, patients were locked away from society and often from each other. Rooms were bare and, to say the least, uninviting. It was often said that these precautions were required in order to protect the patients.

The St. Louis University Medical School staff, which will operate this hospital, wanted an entirely different type of plant, one based on the most valid new principles of treatment now generally accepted. In place of a closed type of hospital, they desired one which would express openness to the utmost degree possible. This type of hospital, they felt, would be most conducive to patient recovery. In it, the patient would not be locked up, constantly watched, and barred from walking through the building. Instead, he would be provided with an atmosphere of freedom, within desirable limits. He would be placed in a pleasant environment, close to the ground, with many everchanging views of gardens, water, and trees. He would have access to varied social and recreational facilities. These things would help in the fight for early recovery, and these are the things the architects have provided in this building.

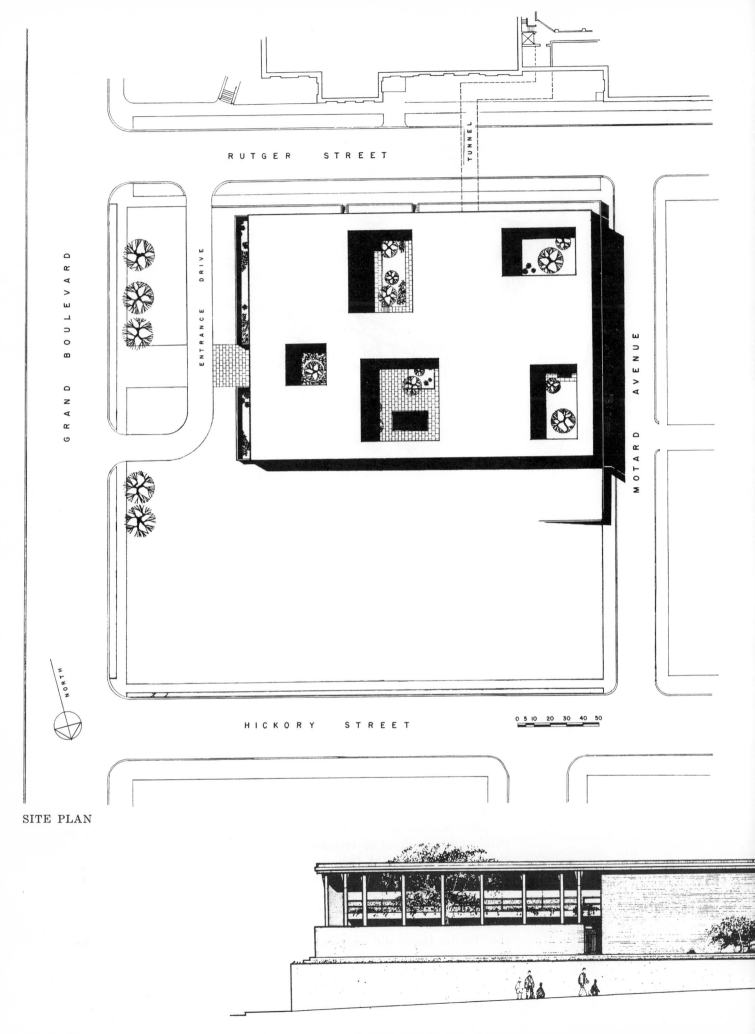

RUTGER STREET

TUNNEL

GRAND BOULEVARD

ENTRANCE DRIVE

MOTARD AVENUE

NORTH

HICKORY STREET

0 5 10 20 30 40 50

SITE PLAN

HOSPITAL BUILDINGS

Of his intentions in the planning of this building, the designer, Gyo Obata, says, "Since the building is in an urban area, without pleasant views to the outside, we attempted to create our own views by using garden courts. Because of the size limitations of the site, we had to go to a two-level scheme. However, to bring the patients as close as possible to the ground, the two-story living-dining room was devised. This room makes access to the ground from the second level seem easy. The inpatient rooms are conceived of as dormitories rather than as hospital rooms, since the patients to be housed here will usually be ambulatory. The 60 patients will be divided into three equal groups. Each group will occupy a two-story wing composed of 20 private bedrooms (or 12 bedrooms and two 4-bed wards), and a centrally located living-dining area. Each of the living rooms will overlook a landscaped court. The nurses' control station is located at the junction of the three wings. This makes easy supervision of the wings possible, yet not too annoying or obvious to the patients. Each room will be furnished with a sofa-bed, desk, chairs, and wardrobe. Each will have a semi-private toilet. Baths and showers will be located within comfortable walking distance, at the ends of the wings.

"Adjoining the corridor connecting the inpatient wings with the other facilities are located areas for patient games, hobbies, and other pursuits. The lounge on the lower level may be furnished as a sidewalk café, where the patients may sit and talk, or simply look out into the garden. An attempt was made to design the lobby to be as attractive as possible. This was considered highly important since many patients are reluctant to enter a psychiatric hospital. It was felt that if we could avoid a "social outcast aspect" at the entrance to the building, and instead make it inviting and warm, much of the patients' natural initial reaction against the institution could be avoided and they could begin their treatment under better circumstances."

In order to achieve an open plan on the small urban site (only half of the lot shown was available for this building), the architects decided on a scheme which resembles a number of small buildings, closely related to each other, but separated by courtyards, under a common roof. In this way, the desired openness was achieved, yet the entire design has been controlled and unified. One of the important program requirements, that of placing the patient facilities as close as possible to the ground, was made quite difficult by the small site, which necessitated a two-story scheme. By the use of enclosed courtyards and a two-story living-dining area in the inpatient areas, many of the desirable features which would have been possible in a single story plan have been retained. The resulting building is in harmony with the surrounding residential area and the St. Louis Hospital buildings. As shown in the site plan, the building will receive its supplies, food, steam, and laboratory work from the nearby Desloge Hospital

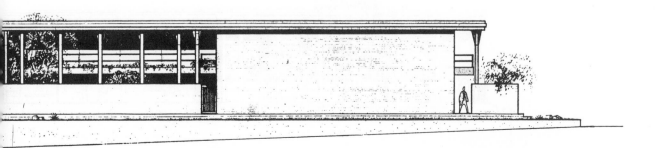

SOUTH ELEVATION

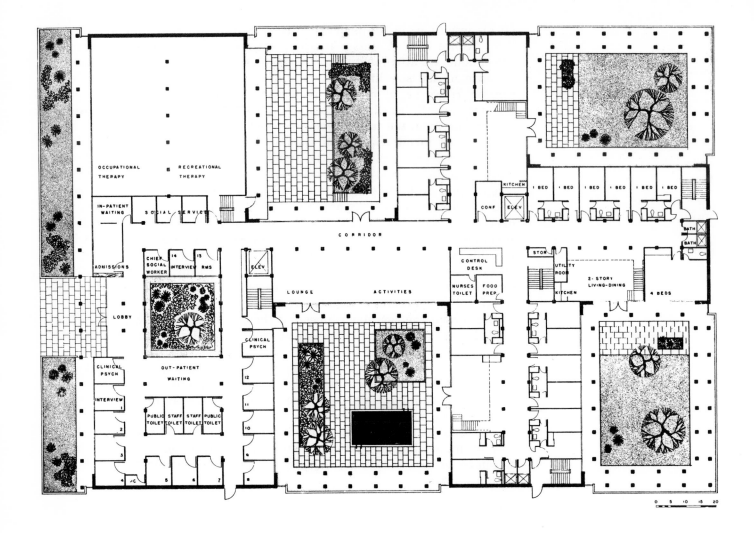

## FIRST FLOOR PLAN

The first floor of the hospital is divided into two major areas, the inpatient portion (consisting of three almost identical wings with similar facilities on the second floor) and the outpatient area. Connecting the two is a corridor containing spaces for activities, lounge, and related functions. All of these areas open onto landscaped courtyards, enclosed by moderately high walls. Each of the inpatient wings together with its upper story functions as a self-sufficient unit. Each contains a two-story living and dining area with a kitchen. These are shared with the patients on the second floor. Thus, each of these units becomes much like a residential dormitory, complete with private areas and communal facilities. By the provision of spaces of this sort, it is felt that the patients can have experiences similar to those they might have in a non-institutional setting or at home, and that these experiences will be conducive to early recovery. The wing across the front of the building is divided into an outpatient department with consultation rooms and a complete occupational and recreational therapy department

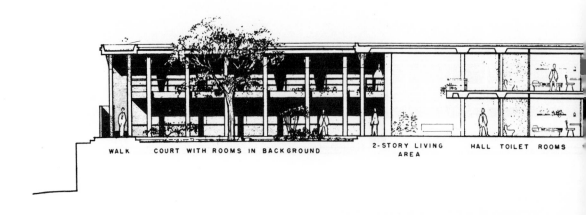

WALK    COURT WITH ROOMS IN BACKGROUND     2-STORY LIVING AREA     HALL    TOILET ROOMS

Dr. Charles E. Goshen of the American Psychiatric Association, who worked closely with the architects on this hospital, says of the principles on which its design is based, "the trend today is toward the liquidation of state and federal hospital psychiatric beds and their replacement by psychiatric sections in general hospitals. Of about 6000 general hospitals now in existence in the United States, about 10 per cent now have in operation efficiently functioning psychiatric facilities. This is an increase of almost 100 per cent within ten years, yet the present number of beds of this type in general hospitals remains only about 15,000 to 20,000 total. This compares to about 550,000 psychiatric beds in state hospitals.

"In spite of the extremely small number of beds available in general hospitals, there were more admissions of patients to these hospitals than to state institutions last year. This phenomenal record was made possible by the extremely fast turnover of patients (the average stay is about 17-21 days) in the general hospital sections. Contrasted with this is an average stay of approximately three years in state hospitals. In terms of costs to the taxpayer, the short-term general hospital stay is considerably cheaper, in spite of higher costs per day of treatment, than the total costs in state institutions.

"In an institution such as this new hospital, many advantages will obviously accrue to patients. Here, the outside which is unattractive, has been shut out and a sort of "captive space" has been created inside. An environment for the best kind of psychiatric treatment will be provided. Less obvious, perhaps, are two other advantages to be gained in a building like this, the provision for training more professionals in psychiatric specialties and the opportunity for research. In addition, we expect that this new, exciting architecture will create the best possible impression of psychiatry on the general public. This will help in many ways, not the least of them being the probability that we can make contact with patients needing psychiatric care earlier. This can only result in better treatment and shorter periods of care."

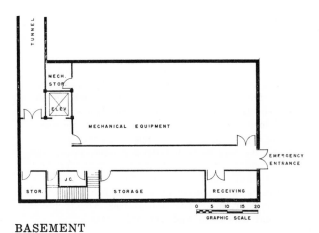

BASEMENT

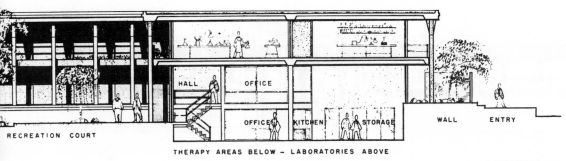

RECREATION COURT

THERAPY AREAS BELOW - LABORATORIES ABOVE

SECTION

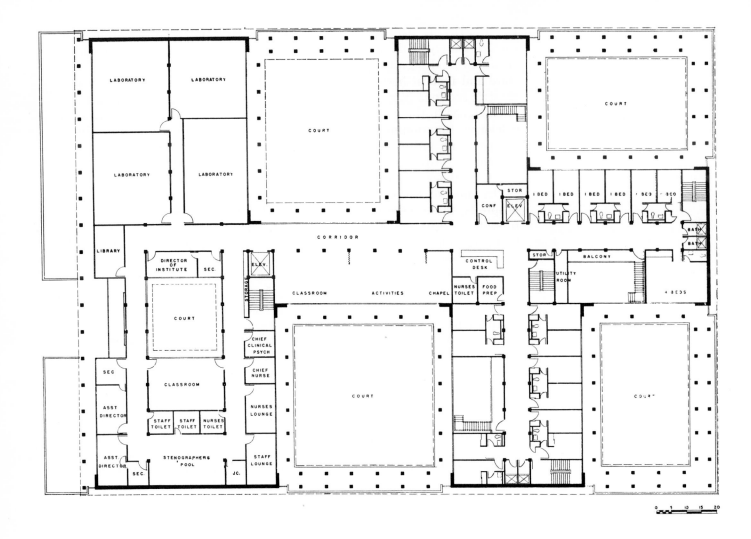

## SECOND FLOOR PLAN

All major areas on the second floor are provided with balconies which may be used by patients and staff for secondary means of circulation. More importantly, these contribute to the atmosphere of openness and freedom which was considered such an all-important program requirement. From them, the landscaped courtyards below may be viewed from all of the important second-floor areas. Thus, the patients are provided with a variety of interesting and satisfying experiences with the spatial concepts of the building on both the first and second floors. As may be seen from a comparison of the two plans, the inpatient portion of the second floor is almost identical with the first floor. The patients are provided with rooms similar to those on the first floor. The two-story living-dining areas are shared by the patients housed on the two floors. Most of the administration spaces are located on this floor, as are the laboratories. Also included here are the library, chapel, and additional classroom and activity areas

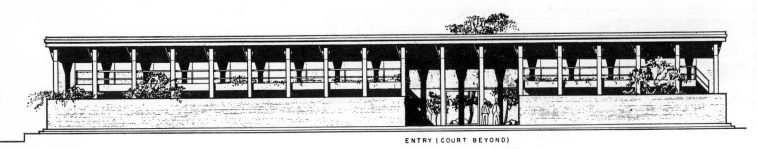

ENTRY (COURT BEYOND)

EAST (FRONT) ELEVATION

# SPECIAL FACILITIES

# Planning the Surgical Suite

*By Aaron N. Kiff and Mary Worthen, Kiff, Colean, Souder & Voss (Office of York and Sawyer)*

*In recent years accepted ideas about planning surgical suites have been suffering some obsolescence. The fabulous surgical procedures of today involve many more people and vastly more equipment. Planning for their smooth functioning, over long, tense hours, is an ever more complicated assignment. This study assembles a dozen or so plans of most interesting surgical suites, with analyses by the architects, surgeons, nurses, administrators and others who have used them. Aaron N. Kiff and Mary Worthen, of Kiff, Colean, Souder & Voss (Office of York & Sawyer) have brought together the material and the comments, and have added their own notes to round out the evaluation.*

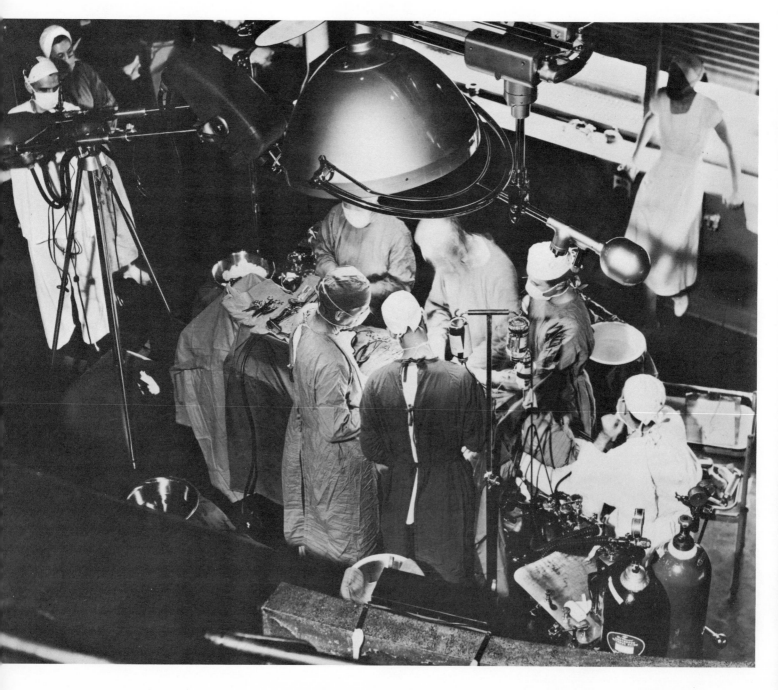

The surgical suite of the general hospital is a very complex workshop. It is one of the most important departments of any hospital, and its planning is complicated by the diversities of opinion and experience of the many persons involved in policy decisions essential to development of a good program of requirements.

We say a "program of requirements" rather than "plan." Before any intelligent planning can be done by the architect, there must be a meeting of minds on the size of department; i.e., the number and type of operating rooms and the work methods to be followed in the supportive areas. Administrators, surgeons, anesthetists, surgical nurses, all must participate in the pre-planning analysis of needs and functional methods. The architect must have a wide understanding of various management procedures to be sure that all are discussed in reaching any conclusions with the particular group involved.

The number and type of operating rooms is the first major decision. In the general hospital, the tendency is to have all major operating rooms as nearly identical as possible to facilitate scheduling of various surgical procedures. Free floor space should be 18 ft by 20 ft, or approximately 350 sq ft. Many surgeons and surgical supervisors recommend 20 ft by 20 ft free floor space.

The planning and equipping of each operating room is based on a series of questions, such as: (a) size, (b) usage, (c) environmental control*, (d) lighting—surgical and general illumination*, (e) intercommunications and signal systems*, (f) electronic equipment and monitoring system*, (g) service lines, such as suction, oxygen, nitrous oxide, compressed air, (h) provision for X-ray, not only X-ray tube stand but control, transformer, and necessary lead protection, (i) provision for TV camera, movie cameras, other recording equipment, (j) safety precaution in hazardous areas, (k) cabinet work, supply cabinets and storage for operating table appliances, (l) need for clocks, film illuminators.

The rapid development of cardiac and neuro-surgery is creating a demand for one or more extra-large operating rooms. This type of surgery calls for a larger team of surgeons, nurses and technicians, plus a great deal of extra equipment, such as heart-lung machines, hypothermia equipment, etc.; also electronic devices for measuring bodily functions, i.e., electro-cardiograph, electro-encephalograph, blood pressure, respiration, body temperature, etc. Today many architects are providing an "instrumentation" room adjacent to or between two extra-

large operating rooms to accommodate such equipment, which is frequently not explosion-proof. The floor of any such room is usually elevated approximately three ft above the operating room floor. Plate glass panels permit vision into operating rooms, and through-wall conduits accommodate wires and other leads of various appliances in the instrumentation room to the surgical field. Such an area can also house the TV control and monitor (if used), X-ray controls, etc.

In the hospital as a whole, the actual patient area is only a very small per cent of the total. The same is true within the surgical suite. The operating rooms themselves will account for only about one-fourth of the total area required for the suite with its supportive functions such as:

Offices and administration areas, scrub areas, work and supply rooms, laboratory, dark room, post-anesthesia recovery, holding or induction areas, lounge, locker and toilet rooms for various personnel groups, conference or teaching rooms, and circulation within the department.

The analysis of various suites illustrating this article show a spread from 1115 sq ft to 1585 sq ft total gross area per operating or cystoscopic room (if included)—and every suite could use more gross floor area for storage, according to comments. Thus, a suite of eight operating rooms averaging 350 sq ft each = 2800 sq ft × 4 = 11,200 sq ft estimated total area required—or 1400 sq ft per operating room.

Within the surgical suite we have three basic zones predicated on three types of activity and circulation involved, and the degree of sterility to be maintained. The pre-planning analysis of these areas is just as important as the determination of the number and type of operating rooms.

*Outer zone*—Administrative elements and basic control where personnel enter the department, patients are received and held or sent to proper holding areas of inner zone; conference, classroom areas, locker spaces, any outpatient reception, etc.

*Intermediate zone*—Predominantly work and storage areas; outside personnel will deliver to this area but should not penetrate the inner zone. The recovery suite, if completely integrated with the surgical suite, is an intermediate or outer zone activity.

*Inner zone*—The actual operating rooms, the scrub areas, the patient holding or induction areas. All alien traffic should be eliminated. Here we want to maintain the highest level of cleanliness and aseptic conditions.

Outer zone administrative areas have increased in importance. Offices are needed for the surgical supervisor, the clerks who manage scheduling and paper work, the clinical instructor (particularly if there is a school of nursing), possibly the chief of staff. There must be provision for surgeons to dictate medical records.

And don't forget the patient. After all, he is the primary concern. Who is responsible for his transportation to the surgical suite, and on whose bed or stretcher? How is he checked in and where does he wait if the room for which he is scheduled is not ready? Who has not seen surgical corridors lined with occupied stretchers for want of adequate holding, preparation or induction areas? Another factor is added if any ambulant outpatient work is to be done. There must be provision for receiving, controlled waiting, dressing rooms and toilets.

A variety of persons must be provided with lounge, locker and toilet space—surgeons (male and female), nurses, technicians, aides, orderlies. Coffee and cola seem to lubricate the entire department; some systematic provision for their supply is warranted.

A conference or classroom for departmental meetings and in-service training programs is easily justified.

The access to all these areas should be removed from strictly surgical areas, as people are entering and leaving in street clothes and should not penetrate into other zones until after changing shoes and clothing.

The planning and equipping of the intermediate zone is based on the method of processing and storing of the thousands of items involved. It is fairly common practice for the central sterile supply department, elsewhere in the hospital, to be responsible for the preparation and autoclaving of all surgical linen packs, gloves, syringes, needles, and external fluids. The storage of these items to be used in surgery becomes the responsibility of the surgical department and adequate space must be provided for a predetermined level of inventory.

The method of processing surgical instruments has been the subject of various research projects, notably at the University of Pittsburgh. New ultrasonic cleaning equipment is eliminating a time-consuming, laborious process. The cost of the equipment discourages duplication and encourages the consolidation of work areas where lay personnel can be trained under close supervision to carry out approved processing techniques.†

The method of packing and sterilizing instruments and utensils will determine the size, type and location of autoclaves needed. Consideration must be given to inclusion of an ethylene oxide sterilizer for cystoscopes, bronchoscopes and delicate surgical instruments which cannot be sterilized by steam or

high temperatures. How and where instruments will be stored is another decision to be made.

Suitable storage space must be provided for: (a) clean surgical supplies such as extra linen, tape, bandage materials, etc.; (b) parenteral solutions, external fluids or sterile water; (c) essential drugs and narcotics; (d) blood supplies, bone bank, tissue bank, eye bank, etc.; (e) radium and isotopes used in surgery.

It seems impossible to provide adequate centralized garage-type spaces for bulky equipment not in constant use. Dr. Carl Walter has estimated that an average of 80 sq ft per operating room is needed.

The intermediate zone also houses the facilities for handling waste, soiled linen, etc., and janitorial equipment for routine housekeeping.

The anesthesia service cannot be shortchanged. It may spread over all zones of the surgical suite. Office space is required, work and storage space for equipment. And most important is the decision on where induction of the patient is to take place: centrally to all rooms, locally in induction areas (sometimes referred to as preparation or holding rooms) or in the operating room proper. There are acknowledged hazards in moving anesthetized patients and equipment. Induction areas should permit quicker turnover in operating room usage, but they also require more anesthetists and nurses to administer.‡

The post-anesthesia recovery room has become an integral part of the surgical suite in most cases. The size will vary from one-and-a-half to two beds per operating room. There is a close relationship between the anesthesia department and the recovery room.

Any frozen section laboratory should be located near the entrance of the surgical suite so that laboratory personnel need not penetrate the inner zone.

Any dark room facilities should be located to serve those rooms generating greatest load of film, normally the cystoscopic, urological and orthopedic services. It should be accessible from a corridor to prevent alien traffic through any operating room.

Inner zone planning includes the operating rooms and their essential supportive elements. Decisions must be made on the type of scrub-up sinks or troughs and their location providing minimum travel to the operating room to eliminate chance of contamination after scrub procedure.

The need for local "sub-sterilizing" rooms is being questioned by many authorities. The trend toward centralization of work areas and sterilizing equipment, and the changing techniques of instrument packaging are reducing the importance of the sub-sterilizing area. Circulation travel distance and work patterns are factors determining the need for decentralized work areas. When such areas are provided there should be staff access for servicing and

---

† Long Island Jewish Hospital and University of California Hospital illustrate a large work area centrally located to serve all the operating rooms.

‡ Experience with various suites indicates that what was planned for induction frequently is converted to other causes. (See Grace-New Haven Hospital, Moffitt Hospital of University of California, Rhode Island Hospital.)

stocking them without going through an operating room.

The program of need dictates the gross area required for the surgical suite. Recent developments indicate that more efficient departments with minimum travel distances can be planned in bulk, squarish areas. This tendency has affected the location of the surgical suite in relationship to the hospital as a whole. The suite has come downstairs to a lower floor where it is more possible to spread out and achieve the desired shape, divorced from the usually narrow structural pattern of a nursing unit. Planning within the squarish areas has been made possible with the parallel development of air conditioning and artificial lighting. Dependence upon windows for ventilation and light is a thing of the past.

The optimum conditions of temperature, humidity, and light level can be controlled by mechanical means far better than by nature.

The surgical suite location must mesh with the total circulation pattern so that patients can be moved to and from surgery with a minimum of travel through other hospital services. Its location is also affected by its close relationship to three other major hospital services—the X-ray department, the clinical laboratories, and the central sterile supply.

One other important factor in the location of the surgical suite is the future. Expansion! Anticipate ways and means to permit growth in an orderly fashion without upsetting basic relationship of internal organization—or without extending lines of travel to unacceptable or uneconomical lengths.

## HARLAN MEMORIAL HOSPITAL, KENTUCKY, Miners Memorial Hospital Association

### MEDICAL BACKGROUND

From John C. Blankenbeckler, Acting Hospital Administrator: "As originally designed, there was inadequate space for the anesthetists to perform their cleaning, storage and general care of their instruments and equipment. However, this has been remedied by enclosing part of the recovery room with a glass wall adjacent to the corridor. This room can be entered directly by the first door on the left as you enter the operating room corridor, or by entering through the recovery room itself.

"'Harlan Memorial Hospital has the best spatial organization of facilities I have seen, and I have no constructive suggestions in that regard.' I am quoting Dr. W. H. Potter, Chief of Surgical Service.

"The four operating rooms should have an electrical circuit so that the portable X-ray unit could be plugged in within the operating room and eliminate an extension cord being run to the corridor. This could be handled by using the electrical panel which is installed in the corner of each room. This cord poses a safety hazard to the operating room personnel.

"The instrument room is used to capacity and possibly 40 per cent more space could be used, if available, for a more ideal arrangement. However, installation of additional instrument poles would solve this problem for all practical purposes.

"All concerned agree wholeheartedly that the arrangement of the operating room, its location being proximal to the cystoscopy room, fracture room, emergency room and the radiology department, are assets to the operating of the department.

"The safety panel mentioned above has many good points. With all elec-

trical cords running to one location, both the patient and the personnel are much safer. The automatic monitor is excellent and contributes much toward the safety of the patient and also, actually and psychologically, to that of the operating room personnel.

"Space for instrument cleaning and autoclaving is very adequate.

"Dr. Potter also commented that an adequate area for pre-operative patients, not so close to the recovery room and more private, could have been provided."

### COMMENT

"1. Little storage space within department, but system of supply eliminates need for a great deal, as all basic supplies are just across corridor. Very little storage space for extra equipment, fracture and orthopedic rooms.

"2. X-ray department adjacent, containing fracture and cystoscopy room, plus developing facilities; portable X-ray used as required in operating rooms.

"3. Relationship to lab remote; no local tissue or frozen section facilities.

"4. Good relationship of emergency facilities to operating rooms and X-ray department.

"5. Note elimination of doors whenever practical, and local building and fire laws permit. Good, as doors are always in the way, particularly where heavy supply line exists within department and where privacy is not essential.

"6. The pre-operative patient will be left in the corridor until room is ready, unless there is very good scheduling."

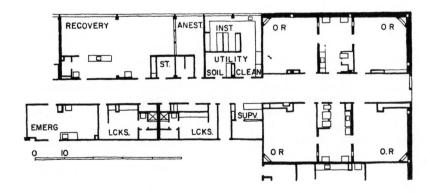

*Sherlock, Smith & Adams, Architects*

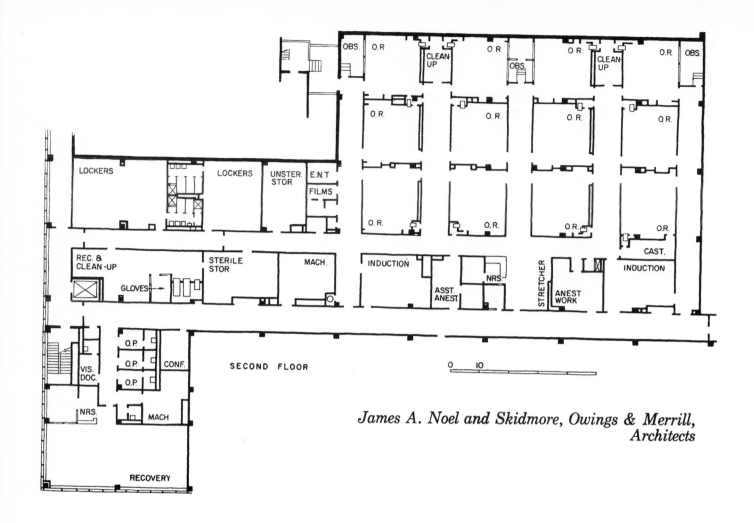

LOCKERS LOCKERS UNSTER. E.N.T
STOR. FILMS

OBS. O.R CLEAN UP O.R. O.R. CLEAN UP O.R. OBS.
OBS.

O.R. O.R. O.R. O.R.

O.R. O.R. O.R. O.R.
CAST.

REC. & CLEAN-UP STERILE STOR. MACH. INDUCTION STRETCHER INDUCTION
GLOVES→ NRS.
ASST. ANEST WORK
ANEST.

VIS. DOC. O.P. CONF. SECOND FLOOR 0 10
O.P.
O.P.
NRS. MACH

RECOVERY

*James A. Noel and Skidmore, Owings & Merrill,*
*Architects*

## TEMPLE UNIVERSITY MEDICAL CENTER, PHILADELPHIA

### ARCHITECTURAL BACKGROUND

From Harold H. Olson, Project Manager: "The planning of the surgical suite at Temple University Hospital was unusually successful because the architects were able to get more exact program information from the staff than was obtainable for any other area of the hospital, and therefore the problem was more fully understood and a plan was developed that fitted these particular needs.

"Being a teaching hospital, the pattern of traffic within the surgical suite must provide easy access and circulation for the department head and other faculty members among the 12 operating rooms. It must also allow easy access for large groups of students and other visitors. Neither of these special traffic patterns should interfere with the normal passage of the patient into and out of the surgical suite, nor should the patient even be aware of their existence.

"Efforts were made to keep every operating room alike in order to achieve maximum flexibility in their use; however, various branches of surgery required making special provision in a few of the rooms. Thus we have one shielded room equipped for electro-encephalography, two rooms equipped for television, one with an observation gallery, and one equipped for orthopedic surgery.

"A square windowless building, instead of a more conventional form with normal fenestration, allowed the development of this unusual plan which meets the special requirements of this institution. All rooms are air conditioned and artificially lighted, making it possible to perform all types of surgical procedures without regard to light-proof shades or the problems normally incurred in rooms with windows."

### COMMENT

"1. Good segregation of patient travel and staff travel.

"2. Induction rooms make good receiving patient-holding area. As-sume attendant with patient must check at 'clerk' to know which induction area is to be used. Some backtracking from induction rooms to center six operating rooms. Moving table and anesthetizing equipment the distance involved seems hazardous, though anesthetists have two schools of thought on the subject.

"3. High-speed instrument autoclaves *within* each room is rather unusual. Would seem that three or four in each substerilizing area serving six rooms would have been adequate. Also would eliminate small heating element from operating room.

"4. Conference room seems small for teaching hospital.

"5. Staff lockers located for pretty good segregation.

"6. Rather unusual to find separate work room geared to take care of surgical pack work which more usually is handled in central sterile.

"7. Good to see some provision for outpatients, but think location—so far removed from control point center of surgical suite—unfortunate."

# LONG ISLAND JEWISH HOSPITAL, NEW HYDE PARK, N. Y.

## ARCHITECTURAL BACKGROUND

From Isaiah Ehrlich, of the office of Louis Allen Abramson, architect: "The special aspects of the suite are —1. Its location on the first floor outside the main mass of the building, to provide for expansion of the operating room suite when the additional floors are added. Also, we did not want the operating rooms to be confined by the dimensions of the typical floors. Placing the suite where we did, we were able to make the rooms of the dimensions we wished, in addition to having the story height a full foot higher than the typical story. Having it on the first floor produced better relations with the emergency unit.

"2. With the double corridor arrangement, we were able to discard the old Goldwater Unit of a substerilizing and scrub-up space between each pair of operating rooms. We felt that this arrangement was wasteful of equipment and in no way guaranteed sterile instruments. We placed the nurses' work room so that it is central to the operating rooms, including those to be added at the westerly end in the future. We provided a continuous conveyor from this work room to central sterile supply on floor

below so as to obviate the need for any personnel circulation between the two points, and by doing this we were able to place central supply at a point readily accessible to the nursing units without the need of help who do not belong in the operating room ever getting in there. A little detail that we added was that the doors to the nurses' work room are pneumatically operated by a foot treadle in the terrazzo floor, so that a nurse coming in holding heavy trays has the doors opened automatically.

"3. All operating rooms are without windows, as we were convinced that outside light interferes with proper light control in the operating room, acts as an annoying distraction to the surgeons, adds to heating and cooling loads and presents the usual problems with double sets of windows.

"4. The operating room has its own instrument washing and handling unit but is remote from central sterile supply.

"5. The post-operative nursing unit is in a tight relation to the operating room suite for ease of control by the anesthetists. The arrangement provides direct access from the operating room suite to the post-operative nursing unit and permits easy

access to the nursing unit from outside the operating room area. This we felt to be important because visitors were to be admitted.

"I sounded out the hospital personnel as to how the above elements have been functioning. The reactions of the chief anesthetist and the operating room supervisor are: 1. They are highly satisfied with location. Partition dividing cystoscopy room into two stations was found to cramp activity somewhat and will be removed. 2. They feel the central core location of the nurses' work room is better than the conventional arrangement. They would, however, have liked to have had more storage space, and 100 per cent more room for anesthetists' offices, anesthesia storage and induction. 3. The doctors are highly satisfied with the operating rooms without windows. Some of the nurses are not, for psychological reasons; these are a small minority. 4. They are satisfied with the nurses' work room arrangement. Doors are not provided in the instrument storage room. Nurses feel there should be doors on the cabinets. The conveyor to central sterile is no longer used. Some of the packs coming from central sterile are too large for the conveyor and it was necessary to send personnel there anyway. Now regular trips are made there. The pneumatic doors are kept constantly open and the operating devices are not used. 5. Recovery unit and its location are highly satisfactory."

## COMMENT

"1. Good circulation and separation of patient and staff.

"2. Good control check-in for both patients and staff.

"3. Ample maneuvering space in and out of operating rooms. Note divided doors, large and small leaf. Both must be opened when moving patient, but for housekeeping chores it is only necessary to open 3-ft door. Reduces swing area.

"4. Good consolidation of clean-up, work, instrument space—but admittedly cramped.

"5. Good pre-operation holding area under supervision.

"6. No access to dark room from areas other than fracture and cystoscopy, though they are the major users.

"7. In two of the operating rooms, the room must be traversed to stock supply cabinets.

"8. Lack of storage space for extra equipment."

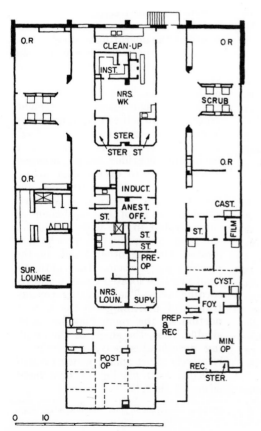

*Louis Allen Abramson, Architect*

# THE NATIONAL INSTITUTES OF HEALTH, BETHESDA, MD.

## Operating Facilities, Cardiovascular and Neurological Surgery*

### ARCHITECTURAL BACKGROUND

From John W. Franklin, of the architects' office, outlining the program requirements: "1. Two operating rooms for heart surgery and two operating rooms for neurological surgery, with all necessary supporting areas, to comprise two physically separated surgical suites, with each serving having complete and independent staffs. 2. Isolated location to eliminate all traffic by unauthorized personnel and visitors, and having convenient access to nursing units, central sterile supply and blood bank. 3. Large operating rooms to accommodate the many equipment items required for the various procedures, plus 18-20 people, plus provision for use of heart-lung machine and hypothermia. 4. If possible, one central recording room for instrumentation for each suite with operating and anesthesia rooms, X-ray and catheterization laboratory grouped around it, avoiding the need for duplication of costly instruments for each recording room, or for moving sensitive electronic equipment from one to the other, risking possible damage. 5. Close relationship between other supporting spaces such as laboratories, dark rooms, heart-lung laboratory, instrument clean-up, sterilizing rooms, work room, recovery room, anesthesia work room and lab, with operating rooms. 6. Observation facilities for visitors and staff. 7. Adequate provision for personnel, including locker rooms, briefing rooms and rest rooms. 8. Extensive means of communication—physical, mechanical and visual—between various areas. 9. Best possible lighting and bacteria-free air, with special attention to methods of air handling. 10. Space for staff consultation and training. 11. Elimination of undesirable wiring and tubing running across floor of operating rooms— more of a problem than normally because of the use of such equipment as the heart-lung machine, hypothermia, EEG, EKG, oscilloscopes, cautery, gas analyses, respirator, defibrillator, anesthograph, blood withdrawal unit with photoelectric cell, and, in addition, the necessary tubing for air, vacuum, oxygen and nitrous oxide. 12. Provision for still and motion picture photography and television.

"The circular scheme, rather than a number of rectangular schemes studied, with a central recording cyl-inder and patient areas on the periphery, proved to be the most direct and logical solution of the problem, from both the functional and structural aspects. With the framing system employed, it also was the most flexible for possible future rearrangement, as there are columns only at the edge of the recording circle and the inside face of the corridor.

"On the neurological floor, the operating table will be located on a radius so that the patient's head is about 7 ft from the recording room. As effective observation in this case must be directly behind and above the head of the operating table, and as few observers will be invited for direct viewing, it was decided to combine the recording and observation area.

"The entire structure will be air conditioned. In the operating rooms, to reduce air turbulence, radiant cooling panels will be installed in the walls supplementing the conditioned air. Studies have proven that turbulence in otherwise clean air introduced into a room quickly picks up and suspends in the clean air many bacteria from the floors, equipment and clothing in the room. As the cleanest air is the freshly filtered incoming supply, it is planned to bathe the operating field with it, thereby pushing aside air which has been in contact with floors, people, drapes.

### MEDICAL BACKGROUND

From Jack Masur, M.D., Assistant Surgeon General and Director, Clinical Center: "The two major factors which led to the decision to construct a new wing to accommodate the research teams in neurosurgery and cardiac surgery were: 1, increasing number and complexity of recording apparatus, and 2, increasing number of specialists and technicians engaged in the surgical procedures in the room and around the operating table. The present array of electronic devices and other recording apparatus in the modern operating room is impressive, but a look-see at what is going on in the nearby laboratories reveals that the best is yet to come. Moreover, the requirements of present-day anesthesiology and the utilization of hypothermia and oxygenators all add up to more men and more machines to be considered in the design and operational approach.

"The recrudescence of the problems of infections reminds us sharply that our much vaunted 'conquest' is not yet complete. In neurosurgery particularly, where one deals with vital tissues that are utterly destroyed by infection, this is an especially crucial problem. Thus, the current debate about recirculation of conditioned air in operating rooms seems futile—rather we ought to be learning a good deal more about setting up stricter specifications for the *quality* of air.

"The presence of so much electronic equipment will call for more attention to improved techniques of shielding; the larger number of persons involved in complex surgical procedures will necessitate the adaptation of flexible intercommunications arrangements; in a period of innovation with more complicated surgical approaches, space for the briefing of the teams is required; the increased length of time that staff is working in operating rooms needs to be reckoned with; the real usefulness of television (close-range and long-range) for true instructional purposes has not yet found clear expression; the proper channeling of all the 'spaghetti' running across the floor is yet to be solved; et cetera, et cetera."

From E. K. Day, Chief, Research Facilities Branch, Division of Research Services, Public Health Service: "The building makes possible the contingence of the operating suite elements in a circular pattern, yet provides one direct and compact instrumentation space contiguous to all of the operating areas. This convenient functional and economical arrangement, from the viewpoint of equipment use, however, requires the sacrifice of additional space since it necessitates a peripheral corridor which occupies almost one-third of the floor area.

"There are other advantages and disadvantages for cardiac surgery, since the bulk of the equipment is concentrated in the wide portion of the room where the patient's head is located. On the other hand, in the neurosurgery room, the patient's head must be located close to the recording area. The resulting concentration of machinery in the narrow portion of the room may be undesirable. Also, the shape of the building necessitates polygonal walls of relatively short spans, which present difficulties in placing of equipment adjacent thereto."

---

* Under construction; no administrative comment possible.

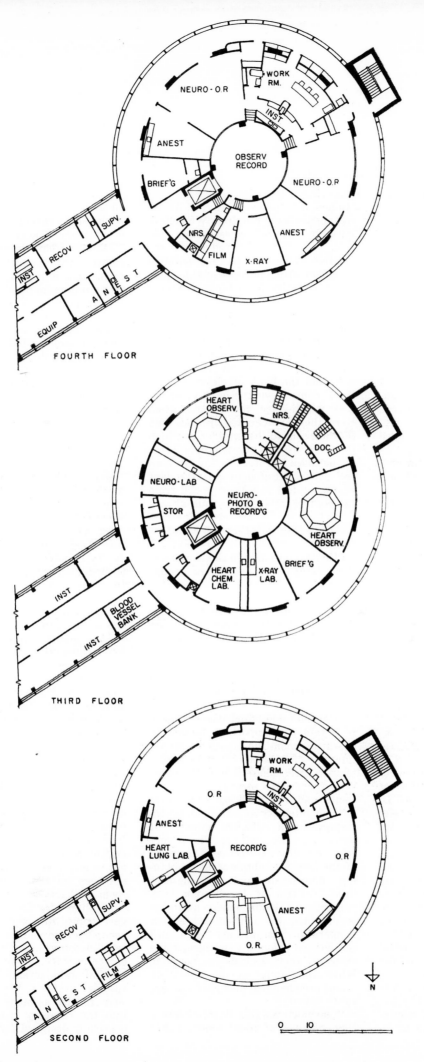

FOURTH FLOOR

THIRD FLOOR

*Kiff, Colean, Voss & Souder, The Office of York & Sawyer, Architects*

SECOND FLOOR

0    10

N

# RHODE ISLAND HOSPITAL, PROVIDENCE

## ARCHITECTURAL BACKGROUND

From Henry R. Shepley, architect: "The layout is not unusual, but was worked out with great care. A few of its features are: 1. A 24-hour special nursing unit on the floor immediately above surgery fulfills some of the recovery functions, which permits a considerably smaller than average recovery room on the surgical floor. 2. The scrub and sterilizing rooms between the operating rooms replace the conventional pattern of two separate rooms. 3. The bed garage at each end of the central core saves clutter in the corridors. 4. Operating Room No. 12 is fully equipped for X-ray.

"There are certain built-in features in the way of equipment which are quite interesting: 1. The doors between the scrub-sterilizing rooms and the operating rooms are equipped with power-operated 'magic' hardware. 2. The scrub sink faucets are operated by electronically controlled temperature and humidity recording devices. 4. The intercom and emergency call systems between operating rooms and control desk are quite elaborate. 5. Operating Room No. 1 is equipped for closed circuit built-in television broadcasting to the classroom on the same floor and the main hospital auditorium."

## MEDICAL BACKGROUND

From Dorothy L. Morrison, R.N., and Meyer Saklad, M.D.: "The operating room suite in this general hospital of 659 beds was designed to care for about 12,000-14,000 surgical procedures yearly. On the operating corridor are 14 operating rooms. In general, their use is as follows: one gynecologic, one genito-urinary, two cystoscopy, two orthopedic, one nose and throat, one alternating nose and throat and dental, one alternating eye and general surgery, one alternating neurosurgery and general surgery, three general surgery and one special function room. All the rooms, with the exception of the two cystoscopy rooms, may serve as general duty rooms, and are not reserved for the indicated service entirely.

"The special function room in this corridor requires comment. The patient in the operating room requiring X-rays should be able to be so studied by whatever heavy duty X-ray apparatus is required. We believe strongly that all anesthetized patients should be X-rayed in the operating room corridor for safety's sake. The prime purpose of this room is for operative procedures requiring X-ray procedures not readily available in the cystoscopic and orthopedic rooms.

"It may be noted that the North corridor is separated from the South and West corridors by the control desk and the bank of elevators. Patients come down the bank of elevators which face the control desk. Here they are checked in and then they are sent to the corridor in which they are to be operated upon. One of the three elevators facing the control desk is staffed by an attendant who is subject to telephone call from the control desk. He is thus always available to serve the operating corridors in case the other two elevators are busy.

"Centrally located in the North and West wings are anesthesia rooms. They serve as distribution centers for anesthesia equipment in these corridors. The anesthesia room in the West corridor also serves as an induction room for tonsillectomies. The anesthesia room in the South corridor serves as a room for the preparation of anesthesia supplies and also as a distribution area for this corridor.

"Considerable effort was expended to obtain two important factors in operating room illumination—proper intensity of light and its correct color temperature. These are *both* necessary for proper observation of patients and for working conditions.

"The intensity is obtained by incorporating a sufficient number of units of proper wattage. The proper color temperature—actually the color of the light—is obtained by combining fluorescent and incandescent light. Control of the Kelvin temperature of the incandescent lights is obtained by a rheostat. Kelvin temperature readings are taken until the desired color is reached and the rheostat then locked in position. When the lamps in the operating rooms are changed, new readings are again taken.

"Inasmuch as this hospital has a large number of night emergencies, all such procedures are concentrated in the South corridor for the purpose of efficiency. The reason is two-fold: 1, this corridor is adjacent to the recovery room, and 2, the operating rooms in this corridor are so placed that a minimum number of personnel can supervise several operating rooms at a given time. There is a telephone extension at the end of the corridor common to that of the desk, so that incoming calls can be handled from either position. This makes it possible to function at night with less personnel than would ordinarily be the case.

"The operating rooms are divided into pairs, with a scrub room between each two rooms, with the exception of the operating rooms in the North corridor. Here one combination scrub and sterilizing room serves the genito-urinary room, the two cystoscopy rooms and the special function room. The scrub rooms between each pair of operating rooms have worked out extremely well. There is enough room for either five or six people at the same time. The sinks are of stainless steel and are built with a slanting portion under the faucet so that the water is less likely to splash.

"The instrument scrub room is so constructed that the dirty instruments come in one end, are cleaned and processed and passed through a window to the central instrument storage room. In this instrument scrub room soiled sponges and debris are discarded.

"Experience has demonstrated that with but few but important exceptions, the operating corridor has worked out very well. A serious weakness is the inadequate size of our recovery room. It had been hoped that inasmuch as the special care unit was in such close proximity to the operating room, the recovery room need not be large. This, unfortunately, has not been the case, and the recovery room as it now stands does not meet our full needs. The volume of surgery (up to 62 per day) and the severity and type of surgery have necessitated that many patients remain on the operating room floor to await the full stabilization of their cardiovascular systems. We have on occasion crowded as many as 13 patients into the recovery room, which was originally designed for five.

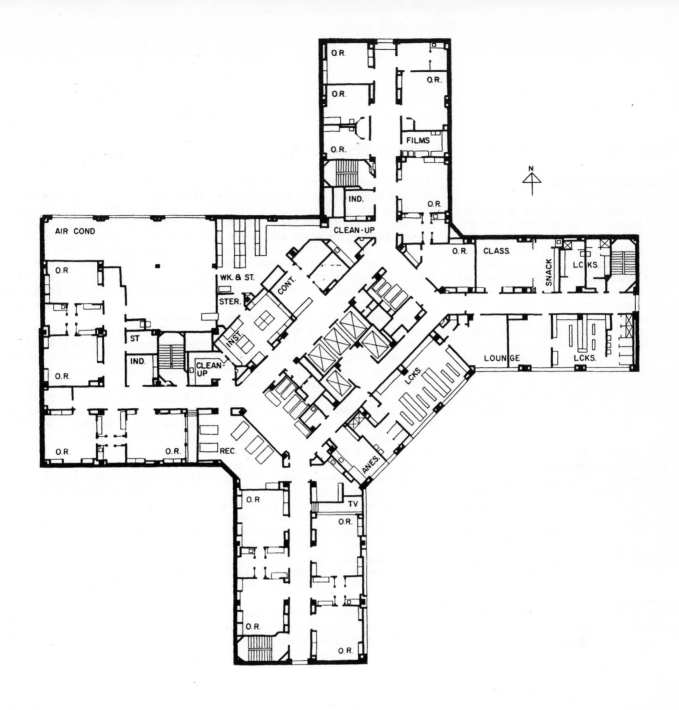

*Shepley, Bulfinch, Richardson & Abbott, Architects*

"The South and West operating corridors, with the recovery room at their junction, are models of efficiency. It is unfortunate that the North corridor is located at such a distance from the center of activity.

"In the planning stage, thought was given to the placement of equipment. With the advent of new procedures, requiring much in the way of large equipment, as monitors, pressure breathing devices, hypothermic equipment and heart-lung machines, we find ourselves bulging at the seams. We strongly suggest that in new construction there be made generous provision for storage space. The use of equipment as enumerated above makes it imperative that in a hospital the size of ours doing the type of surgery we do there be at least two rooms 1.5 times as large as any we have.

## COMMENT

"1. Zoning excellent, though certain amount of back-tracking for staff to control point if they enter from opposite side elevators.

"2. The two clean-up areas, work and instrument room could have been consolidated, with savings in equipment and possibly in personnel, with better supervision.

"3. Usual problem of extra equipment storage.

"5. Operating rooms seem to have excessive cabinet space; questionable if it is good policy to store so much in operating rooms.

"6. Classroom-snack bar excellent idea.

"7. Glad to see the usually forgotten orderlies and aides given locker rooms."

# STUYVESANT PAVILION, ST. LUKE'S HOSPITAL, NEW YORK

## ARCHITECTURAL BACKGROUND

From Kiff, Colean, Voss & Souder, architects: on the program—"1. Extension of existing operating suite of 10 rooms in general voluntary hospital of 523 beds. 2. To provide five new operating rooms for general and special surgery. 3. To provide common instrument and work room suite to serve five new operating rooms; all surgical packs will have been prepared and autoclaved in central sterile supply. 4. Nurses' and surgeons' locker rooms, teaching facilities, post-anesthesia recovery room, etc., existing elsewhere on floor serving existing and new surgical suites. 5. Two of new operating rooms to be larger than standard rooms for special surgical techniques involving extensive instrumentation, and large number of persons on team; i.e., surgeons, nurses, technicians. 6. Holding areas to serve as anesthesia induction rooms or waiting space for patient out of corridor circulation. 7. Surgeons wanted windows, even if small, for eye relief. Sills are 4 ft 6 in. from floor. 8. Not a teaching hospital, so no need for direct observation galleries; TV on closed circuit to large lecture hall on another floor."

On site problems: "1. Very limited building site so that shape of addition was governed by surrounding existing buildings, building code restrictions, etc. 2. Access from existing building limited to two: one for general patient approach and one to balance of floor and related services. 3. All agreed that corridor access for patients to operating rooms should have been around perimeter, so operating rooms could have direct access to central work area, but limitations of structure did not permit."

On special equipment: "1. Two large operating rooms equipped for TV, ceiling mounted X-ray tube, hypothermia, conduits from instrument control room for various leads of ECG, EEG, blood pressure, body temperature, etc. 2. Electric-controlled light-proofed shades in operating rooms. 3. Built-in X-ray illuminators, clocks, stainless steel supply cabinet. 4. Stainless steel scrub-up troughs—as it turned out, too narrow and heads too close together, inadequate elbow room; also proved to be very noisy—like drum—and had to be insulated with sound-absorbing material; had problem of water on floor from elbow drip as troughs too shallow front to back. 5. Common work room with all sterilizers for instruments in one location; wrapped autoclaved standard instrument trays prepared for day's schedule; special instruments autoclaved as required; room planned with idea that instrument tables from operating rooms would be set up in work room and sufficient number of such tables in use, so ready to move into operating room as soon as room cleaned up after each case. 6. Piped gases, oxygen, nitrous oxide and compressed air in-drops from ceiling in two locations; two vacuum-suction lines wall-mounted in each operating room. 7. Small dark room for developing; small frozen section lab with provision for refrigerator for blood and deep-freeze for bone and tissue bank. 8. Conductive ceramic tile floor. 9. Recess in ceiling for surgical lights was necessary because of existing floor-to-floor heights, structural beams and duct work."

## MEDICAL BACKGROUND

From Harold A. Zintel, M.D., Director of Surgery: "The general operating room size and the size of the ancillary rooms, including the hold or anesthesia rooms and the central make-up room, appear to be quite satisfactory. The general make-up room is not used entirely as we had anticipated . . . it was our original idea that tables be made up here, covered and delivered to the individual rooms. Prior to our moving into this area, we went to a complete pack system, whereby all of the drapes and instruments are prepared, the drapes in the laundry room and the instruments in the operating room, and sterilized in the very large autoclaves in the central supply. These are stored temporarily on the very adequate shelving of the central make-up area and here they are disbursed to the individual operating rooms. The autoclaves of the make-up room are used mainly for sterilizing individual instruments of a specific nature not included in one of the regular packs.

"We have had some difficulty with the scrub sinks in that there was considerable noise and splashing. Although we had requested a stainless steel trough and inner dimensions are very similar to those of the porcelain sinks in the Lyle operating room, we ended up with troughs which were considerably narrowed and more shallow.

"The instrument storage room with the adjustable peg bars and shelves has been very satisfactory as far as I know."

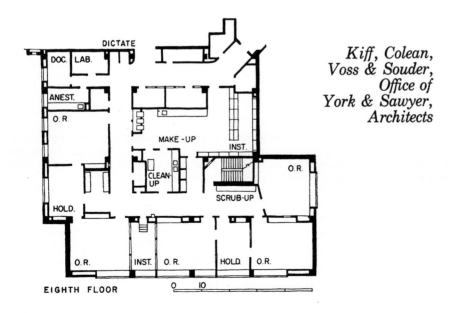

*Kiff, Colean, Voss & Souder, Office of York & Sawyer, Architects*

EIGHTH FLOOR

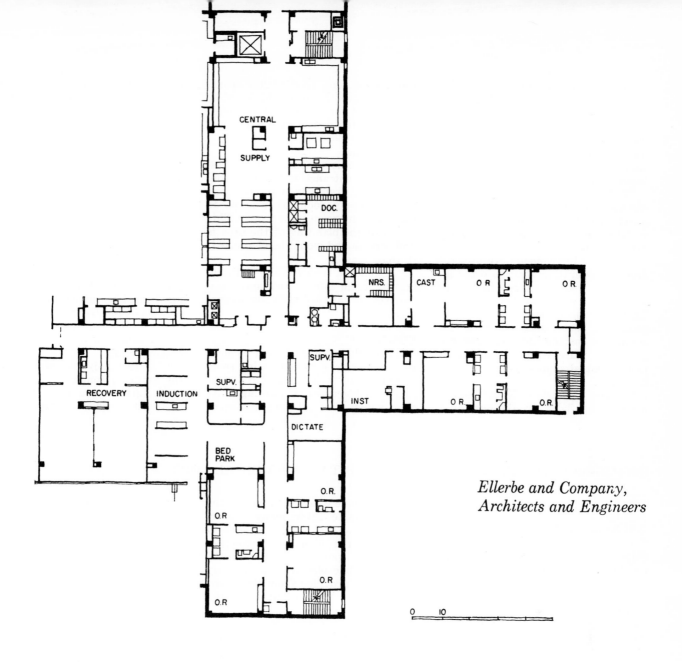

*Ellerbe and Company,*
*Architects and Engineers*

## OCHSNER FOUNDATION HOSPITAL, NEW ORLEANS

### ARCHITECTURAL BACKGROUND

From Edwin Larson, Ellerbe and Company: "1. The surgical suite in this instance consists of eight major operating rooms; except for some special features incorporated in the orthopedic operating room, all operating rooms are identical in layout and equipment. In this layout we have incorporated the conventional scrub-up and utility area between each pair of operating rooms.

"2. The hospital has central instrument cleaning and sterilizing for the operating room, with all other sterilizing and pack work for operating room done in central supply, which is adjacent to surgery and has a direct connection to surgery.

"3. This layout incorporates a centralized pre-induction area which makes for more efficient use of the operating rooms.

"4. We have an unusually large post-operation recovery room. Its capacity is 16 beds with two special alcoves for possible terminal cases. These alcoves have direct access from the corridor for relatives. This post-operation recovery room is operated 24 hours a day.

"5. One special feature that the owners feel very valuable is the hostess lounge adjacent to surgery. Relatives of patients undergoing surgery are brought to this lounge. There is a nurse in constant attendance in this lounge who can talk to relatives and allay their fears and so forth. There is a coffee bar in this area also. After the surgeon has completed the operation, he comes into this room and is able immediately to inform the relatives of the condition of the patient and the success of the operation. There are two private cubicles in this area for such consultation. The own-

ers feel that this room is invaluable from the public relations standpoint.

"6. The expansion of this surgical layout is planned to go horizontally and provisions have been made for such expansion; however, we are in the process of adding additional beds to this institution, in fact, about doubling or tripling the capacity. In spite of the fact that a very large proportion of work in this institution is surgical, the efficiency is such that the owners do not feel it is necessary to add operating rooms at this time; however, if it does become necessary, it will not be difficult and can be accomplished without interrupting the existing operation of the surgical suite."

### MEDICAL BACKGROUND

From Edward H. Leveroos, M.D., Director: "1. Patients are anesthetized in an area outside the operating room suite on an operating table; the table and patient are then moved into the room designated for surgery.

"2. Storage space for operating room equipment is not adequate. We have incorporated plans for additional space in the next phase of our building program.

"3. Ultrasonic equipment for cleaning instruments has not been purchased. We are considering the installation of such equipment, however, in the near future.

"4. Dirty instruments are brought from the operating room into the instrument room where they are washed by a maid and then sterilized. They are then dried, checked and placed in instrument cabinets. Instruments for the following day are set up in pans, wrapped and taken to the central supply room for autoclaving.

"5. The following X-ray equipment is available in the operating room area: one 15-milliamp spark-proof diagnostic unit which, while portable, is for all intents stationed in one of the operating rooms; one 30-milliamp portable unit in the recovery room.

"6. There is considerable congestion at the entrance to the operating suite, with traffic to and from the central supply room as well as to the operating room suite proper. This aspect of the planning of the area is undesirable and would be changed if it were feasible to do so.

"In general, however, the staff, operating room nurses and anesthesiologists are satisfied with the present layout."

## COMMENT

"1. Though balance of floor is bulk rectangular area, the operating room suite is pretty well confined to limitations of ribbon plan of nursing units over, which does not permit concentration that a squarer area does.

"2. Entrance for surgeons and nurses in middle of patient and service traffic; might produce congestion.

"3. There may be some cross-traffic to issue point of central sterile supply opposite induction area.

"4. If patients are received in induction center, it seems remote from control area for checking in.

"5. Even though central sterile supply is responsible for all surgical pack work, would seem better if the storage for surgical sterile supplies were within operating room suite proper. A lot of back-and-forth movement must be mixed with movement and issue for balance of hospital.

"6. Instrument area seems far removed from one wing with four operating rooms.

"7. Practically no storage space for extra equipment.

"8. Little space for collecting all the waste products, linen, etc."

# GRACE–NEW HAVEN COMMUNITY HOSPITAL, MEMORIAL UNIT, NEW HAVEN, CONN.

## ARCHITECTURAL BACKGROUND

From the Office of Douglas Orr, architect: "The operating suite was placed on the second floor of the building directly under the mechanical floor, so that air conditioning could be handled with small units rather than through a central system. This provided much greater flexibility, particularly as radiology suite was on the same floor. It may be noted that all services are centralized in the center core area with patient elevators operating independently of staff or public elevators. In passing from the elevator lobby to the operating suite, the control is immediate because of the location of the nurses' station. This gives visual control down both corridors. Supplies coming to this floor from central sterilizing are by dumbwaiter to the supply room, the unloading being automatic.

"It was the intent of the plan that the patient be brought to the operating room in bed, not in a stretcher. All openings and clearances were provided to make this possible. Anesthesia is administered in the anesthesia rooms in the general operating room area. It was planned that the patient be transferred after anesthesia from the bed to the operating table, the bed remaining in the anesthesia room. After the operation, the patient was to be returned directly to his bed, going to the recovery room before returning to the nursing floor.

This technique was determined as the most desirable after many conferences and was the established criteria on which the plan was developed. Ambulatory patients arrive on the floor on public elevators, a dressing room being provided from the lobby, and they are then admitted to the operating room suite at the nurses' station.

"The recovery room was provided for nine beds under the supervision of nursing care and with the anesthetist's office adjoining. Recently, an 'intensive care' unit has been designed to which some patients will go after operation, thus providing more efficient service and lightening the load on the regular nursing floor.

"All of the regular facilities such as scrub-up rooms and sterilizing units are provided between each pair of operating rooms with direct access from corridors so they may be reached and supplied without going through the operating room. Locker rooms for nurses and doctors are arranged so they are accessible from the public elevator lobby but also have direct access to the operating suite.

"All instruments are sterilized in the sterilizing rooms adjacent to the operating rooms, where high-speed sterilizers are installed. There is a small food pantry to provide nourishment if needed. A soiled linen sorting area is provided at the linen chute.

"The plan as laid out makes a very flexible arrangement with minimum traffic interference for the various functions. Provision has been made in the structure to enlarge the operating area between the two rear wings behind the core section, should future need require it."

## MEDICAL BACKGROUND

From John D. Thompson, Research Associate, Hospital Administration Section, Yale University School of Medicine: "A review of the original plans of the operating room with the present way the spaces are now being used results in a critical appraisal of the suite—which is somewhat valid, though not as objective an evaluation as one would desire. This review reveals a change in the function of three spaces. All of these rooms were designated as 'anesthesia' rooms (induction rooms) and have never been so used. One is now used as another anesthesiologist's office, one is the operating room supervisor's office (she claims she can't work in the 'gold fish bowl') and the other is used as an extra storage room. All other areas are used as indicated on the plans.

"Still another evaluation approach is the opinion of the operating room supervisor as to the design of the unit. Her main criticism is the lack of storage space in the area and the location of the storage cabinets in the operating rooms themselves. They are now on the outside wall, which means that the room has to be entered to replenish them. She sug-

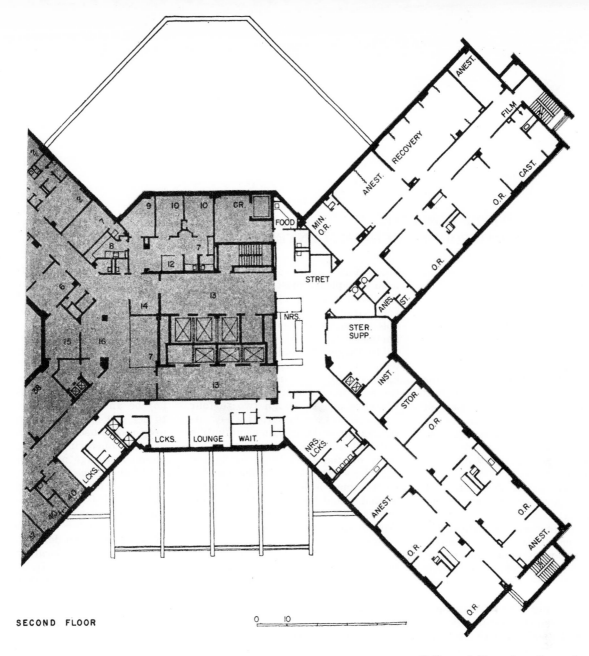

SECOND FLOOR

0   10

*Office of Douglas Orr, Architect*

gests lockers in the corridor wall with double doors front and back, so they can be replenished from the corridor. She also complained of the inadequate size of the nurses' locker room. This designation is a misnomer, since maids, EKG technicians, female physicians in pathology and surgery all use this area.

"Some of the less commonly seen good features of the area are the ambulatory patient waiting and dressing area and the arrangement of the cystoscopy suite between X-ray and the operating room. The location of this suite is always difficult, since both services feel the area belongs to them. Its placement between the two services is, I believe, as good a solution to this conundrum as can be attained.

"On the whole, I would say the op-erating suite in the Memorial Unit is a good example of fitting such an area into a basic shape determined by the needs of the patient floors above it."

## COMMENT

"1. Memorial Unit is one portion of a large teaching hospital. Certain special facilities, therefore—cardiac and neurosurgery—are in older buildings.

"2. Though planned for, induction rooms are not used. This seems to be a trend—particularly if operating rooms removed, involving long movement of anesthetized patients. Static hazard even with conduction flooring. Space reverts to other usage.

"3. Good control for checking in patients, but with anesthesia rooms taken for other use, patients must be left in corridor unless excellent organization in timing of patient's arrival in surgical suite.

"4. Local instrument sterilization used instead of central pack.

"5. Perhaps more consolidation of 'utility,' 'instruments' and 'sterile supply' could have saved personnel and given better supervision.

"6. Too bad dark room accessible from plaster room only, unless policy is that all other film goes to main X-ray department, on same floor, for processing.

"7. No provision for laboratory-frozen section.

"8. Classroom and food service—good.

"9. Soiled linen and trash collection—good.

"10. Provision for ambulant outpatients—good."

# HERBERT C. MOFFITT HOSPITAL,
# UNIVERSITY OF CALIFORNIA MEDICAL CENTER, SAN FRANCISCO

## ARCHITECTURAL BACKGROUND

From Milton T. Pfleuger, architect: "The 500-bed Herbert C. Moffitt Hospital at the University of California Medical Center in San Francisco is the teaching hospital for the center. . . . It is a 15-story building. The operating department is on the fourth floor with X-ray on the third and laboratories on the fifth. Each of the service floors has a gross area of over 26,000 sq ft, and these are more or less in block form upon which the 'cross' of the typical bed floor is superimposed.

"The large service floors in block form were developed to permit efficient departmental layouts as opposed to 'strung-out' departments.

"The operating floor is a complete department, with operating rooms, etc., in the large block, cystoscopy in one wing, locker rooms, etc., in another wing, and departmental offices in the third wing. The latter wing is the 'tie' between the hospital and the adjoining Medical Sciences Building, the doctors serving, of course, both hospital and medical sciences.

"In the main operating block, great thought and consideration was given by the staff to methods of teaching and facilities which would enable most efficient and speedy use of rooms. The individual prep rooms are a case in point.

"The centralized work area provides shorter travel, speedy clean-up and good supervision."

## MEDICAL BACKGROUND

From Mary K. Vickery, Operating Room Supervisor: "Having the entire fourth floor devoted to the department of surgery, anesthesia, urology and the operating rooms has cut down on the traffic of personnel and patients not directly concerned with this part of the hospital.

"In the cystoscopy wing: 1. The complete X-ray unit next to cystoscopy has worked out very well for both cystoscopy and the operating room. 2. The four cystoscopy rooms seem to be the correct number in proportion to the hospital. Being a combined X-ray and urology unit, it is used to capacity most of the time. 3. The head nurse in cystoscopy seems very satisfied with the layout and is able to run an efficient and busy department.

"In the locker and dressing room wing: 1. The surgeons' locker area has been difficult to manage, because there is not adequate locker space. We have had to assign two to four surgeons to each locker. If a key arrangement, rather than combination locks, whereby the surgeons could not carry off the keys, could be figured out, the surgeons would not have to be assigned a locker. The number needed would be less, but would necessitate a place for shoe storage. 2. Women surgeons' and nurses' locker rooms OK.

"In the office wing: 1. Much doubling and tripling up has been necessary to house the full-time staff in the office area. Offices are large enough to do this unless the number increases. 2. Nurses' demonstration room, which is a 'mock-up' operating room, has been a most valuable teaching aid for student nurses. 3. The post-anesthesia room is inadequate in size, but is an especially efficient unit with the space limitation. Patient flow is the most difficult part of this unit to manage, since there is no exit.

"In the operating room wing: 1. The cul-de-sac plan is better than an open plan because it tends to limit unnecessary traffic. 2. The centralized work area is excellent. This makes possible faster and easier case preparation and disassembly, following case completion. Also, it concentrates the auxiliary help so that it can be better controlled and supervised. Cabinet design should be planned in detail for this area. This was not done here, so that we have had to use the sterile storage area for instruments. The unsterile storage area is about one-quarter the space needed for large equipment such as extra instrument tables, hypothermia equipment, cardiac by-pass equipment, monitors, etc. We have had to use the east corridor for this type of storage.

"The prep rooms, I feel, are a luxury. They make it possible to get the patients to surgery somewhat in advance and furnish a place for waiting patients other than the corridor. Another purpose of these rooms is to decrease the time between cases. This requires extra anesthetists and nurses, however, and unless there are more anesthestists than one per operating room, the waiting patient cannot be anesthetized. I would prefer to see the space taken up by these prep rooms used to increase the size of the operating rooms and for planned storage of equipment.

"I believe the minimum size of an individual operating room should be 20 ft by 20 ft. In a university medical center, in which many large procedures requiring many large pieces of equipment are done, there should be at least two operating rooms 25 ft by 25 ft in size. It is difficult to maintain aseptic technique for these cases in such cramped quarters."

## COMMENT

"1. For 10 operating room suite, entrance seems cramped, though good patient control for double-corridor layout.

"2. Ingenious method of taking care of X-ray transformer and control units outside of operating room.

"3. Appears to be excessive amount of cabinet storage within operating rooms and prep areas.

"4. As teaching hospital, seems to have too few facilities for observation. Also, there might be at least one larger operating room for complicated surgery requiring larger team and more equipment.

"5. Anesthesia storage and work room seem very small for department of this size, but perhaps local prep rooms take portion of supplies.

"6. Efficiency of dumbwaiters from central sterile supply debatable when removed from any central control. Must have good intercom system to have person at dumbwaiter to receive when needed.

"7. Long haul to dark room in cystoscopy suite from orthopedic and plaster room, where perhaps major portion of film originates."

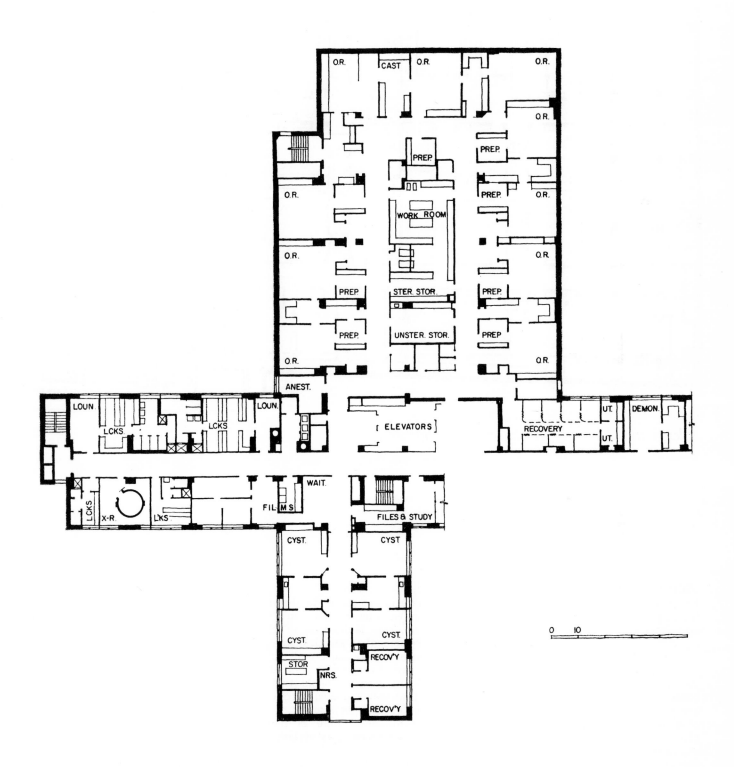

*Milton T. Pfleuger, Architect*

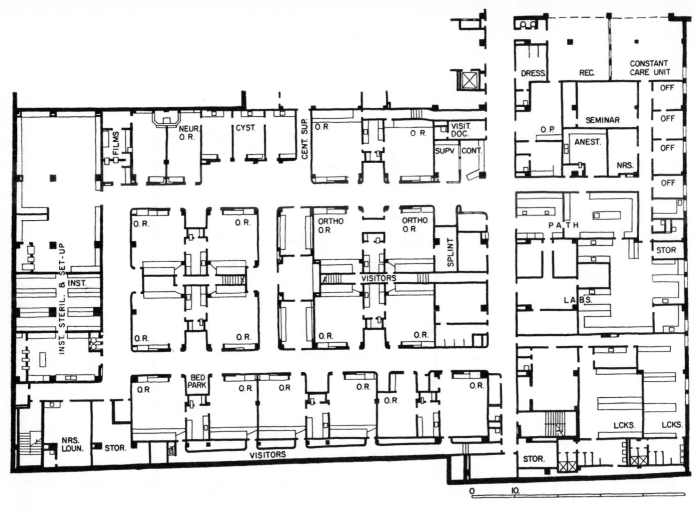

*Ellerbe and Company, Architects and Engineers*

## CLEVELAND CLINIC HOSPITAL, CLEVELAND

### MEDICAL BACKGROUND

From James G. Harding, Superintendent: "1. The surgical suite is large because of the fact that ours is a referral type practice, in that the more complicated type surgery is referred here. Therefore, not only is our volume high in comparison to other places, but the type of cases are much more time-consuming and difficult than the average 450-bed hospital. The hospital is not primarily engaged in surgical work. However, the proportion is about 55 per cent surgical and 45 per cent medical. Since our men work in two rooms at one time because of the type of practice, we definitely do not feel that the number of rooms in our surgical suite is out of proportion. Here again, it is impossible to compare one hospital with another on the basis of a conception of how many operating rooms should be built per bed.

"2. There is no disadvantage to the substerilizing rooms not being accessible from the corridor.

"3. There is not adequate storage space for equipment, but, on the other hand, this is because of the rapid development in surgical procedures which require more and more storage space. We would be very surprised if any hospital could truthfully say that they had adequate storage space for any purpose.

"4. The nurses' lounge is more than adequate since it is strictly a lounge and not a locker room. The locker room is located very close to the surgery suite.

"5. We haven't been aware of any problem regarding floor space since I believe our floor space is fine for any major procedure, even including the open heart operations performed so often here.

"All in all, I would say that our operating pavilion has been one of the best from a practical standpoint. In fact, we have had visitors from all over the country, and they have been very impressed with the layout, etc. You will note that we have viewing galleries for visitors in each major operating room. Since times have changed, we do not believe these will be necessary in the future. Also, the central scrub room is somewhat controversial, but works well for us due to the fact that we have a closed staff, and the scrub rooms are located centrally with wide corridors leading to the operating rooms. I would say that the layout and everything about the suite has proven to be excellent, and the fact that we have the pathology department on the same floor has proven to be a wise feature also."

### ARCHITECTURAL BACKGROUND

From Ellerby and Company, architects: "1. In studying this plan it must be borne in mind that the Cleveland Clinic Hospital has a closed staff, and had been operating a surgery for several years. A great deal of time was spent in study on the layout, both as to staff requirements and the flow of patients, supplies and staff.

"2. The suite consists of a total of 21 operating rooms. Sixteen of the rooms are typical as to size and equipment, making it possible to schedule any type of major surgery in any one of them.

"3. All major operating rooms have view galleries. Access to all view galleries is from the corridor entering the surgical suite, thus any visitor can get into any view gallery without entering the surgical area.

"5. Centralized scrub-up and gowning area is incorporated in this plan. This is unusual for an operating suite of this size. However, the owners had some 20 years experience with this procedure and they were convinced it was the best procedure for them with their closed staff.

"6. Considerable area is devoted to centralized instrument washing, storing, sterilizing and set-up.

"7. Except for instrument steriliz-ing, all other packwork and steriliz-ing for surgery is done in central supply. Central supply is adjacent to surgery and has a direct connection.

"8. Directly adjacent to central supply is a very extensive surgical-pathological laboratory.

"9. X-ray facilities in this surgical suite came in for very special studying. The neurological operating rooms have their own X-ray facilities. Six of the other major operating rooms have special X-ray facilities. These facilities basically consist of a portable tube stand, which is plugged into a jack in the operating room and the control panel being in an alcove outside of the operating room, which enables the use of X-ray equipment that is superior to normal portable unit, and also provides the utmost in explosion-proof equipment.

"10. Surgical section has its own library.

"11. Adjacent to surgery is the surgical recovery area and the constant care unit.

"12. A very complete signal sys-tem and intercom system has been installed, enabling the personnel in the operating room to call any of the staff or personnel as may be required, and special signals in case of emergencies."

## COMMENTS

"1. Interesting, but very special.

"2. Nurses' lounge seems very small for such a large unit.

"3. No access to sub-utility rooms except through operating room; this is a drawback.

"4. Supply cabinets in operating rooms can be stocked without going through operating room.

"5. Organization of total 21 rooms very compact.

"6. Lack of storage space.

"7. Good administrative control—secretaries, dictating, etc., and check-in point for patients.

"8. Doubt if central scrub acceptable for other institutions, with 55-ft corridor travel to farthest operating room door."

# CHUQUICAMATA HOSPITAL, CHILE*

## ARCHITECTURAL BACKGROUND

From J. J. Souder, architect: "The operating pavilion of the Chuquicamata Hospital, a 250-bed general hospital, company-owned and operated in connection with a large mining enterprise in northern Chile, is designed around two basic considerations: (a) a shortage of highly trained working personnel dictates the concentration of all skilled tasks in a simple, easily supervised area; (b) the complete separation of patient traffic from staff traffic has enthusiastic precedent in Chile and was desired by the staff.

"The result is an inner core of work space, sterile storage, instrument storage, sterilization and post-operative recovery which is directly related by dumbwaiter to central sterile supply. This core is surrounded on three sides by doctors' and nurses' lockers, five operating rooms with scrub facilities, anesthesia space, the usual small laboratory and dark room, and, at a point which controls a view of both incoming patients and the work area, a supervisor's station. Beyond this intermediate ring is a peripheral corridor which brings patients from the elevator lobby to the operating rooms.

"Four of the operating rooms are typical major surgeries in size and equipment. One of the four has a small gallery with ports provided for leads to data-recording equipment, but highly specialized surgery will not be done at Chuquicamata except in emergency. (Chuquicamata is 800 miles from medical centers in Santiago or Lima.) The fifth room is a urological room, and is so located that patients not to be anesthetized can be brought in and out quickly.

"Scrub facilities are immediately inside from the two pairs of major rooms. Only one battery of sterilizers, within range of the supervisor's eyes, is used for all sterilization in the suite.

"The work room is primarily an instrument and assembly room. All packs are to be prepared in central sterile supply and sterilized under supervision of the pharmacist. (Central supply is located adjacent to the manufacturing pharmacy, shares steriliz-

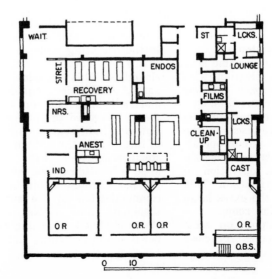

*Kiff, Colean, Voss & Souder, Office of York & Sawyer, Architects*

*Under construction; no administrative comment possible.

ing facilities with it and is administratively supervised by the pharmacist.)

"A glazed wall separates the work room from the recovery room so that, again, the supervisor and anesthetist can readily observe the type of care being given to post-operative patients without long absence from other duties.

"Doctors and staff, who are full-time employes, have already changed from street clothes to hospital clothing before going on to their work sites.

"Patients are brought to a waiting space outside the supervisor's office and then by private corridor either to anesthesia induction rooms or direct to the operating room. They neither see nor hear the preparatory activities between work room and surgery. They follow the same route back to recovery, which adjoins the waiting room, and after recovery go directly out of the suite."

## COMMENT
"1. Very compact plan.
"2. Good circulation; patient travel separated from staff travel.
"3. Circulation between doctors' lockers and nurses station control point remote.
"4. Lack of free floor space for additional equipment storage.
"5. Interesting corner cabinet for suction lines, illuminators.
"6. Supply cabinet can be stocked without crossing operating room."

# M. D. ANDERSON HOSPITAL AND TUMOR INSTITUTE, UNIVERSITY OF TEXAS, HOUSTON

## ARCHITECTURAL BACKGROUND
From MacKie and Kamrath, architects: "Cancer treatment requires extensive surgical services—much more than the general hospital.

"Eight major operating suites were grouped in units of four each, with adjoining preparation rooms, so that patients could receive pre-operative anesthesia while other patients were on the operating table. Prep rooms also used for post-operative recovery. Anesthesia banks built into common wall between operating room and prep room. Cabinets built into corridor walls, so that operation packs could be inserted from corridor side and removed from operating side, omitting traffic through operating room.

"View gallery and television projection room dropped to 7 ft above main operating suite floor for close vision and enlarged TV projection in color to various conference rooms and auditorium in the main building. Colors selected for contrast in TV projection.

"Special operating room lights were designed by the hospital. Every effort was made to eliminate equipment, cords, extra lights, etc., from cluttering up the operating room floors. Provisions made for use of X-ray and radioactive isotopes.

"Pathologist located on same floor with two-way communication with surgeons, so that frozen sections could be viewed and reported on during surgery. Large amounts of surgical instruments are used in the eight major and two minor operating rooms, as each instrument is used only once during an operation to avoid cancer cell distribution. This feature accounts for the extra large instrument sterilization room.

"Central sterile supply on same floor as operating rooms for close supervision by surgical supervisor and immediate access for supplies to both the surgical unit and the main hospital.

"A private elevator direct from the surgical floor to the betatron and cobalt room located 20 ft below ground gives ready access as required for treatment with high voltage beta and gamma rays.

"Main hospital sound control room is located immediately above main surgical suite for close supervision of TV projection and lecture recording."

## MEDICAL BACKGROUND
From R. Lee Clark Jr., M.D., Director and Surgeon-in-Chief: "The surgical suite at the University of Texas M.D. Anderson hospital and Tumor Institute was designed after 15 years of experience in evaluating surgical pavilions at the principal medical centers in America and Europe. Basically, the surgical suite is designed to minimize traffic through the operating rooms and operating suite and to provide maximum utilization of space, equipment and personnel to save the time of the surgeons and preserve the safety of the patient.

"Unique in this design is a utility panel in one wall where there is concentrated the major equipment used in the operating room in order that it can be supervised by the anesthesiologists. This includes anesthetic gases, anesthesia supplies, cautery and radio-knife, suction and instruments to record the patient's condition, and light control. Other factors of interest are the combination quick sterilization room with a scrub-up area, utilization of the corridor wall for pass-through cabinets, two-way communication to the surgical pathologists and nurse supervisor, static electricity warning devices, a newly designed ceiling light controllable by the surgeon, provision of color-compatible television, observation galleries, pre-anesthesia preparation rooms and post-anesthesia recovery room, provision for the use of X-ray therapy and radioactive isotopes in the operating room, complete separate air conditioning and humidity control for each individual operating room, and finally, a carefully designed flow plan for the preparations of sterile linens, materials, supplies and instruments under the supervision of the central control of the nurse supervisor."

## COMMENT
"1. Through-wall cabinets excellent, but their use must always be checked for approval by local building codes an dinsurance underwriters, as corridors are usually legal fire exists.
"2. Prep rooms give good holding space for pre-operative patients, even if they may not be used for induction. Manpower—enough nurses and anesthetists—is a problem.
"3. Good control of patients and staff entering department, with check-in point centrally located.
"4. Is there enough equipment storage space?
"5. Assume the access to pathological lab and isotope labs via stair and elevator within department, to avoid major portion of traffic to and from these serves through sterile surgical corridor.
"6. Ingenious method of providing small observation galleries in certain rooms as distinct from observation dome over one major room.
"7. Are there adequate facilities for handling waste, soiled linen, etc.?
"8. Hospital of this nature should need some facilities for teaching and conference within or adjacent to surgical suite."

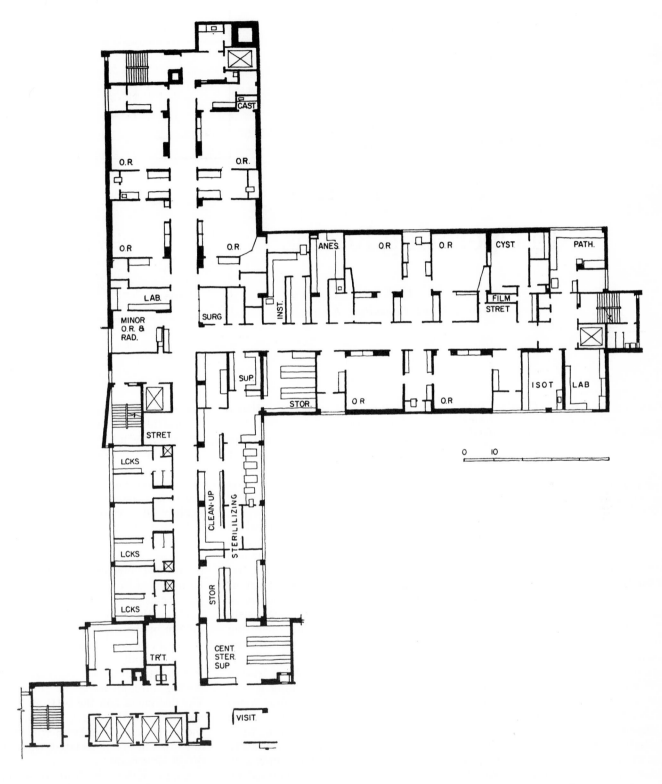

*MacKie and Kamrath, Architects; Schmidt, Garden & Erickson, Consulting Architects*

Theoretically, an ideal form of air flow (top) would be from the ceiling as a supply to the floor as an exhaust. Since this is impractical, the engineers have used portions of the ceiling for supply outlets, and registers on sidewalls for exhaust. The center sketch shows how a portion of the ceiling is used for air supply in the neurological operating rooms. The bottom sketch shows air supply from the periphery of the observation dome for cardiac operating rooms

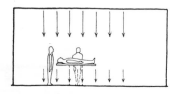

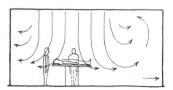

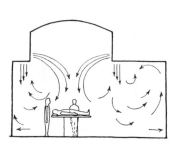

# A New Approach to Air Distribution In Operating Rooms

*by Edward A. DeVan*
*Krey & Hunt, Consulting Engineers*

*Operating Facilities for Cardiovascular and Neurological Surgery, Clinical Center, National Institutes of Health, Bethesda, Md., Jack Masur, M.D., Director; D. L. Snow, Chief, Sanitary Engineering Branch*

*Kiff Colean, Voss & Souder, The Office of York & Sawyer, Architects; Krey & Hunt, Consulting Mechanical and Electrical Engineers; Bolt Beranek and Newman Inc. (Instrumentation)*

A novel approach to the distribution of conditioned air has been developed for new operating facilities at the National Institutes of Health in an effort to improve the sterility of the air, especially in the vicinity of the operating table. This is particularly significant in light of the medical profession and hospital authorities' taking a new look at aseptic techniques to minimize infection.

Essentially, the idea is to bathe the patient in a current of fresh supply air so that this clean air provides a protective curtain about the operating field. The thinking behind this is that outdoor air generally is free of pathogenic organisms, so if proper precautions are taken in the design of the air supply system, the conditioned air that enters the room will have a very low bacteria count.

But actual studies indicate that if supply air is introduced into the operating room in such a way that a turbulent pattern is created, this air can wipe the room surfaces, equipment and clothing, and pick up sufficient pathogens to create an unsatisfactory condition, particularly for cardiovascular and neurological surgery.

Based on this premise, the ideal air distribution would be one in which the entire ceiling is an air supply and the entire floor is an exhaust, resulting in a complete and constant purge of the room, with minimum local recirculation. But obviously this is impractical. The operating facilities at NIH will have instead a modified version in which the air supply is directly over the operating table and an exhaust opening is provided near the floor on all four walls.

In the new operating rooms at the National Institutes of Health, 65 F air will be directed at the operating field, but the ceiling air supply covers a larger area than the operating table itself.

In the case of the cardiac operating room, the placement of supply outlets was dictated by the perimeter of the dome required in the ceiling for observation, for television and camera ports, and for the mounting of a circle of 24 recessed incandescent fixtures. These lights are directed at the operating field, and can be individually controlled at a console by the surgeon.

In the neurological operating room, no dome was required, since observation will be from the recording room. The air supply issues from perforated metal pans with air valves, set in a dropped ceiling. Recessed fixtures for general illumination are interspersed with the pans. Suspended surgical lights also will be provided in both types of operating rooms.

While the supply air is the cleanest air in the room, its temperature, at 65 F, makes it also the coldest and a normally clothed person might feel drafts. However, there are mitigating circumstances in this case. The designers and the NIH staff are hoping that the heavy gowning of the surgeon and his team will offset any discomfort associated with the direct air stream.

Supply outlets are designed so that air quantities can be varied to achieve an optimum combination of cleanest air and least objectionable drafts. Layout of the rooms made it impossible to have four-wall exhaust; instead, two walls are used. The system is designed to permit all bottom exhaust if tests should prove this desirable. Top exhaust also is available to modify the air distribution pattern, if necessary.

The maintenance of a sterile atmosphere is not a function of any one item, but several: (1) cleanliness of air supply, (2) method of air distribution and air change rate, (3) operating room cleaning, (4) operating procedures and techniques. *1. Cleanliness of Air Supply.* It was mentioned that outdoor air is generally free of pathogens, which is the prime reason 100 per cent outdoor air is used for operating suites. If, however, fresh air intakes are too close to exhaust outlets, the fresh air can become contaminated.

Studies have shown that air also can become contaminated in the air handling system due to build-up and accumulation of bacteria on cooling and/or heating coils, and air leakage from fan room into the casing (which cannot be made air-tight) due to negative pressure. These studies indicate the need of filters immediately before the air outlets to operating room suites, regardless of the type of air conditioning system used. *2. Method of Air Distribution and Air Change Rate.* Air distribution has been discussed earlier. Air change rates for operating suites published in the literature vary from 10 to 20 changes per hour, even though in many cases a rate of 6 to 7 a.c. will handle the heat gain. While the higher air change rate will produce the greatest dilution of bacteria, at the same time it can create excess air motion and pick up bacteria clusters on linen, equipment, etc. For the present, until further studies are made, 10 to 12 a.c. are recommended as a compromise.

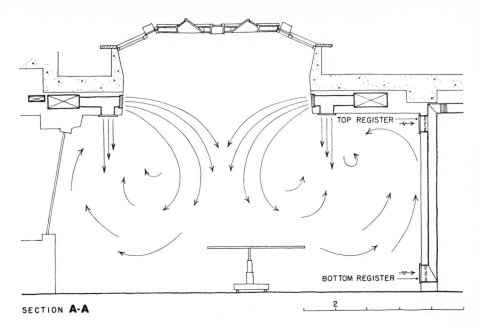

SECTION **A-A**

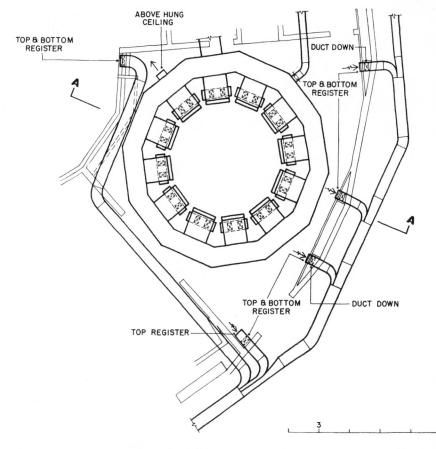

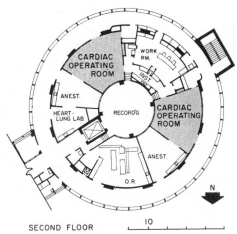

SECOND FLOOR

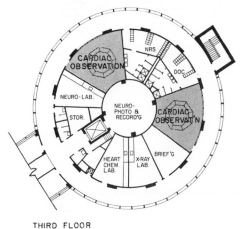

THIRD FLOOR

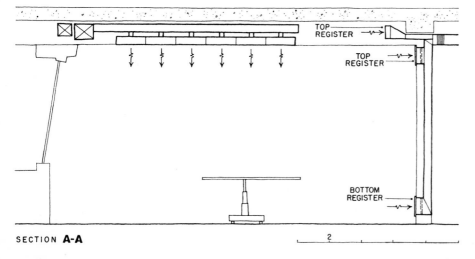

SECTION **A-A**

2

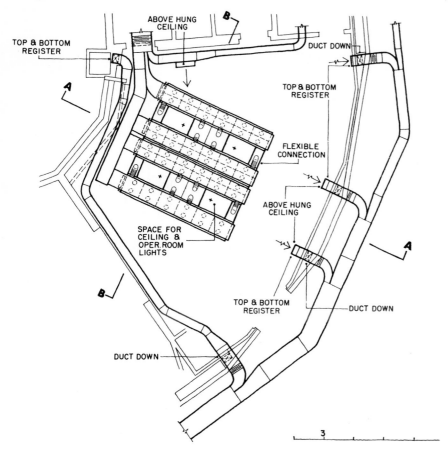

ABOVE HUNG CEILING

TOP & BOTTOM REGISTER

DUCT DOWN

TOP & BOTTOM REGISTER

FLEXIBLE CONNECTION

ABOVE HUNG CEILING

SPACE FOR CEILING & OPER. ROOM LIGHTS

TOP & BOTTOM REGISTER

DUCT DOWN

DUCT DOWN

3

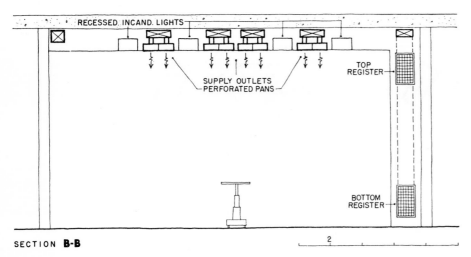

RECESSED INCAND. LIGHTS

TOP REGISTER

SUPPLY OUTLETS PERFORATED PANS

BOTTOM REGISTER

SECTION **B-B**

2

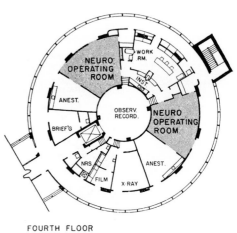

FOURTH FLOOR

3. *Operating Room Cleaning.* It is common practice in operating suites to wash the floors, part of the walls and furniture after every operation, or at least once a day. In some hospitals, however, scant attention is paid to the higher parts of the walls and ceilings, and in particular to the air conditioning outlets. Air conditioning outlets, both supply and exhaust, can be focuses of dust collection.

4. *Operating Room Procedures and Techniques.* Recent tests in a neurosurgical suite showed that the supply air contributed only 18 per cent of the bacteria count during surgery and only 10 per cent during draping. It was deduced that contamination of air was due to partially sterilized linen and equipment, carelessness on the part of personnel and inadequate cleaning of rooms. Historically, all physiological data collecting in cardiovascular and neurological surgery has been done in the operating room. However, this will be done in a separate room, the recording center, at the new operating facilities at the National Institutes of Health. This remote location of instruments and centralization of gases, vacuum and hypothermia lines achieves an operating room requiring a minimum of personnel and machines. This is accomplished by the use of a console unit to which the patient (anesthesia and instrumentation lines) is attached.

*Air Distribution in Operating Rooms*

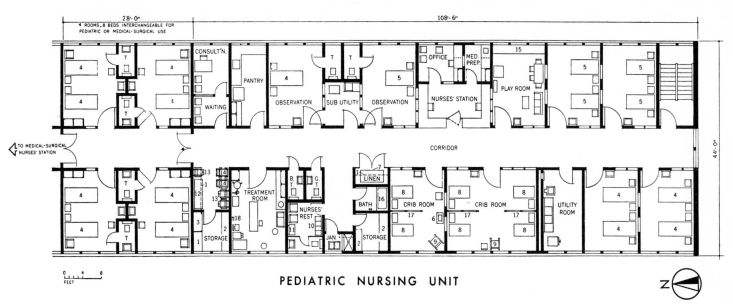

PEDIATRIC NURSING UNIT

**NURSING UNIT**

1. Shelf, 5 ft. 3 in. above floor
2. Shelving
3. Storage Cabinet
4. Adjustable Hospital Bed
5. Adjustable Youth Bed
6. Infant Scale
7. Linen Cart
8. Crib
9. Rocking Chair
10. Lockers, 12 x 15 x 60 in.
11. Table with Mirror over
12. Stretcher
13. Wheel Chair
14. Stroller
15. Toy Storage
16. Raised Bath Tub, with controls on wall
17. Cubicle Partition, 7 ft. high with bottom of clear glass 36 in. above floor
18. Oxygen and Suction Outlets, 5 ft. 3 in. above floor

*This material was abstracted from the chapter of the same name which appears in the manual "The Care of Children in Hospitals", published by the American Academy of Pediatrics. The chapter is the work of the Committee on Hospital Care for the American Academy of Pediatrics under the chairmanship of Dr. Lendon Snedeker, Assistant Administrator of the Children's Medical Center, Boston. The architectural consultant to the committee was Mr. Walter E. Campbell, A.I.A. of the firm of Campbell and Aldrich of Boston, Massachusetts.*

*Planning is by O. B. Ives, Hospital Architect of the Architectural and Engineering Branch, Division of Hospital and Medical Facilities, Public Health Service.*

# Planning the Pediatric Nursing Unit

**T**HIS SCHEME for a pediatrics nursing unit, the Public Health Service architects make clear, might have been done in many other dispositions. It is intended, like all similar schemes issued by the Service's architectural department, merely to illustrate a possible arrangement of rooms and facilities considered desirable. This one, for example, is drawn for a fairly typical hospital wing, on the assumption that it would be part of a conventional hospital; but for that imposition the facilities might be still more conveniently arranged. It does, nevertheless, illustrate desirable planning as well as facilities and equipment needed.

Flexibility is the first important objective. The four rooms at the left of the plan, with their own toilets, are intended to be part of the pediatrics nursing unit, or part of an adjoining adult medical or surgical nursing unit, as occasion demands. Double doors are positioned so that the corridor can be arranged as desired. In use presumably older children would be assigned to these rooms, and nurses would not have to exercise close supervision here.

Notice that nurses' station and utility rooms are centered for the shorter corridor, without these four rooms.

The smaller unit, with 16 beds, is close to a minimum, incidentally, for a special pediatrics wing, the number 14 being cited in the manual of which this plan is a part. A

pediatrics nursing unit could be larger, but should not be as large as an adult unit, since children need more care.

### Bed Rooms

The one-bed rooms are required for critically ill patients, those who need quiet or those who are disturbing to other patients. When appropriately equipped, they may be used as isolation rooms for patients with known or suspected infection. They are useful also for very short-stay patients and for new admissions.

Preferably all, but at least some of the one-bed rooms, should be large enough to accommodate two beds, to provide over-night accommodations for parents. Infants and younger children, in particular, need their mothers during an illness.

It has been recommended that the minimum floor area for a one-bed room be 100 square feet and that for a two-bed room 160 square feet. It has been found in practice, however, that these areas are minimal and do not provide sufficient space for working around the patient and moving beds and stretchers. Recommended areas are 125 square feet for single rooms and 190 square feet for two-bed rooms.

Each room should be equipped with an adjustable hospital bed and an over-bed table for trays or toys. The hospital bed can be replaced by a crib or bassinet as required, but such

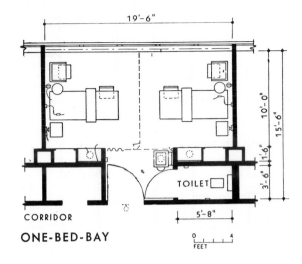

**ONE-BED-BAY**

**BED ROOM**

1. Sliding Window Curtain
2. Straight Chair
3. Duplex Convenience Outlet
4. Nurses' Calling Station
5. Wall Light
6. Bedside Cabinet
7. Oxygen Outlet, 5 ft. 3 in. above floor
8. Telephone Outlet
9. Suction Outlet, 5 ft. 3 in. above floor
10. Curtain
11. Clear Wire Glass in Steel Frame (1296 sq. in. max.) bottom of glass 36 in. above floor
12. Waste Paper Receptacle
13. Lavatory, Gooseneck spout, Knee or Elbow Control
14. Wall-bracket light, switch controlled
15. Corridor Dome Light
16. Door, upper panel clear wire glass
17. Night Light, switch controlled
18. Adjustable Hospital Bed (Youth beds and cribs may be substituted as required)
19. Overbed Table
20. Cubicle Curtain
21. Clear Glass, bottom 36 in. above floor

**UTILITY ROOM**

1. Sanitary Waste Receptacle
2. Double Compartment Deep Sink in Counter
3. Clinical Sink
4. Dome Light and Buzzer, 5 ft. 3 in. above floor
5. Bedpan Washer and Disinfector
6. Bulletin Board, 26 x 24 in.
7. Clear Wire Glass Vision Panel
8. Duplex Convenience Outlet
9. Drying Rod
10. Cabinet Pressure Sterilizer 16 x 16 x 24 in.
11. Ceiling Light

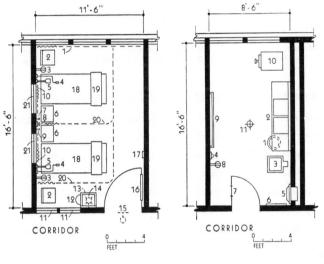

**BED ROOM**   **UTILITY ROOM**

flexibility is predicated on really adequate storage space. Two nurses' call panels should be installed for use when the room is occupied by two children. The call panel should be placed where it is not within too easy reach in rooms which will be used for pre-school children. There should be a bedside cabinet for articles needed in the nursing care of the patient on one side of the bed, possibly a cabinet for favorite toys or other familiar articles on the other side of the bed. This plan shows only the former. Clothing can be stored, to some extent, in this limited space, but it will be preferable in most instances to provide closet space or lockers for such articles.

Every room should have running water. An adult-sized lavatory with gooseneck spout, with either knee or elbow control, should be installed near the entrance. It is desirable that there be a toilet with bedpan flushing attachment and also a clothes closet for one-bed rooms. Cubicle curtains should be available when the room is occupied by two patients. Every one-bed room should have a comfortable chair and a waste paper receptacle.

### Cubicles and Partitions

The use of partitions and cubicles in multiple-bed rooms is quite common but, if they are installed, those in charge of the pediatric unit should be aware of the reasons for their use.

Cubicles are undesirable in that they separate children who otherwise would be able to fraternize and have a happier hospital experience. At the same time it should be recognized that not all children benefit from this social approach.

Cubicles demarcate areas of potential infection, and facilitate the maintenance of precautionary technique, but they cannot be said to decrease airborne infection significantly. The practice of throwing toys from one area to another is discouraged, and visitors are encouraged to confine their attentions to one patient but cubicles increase the difficulty of moving patients. They are relatively expensive to install and keep clean, and in hot weather they greatly reduce air circulation and contribute to discomfort.

If cubicles or partitions are to be used they should permit visibility of patients by nurses and by patients in the same room. They should be made of shatterproof glass above the height of the mattress (36 in.). It is recommended that they be seven feet high and that they extend seven feet from the wall.

### Isolation Rooms

It is essential that each pediatric unit be provided with one or more isolation rooms. These should be equipped in the same way as ordinary single rooms, except that they require facilities for maintaining isolation technique. When not utilized for this purpose they serve as part of the regular unit, for severely ill children, for patients who need quiet, or for new admissions. It is desirable that they be remote from rooms for non-infectious cases but convenient to the nurse's station.

Each isolation room should have an adult-sized lavatory with knee action control, a hook strip for gowns near the corridor door and an individual toilet with bedpan-flushing attachments. It should be connected with a sub-utility room equipped with a sink and utensil sterilizer. The isolation room should be large enough to permit the use of an additional full-sized bed for a second patient with the same infection or for a mother to stay with her child.

### Nurses' Station

Every pediatric unit will have its own nurses' station, preferably situated centrally within the unit. As a general rule, rooms designed for the use of the sickest patients and for young infants should be nearest the nurses' station. The location of the nurses' station may also be determined by the hospital's general plan for controlling visitors.

The requirements for the nurses' station in the pediatric unit are much like those in other parts of the hospital. A chart desk and rack, clock and bulletin board should be provided. The nurses' call system will need to be one which can be used by younger children. A television monitoring system for each room would be even more desirable if finances permit. This will, of course, allow visual as well as auditory control of the situation in each room. A medicine preparation room should be provided directly off the nurses' station. It should contain a counter with an acid-resisting sink, cabinets with a locked narcotics compartment above the counter and refrigerator and cabinets below.

A small private office for the supervising nurse should be provided off the nurses' station.

### Examination and Treatment Room

Separate examination and treatment rooms but, more often, a combination of both, should be provided. A more satisfactory examination can be done in a quiet room with a good light, where the necessary equipment is easily available, and there are fewer distractions for both the child and the examiner.

It is important that all treatments, dressing or other procedures which are painful or disturbing be done where other children cannot watch. For this reason, the treatment room should be located away from patient rooms. If it is also to be used for doing admitting examinations, as will often be the case in the smaller pediatric unit, it should also be near the entrance to the unit.

Two requisites for a good treatment room are an adequate examining-treatment table and ample lighting fixtures. Pediatric diagnosis and treatment procedures are often difficult at best and next to impossible if these requirements are not met. Sound-proofing is another requisite.

Necessary equipment should include supply cupboard, instrument cabinet, bulletin board, nurses' call, clock, dispenser for soap or detergent, and a combination instrument and scrub sink with gooseneck spout and knee or elbow control.

### Waiting and Consultation Room

A waiting room for the pediatric unit is desirable. It should be located close to stairs and elevators and its entrance should be visible from the nurses' station. Comfortable furnishings, soundproofing, and reading matter all should be provided. If possible toilet facilities should be nearby.

Wherever possible, there should be a consultation room for privacy in dealing with parents or children. This may be located near the waiting room and can serve as an office for resident or staff physicians.

The consultation room will often be the only place where nurses can demonstrate the care which the child will need when he goes home. Parent teaching is a very important function of the professional staff, and space must be provided for it. The visitor's room and the consultation and treatment rooms are usually grouped together for convenience in the admission and discharge of patients, but should be shielded from each other.

### Playroom Space

Every pediatric unit should have a playroom. It should not be looked upon as a luxury or as a space where more beds may be placed in an emergency, but as a therapeutic adjunct for patients who are convalescent or ambulatory.

The present plan puts the playroom next to the nurses' station for control. If the hospital is able to provide adequate supervision, possibly by volunteers, the playroom might better be a porch at the outer end of the unit.

The playroom can be used for group activities and recreation — as a playroom for younger children, for games, occupational therapy and school work for older children, and a social room and library for adolescents. At meal time it is an ideal place for group feeding. There should be tables and chairs suitable both for food service and play activities. Storage closets and shelves for toys and other materials should also be provided.

### Utility Room

The utility room should be centrally located in each nursing unit. This room requires ample cupboard and counter space, sterilizer, utensil cabinet, sink with drainboard, hot and cold water supply with elbow or knee control. Space will be required for a hot plate and a container for crushed ice for non-drinking purposes.

A bedpan washer and disinfector and a clinical sink should also be provided with a recessed cabinet for specimens near at hand. Since individual bedpans and urinals are provided at each bedside, no rack is necessary.

### Storage Rooms

Each nursing unit should have separate storage space for linen, supplies, cleaning equipment and such articles as stretchers and wheel chairs.

If the central linen room is large enough, that on the unit need only be large enough to accommodate one day's supply of linen. In the case of infants, a day's linen supply can often be kept in the bedside cabinet.

The stretcher closet should be adequate for the transportation needs of the unit. In a small hospital this area might even be used for the storage of beds of different sizes. A cupboard with shelving may be provided above the level of the stretchers and wheel chairs for additional storage space.

### Oxygen Supply

In spite of additional expense in construction, some hospitals, even small ones, are providing an oxygen and suction outlet for each patient room because of the obvious advantage of having them where they are needed without having to move patients to an oxygen outlet. If only certain rooms can be so provided, those to be given high priority are isolation rooms and one-bed rooms where the sickest children are apt to be placed.

# Diagnostic X-ray Suites for the General Hospital

*by Wilbur R. Taylor,*
*Clifford E. Nelson, M.D.,*
*and William W. McMaster\**

Programming for better medical and surgical care frequently depends on the availability of prompt, thorough, and skillful diagnostic services. Among the many modern diagnostic techniques, x-ray examinations contribute vitally to facilitating effective medication and treatment. A carefully planned diagnostic x-ray department assures an efficient flow of service that may be scheduled promptly and expedited with a minimum of movement and distance for the staff and the patients.

The plans for diagnostic x-ray facilities (pages 141 and 145) were designed to handle daily average workloads of about 35 and 20 patient examinations. The number of x-ray machines to be installed is based on the number of patient examinations and not solely on the number of beds in a hospital. The type of hospital, community need, proportion and extent of outpatient and inpatient examinations, the increasing number of older people in our population, and the patterns of facility usage will affect the number of patient examinations and determine the number of x-ray machines needed.

Flexibility in design is important in planning x-ray facilities, particularly in a small hospital, and it is a requisite in providing for an increase in the workload volume and for expansion of x-ray services. This can be done by adding to the staff or by installing another machine in space planned for future use. When expanding into an adjoining space, the area and shape should be adequate to permit an efficient layout.

In a recent study it was found that many hospitals allotted inadequate space to the x-ray department, and expansion was often impractical. Adequate space for waiting, toilets, and dressing rooms helps insure continuous routines in handling patients. The lack of adequate space results in needless waste of effort and time in efficiently scheduling examinations. An unsatisfactory layout is a handicap to both the hospital and the radiologist since the hospital loses potential revenue, and the radiologist's time, as well as that of the staff, is needlessly wasted. This is particularly important to a small hospital which has a visiting radiologist, for it is to the advantage of the hospital and radiologist to schedule as many examinations as possible during his visit.

## LOCATION

The diagnostic x-ray department should be located on the first floor, conveniently accessible both to outpatients and inpatients. It is also desirable to locate the department close to the elevators and adjoining the outpatient department and near other diagnostic and treatment facilities.

The functional requirements of the department are usually best satisfied by locating the x-ray rooms at the end of a wing. In this location, the activity within the department will not be disturbed by through traffic to other parts of the hospital, and less shielding will be required because of the exterior walls.

## PLAN A

Plan A illustrates an x-ray suite that will provide an efficiently operating service for about 8400 patient examinations yearly, or an average of about 35 examinations daily. This average workload is typical in a hospital of approximately 100 beds (or somewhat more) with an outpatient x-ray service. Unforeseen scheduling problems, of course, will occasionally cause the average of 35 examinations per day to be exceeded.

The staff needed for this volume of work usually includes: 1 radiologist, 2 or 3 technicians, 1 secretary-receptionist, 1 secretary-file clerk, 1 orderly (as needed).

This plan will permit the workload to be augmented at least 50 per cent by increasing the staff, if no more than 20 per cent of the x-ray work is fluoroscopic.

Among the desirable characteristics that this plan attempts to provide for is the need for correlating the functions of the working group to obtain maximum efficiency. The arrangement of patient areas and examination rooms around the perimeter, with the administrative staff in the center, makes it possible for these units to operate more efficiently. The technicians' corridor in the rear of the department provides for easy access to the x-ray rooms, film processing rooms, and distribution areas without interference from patients' cross traffic.

## ADMINISTRATION SPACES

Every radiologist has specific ideas on the most suitable ways for arranging and operating the administrative functions of the x-ray department. Some of the variables involved are assignment of personnel and functions, reception of patients, sequence of patient examinations, film distribution, and staff viewing facilities. This plan provides for flexibility of space arrangements by allowing for variation of several of the operations within the administrative unit.

*Waiting room.* General waiting space for about ten patients is located at the entrance to the department. From here the patient is directed to an assigned dressing room. A separate area, to the left of the entrance and in sight of the secretary-receptionist, is provided for wheelchair and stretcher patients. This section is partitioned off by a curtain which may be partially drawn to provide privacy, yet afford the necessary surveillance of unattended patients from the secretary-receptionist's desk. Additional chairs in this area can be used to ac-

---

*\* The authors are all engaged in work for Public Health Service, Mr. Taylor and Mr. McMaster as architects in the Architectural and Engineering Branch, Division of Hospital and Medical Facilities, Bureau of Medical Services, Dr. Nelson as a radiologist, Division of Radiological Health, Bureau of State Services.*

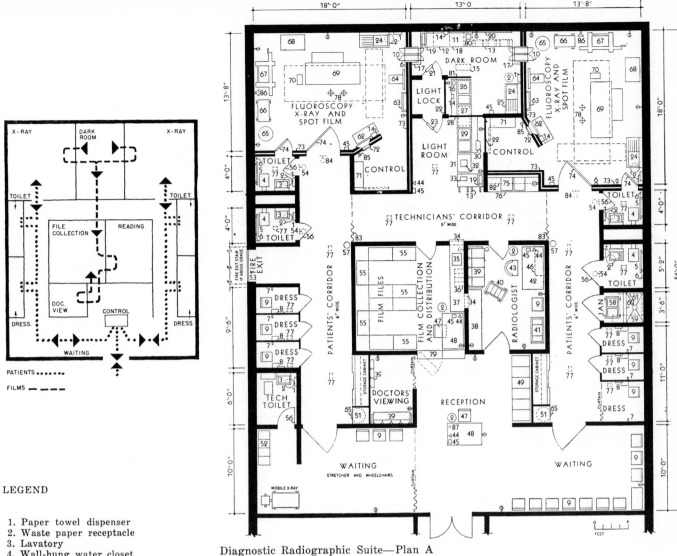

Diagnostic Radiographic Suite—Plan A

## LEGEND

1. Paper towel dispenser
2. Waste paper receptacle
3. Lavatory
4. Wall-hung water closet
5. Continuous grab bar
6. Emergency calling station (push button)
7. Hook strip
8. Mirror and shelf below
9. Straight chair
10. Cassette pass box
11. Film loading counter
12. Film storage bin
13. Film hanger racks under counter
14. Safelight
15. Ceiling light, white and red
16. Timer
17. Counter with storage cabinets below
18. Cassette storage bins
19. Trash deposit cabinet
20. Cassette cover retainer and wall guard
21. Door with light-proof louver in upper panel
22. Access panel
23. Door with light-proof louver in lower panel
24. Utility sink with drainboard
25. Refrigerating unit under drainboard
26. Developing tank with thermostatic mixing valve
27. Through-the-wall fixing tank
28. Light-proof panel
29. Washing tank
30. X-ray film illuminator (wet viewing)
31. Film dryer
32. Film dryer exhaust to outside
33. Film corner cutter
34. Film pass slot
35. Flush-mounted counter illuminator
36. Film sorting bins above counter
37. Film sorting counter
38. Counter with cabinets below
39. On-wall or mobile film illuminators
40. Temporary film file cart
41. Stereoscope
42. Executive type desk
43. Executive type chair
44. Telephone outlet
45. Intercommunication system outlet
46. Bookshelves, 42 in. by 14 in.
47. Typist chair

48. Typist desk
49. Filing cabinet, letter size
50. Gown storage, open shelves, storage cabinet above
51. Gown storage, open shelving with laundry hamper below
52. Technicians' lockers
53. Fire door
54. Dome light, buzzer and annunciator at receptionist's desk
55. Closed metal film files, 5 shelves high
56. Hook on toilet side of door
57. Fire extinguisher
58. Mop truck
59. Shelf
60. Curb and receptor on janitor's sink
61. Mop hanging strip
62. Storage cabinet and writing counter
63. Fluoroscopic apron and glove holder
64. Fluoroscopic chair
65. Laundry hamper
66. Clean linen cart
67. Cassette changer
68. Transformer
69. Radiographic fluoroscopic unit with spot film device
70. Foot stool
71. Control unit
72. Leaded glass view window
73. Lead lining (or other shielding material) as required
74. Lead-lined door, light proofed
75. Barium sink
76. Barium storage (below counter)
77. Red light for dark adaptation
78. Fluoroscopic ceiling light
79. Counter with gate
80. Film identifier, cabinet below
81. Anti-splash panel
82. Wall cabinet over sink
83. Curtain, floor to ceiling
84. Warning light
85. Microphone
86. Loudspeaker
87. Annunciator (for emergency calling station)

commodate the attendants of these patients or for an overflow of waiting patients when needed.

*Secretary-receptionist.* The administrative functions and business records of the department, scheduling of appointments, receiving of patients, typing of the necessary identification forms and requisitions for examinations, and assigning of patients to dressing rooms are handled by the secretary-receptionist. If time permits, the secretary-receptionist assists in typing the radiologist's reports. The desk is centrally located, directly in front of the entrance between the waiting room and administrative area, so that the secretary-receptionist may supervise waiting patients and have access to correspondence and report files.

*Secretary-file clerk.* The secretary-file clerk assembles, sorts and files all films and reports, assists the secretary-receptionist when needed, and transcribes and types the radiologist's reports. These functions are not rigidly fixed and can be interchanged, if desired. For example, a technician may be assigned to assist the file clerk with film assembling and sorting, or the file clerk may be given other functions as needed. The desk is located near a counter-partition in the film collection and distribution area. The low counter and the gate (No. 79) are designed so the entrance to the department can be observed and patients directed when required.

*Doctors' viewing room.* The doctors' viewing room is located near the office of the radiologist so that he may be immediately available for consultation. The room is near the film files, convenient to the secretary and file clerk, and situated so as not to intrude upon the functional flow of the work. Its location within the administrative unit provides privacy so that diagnostic comments and discussions will not be overheard by patients.

*Radiologist's office.* This office is conveniently situated near the x-ray rooms, the secretary-receptionist's desk and the filing distribution area, and is not too easily accessible to the public; it is also provided with a door which opens directly to the technicians' corridor. The fire exit which is located off the technicians' corridor provides a second exit from the department for the radiologist.

*Film files.* The film files are located in the collection and distribution area and convenient to the radiologist's office. Since it is desirable to keep active films for at least five years, approximately 125 linear feet of filing space is provided. After that time, additional storage space elsewhere will be needed for the less active files. Closed front metal x-ray files are recommended (see Fire Safety, page 146). Teaching files may not be needed in a hospital of this size, but if desired, a section of the active files may be allotted for this use.

## GENERAL FACILITIES

*Dressing rooms.* Three dressing rooms for each x-ray machine should be provided so that the equipment and staff can function without delay. Each dressing room should be equipped with a straight-back chair, clothes hook, mirror, and a shelf below the mirror. For the protection of patients' valuables, the doors may be equipped with locks, or centrally located lockers may be provided. Where doors are installed, they should swing outward to avoid the possibility of being blocked by a patient and should be at least 12 inches from the floor.

For the convenience of patients in wheelchairs, an out-sized dressing room is provided. Instead of a door, it is equipped with a curtain so that the patient can maneuver easily.

*Patients' toilet rooms.* Toilets should be immediately available for patients undergoing fluoroscopy, and similar facilities should be conveniently available for waiting patients. A minimum of two toilets should be provided for each x-ray room. All toilets should be located near the x-ray rooms.

At least one toilet room should be directly accessible to each x-ray room and have an opening into the corridor. To prevent the patients from accidentally opening the door between the toilet and x-ray room, this door should be equipped with hardware which is operable only from the x-ray room. The doors of the toilet rooms which open into the patients' corridor should be equipped with bathroom locks, which are operated by knob latch bolts and dead bolts from both sides.

One of the patients' toilet rooms is designed to accommodate a patient in a wheelchair. The room is larger than the others, for easy maneuvering, and has a 3 ft door. The lavatory is set on wall brackets 6 in. out from the wall and 2 ft 10 in. from the floor.

One toilet should be provided with a bedpan flushing attachment. Water closets should be suspended from the wall to simplify cleaning. Each toilet room should be equipped with a grab bar for use by elderly or weak patients. A dome light and buzzer system with an emergency call station in each toilet room and an annunciator at the secretary-receptionist's desk is recommended.

*Technicians' toilets and lockers.* During busy periods it is essential that the staff be available at all times. Separate toilet and locker facilities are provided for technicians. This reduces the time technicians must be absent from the area and contributes to the efficiency of the department.

## STORAGE FACILITIES

*General storage.* For bulk supplies, a storage cabinet equipped with sliding doors and adjustable shelves is located inside each patients' corridor near the entrance. Materials such as films, opaque solutions, developing solutions, and office supplies are stored here.

*Daily linen supplies (x-ray rooms).* Clean linen, requisitioned from the hospital central supply, is stored on a cart (No. 66) in each x-ray room; soiled linen is placed in a hamper (No. 65).

*Gown storage.* Open adjustable shelves for gown storage are placed next to each general bulk supply cabinet, just inside the corridor entrance. The shelving for clean gowns starts about 4 ft from the floor, leaving space beneath for a linen hamper (No. 65) for soiled gowns.

*Janitor's closet.* The janitor's closet must be readily available for emergency cleaning and it should be convenient to the x-ray rooms and toilets. The closet should contain a floor receptor with a curb or a janitor's service sink, a mop-hanging strip and a shelf, and provide space for parking the mop truck.

## DIAGNOSTIC X-RAY ROOMS

*X-ray equipment.* Both rooms are equipped with combination x-ray and fluoroscopic machines with spot film devices. An overhead type tube support is indicated in the plan, as this facilitates x-raying a patient in bed or on a stretcher. For reasons of economy, however, it may

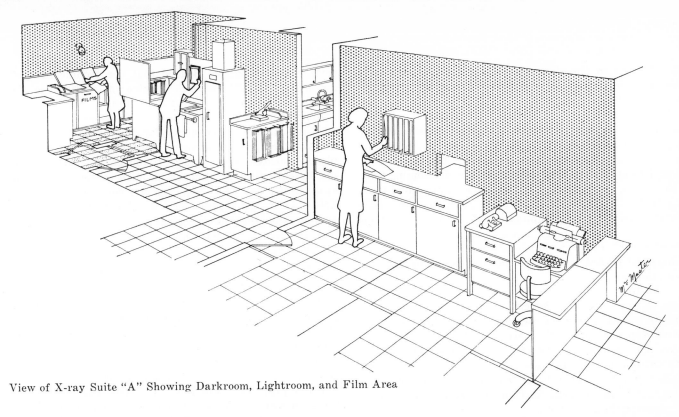

View of X-ray Suite "A" Showing Darkroom, Lightroom, and Film Area

be desirable to equip one room with a floor-ceiling track. If an overhead mounted track is used, it may be supported from the floor by columns or may be bracketed from the wall, although a ceiling suspension makes a neater installation.

The optimum size of the x-ray room is about 14 by 18 ft. Ceiling height requirements vary for different x-ray machines, but a minimum of 9 ft 6 in. is recommended. The machine and transformer should be placed so as to allow adequate space for admittance of a bed or stretcher in the room. Mounting the transformer on the wall is recommended to save floor space. However, sufficient clearances (at least 2 ft above the transformer) for servicing the transformer should be provided.

The sink and drainboard, for handwashing and rinsing utensils and barium equipment, is equipped with a gooseneck spout. It is located near the foot of the x-ray table. The drainboard can also be used as a barium counter.

It is recommended that the control panel be wired to a signal outside each x-ray room to indicate when the machine is on, to prevent other personnel from inadvertently entering the room. A red light bulb will be satisfactory as a signal for most installations.

*Control booth.* It is essential that the control booth be located to the right of the machine so that the patient may be observed when the table is inclined, since machines with end-pivoted tables tilt to the right. In the plan, no door is shown on the control booth as the radiation will have scattered at least twice before it reaches the control booth area. This is in accordance with Handbook 60, as amended, issued by the National Bureau of Standards. The arrangement of the control booth to the right and the cassette changer to the extreme left, as shown in the plan, fully meets this requirement. In addition, since the beam is directed toward the outside wall, radiation exposure to other personnel is lessened, and the amount of shielding required is decreased.

If the cassette changers are placed to the right of the machine (on the wall opposite to that indicated on the plan), a door on the control booth or a baffle placed in

the room is required to protect the technician in the booth. Furthermore, additional shielding is required to protect films and personnel in the department because the primary beam would not be directed toward the outside wall. In the present scheme, the shielding necessary in the interior walls is principally to safeguard against the scatter radiation.

*Storage cabinet and writing counter.* A storage cabinet (No. 62), with a safety light above, serves also as a writing counter for the radiologist and technicians. Shelves in the cabinet provide space for storage of accessory items such as sandbags, measuring devices used with x-ray machine, and disposable items needed for patients' examinations.

FILM PROCESSING AND DISTRIBUTION AREAS
*Darkroom.* This room is located between the two x-ray rooms to facilitate handling of films. Cassettes are loaded and unloaded on the counter (No. 11). Space is provided for loading and stacking cassettes at both ends of the counter.

A utility sink with a drainboard (No. 24), located opposite the processing tank, is provided for mixing chemical solutions and handwashing. A refrigerating unit (No. 25) for the tank is located in the space beneath the drainboard.

X-ray films are processed in an area separated from the loading counter by a partition (No. 81) at the end of the developing tank which helps to avoid accidental splashing and damage to the screens and films on the loading counter. A through-wall processing unit tank permits the radiologist or staff doctors to read the wet films in the lightroom area without interrupting darkroom procedures.

A lightlock between the darkroom and the lightroom, equipped with interlocking doors, is necessary to allow entrance into the darkroom of other personnel during film processing. Although a maze has some advantages over the lightlock, the additional space needed is not justifiable in a facility of this size. Access panels (No.

22), located in the lightlock and in the control space, are provided to simplify installation and servicing of the processing tanks.

*Film processing area.* To reduce unnecessary traffic, the film processing rooms are located near the collection and distribution area. This layout allows the technician to work without interruption during the processing routine. Processing of films begins at the developing tank (No. 26) in the darkroom, and continues to the final rinsing tank (No. 29) in the lightroom where the films may be wet-viewed at an illuminator, if desired, and then dried. After the films are dried, they are brought to the counter (33) in the technicians' corridor for final trimming, and passed through to the film collection and distribution area.

*Collection and distribution area.* Film sorting bins (No. 36) are provided above the counter in the collection and distribution area for temporary filing. After all films have been assembled, they are passed through the film pass slot (No. 34) to the radiologist for interpretation. He returns the films in a file cart or through a slot which leads into a box under the distribution counter. The films may then be temporarily filed for viewing by staff doctors or placed in the active files.

## BARIUM MIXING FACILITES
A two-compartment sink (No. 75) in a counter, located in the technicians' corridor and accessible to both x-ray rooms, is provided for mixing barium. A duplex outlet for plugging in an electric mixer or a heating element is located above the counter unit. Barium supplies for daily use are stored in cabinets under the counter; the bulk supplies can be stocked in one of the general storage cabinets located in the patients' corridors.

## DARK ADAPTATION
Patients must be allowed to become accustomed to the low lighting level in the x-ray rooms and the staff must retain their dark adaptation despite the opening of the doors of the fluoroscopic rooms between patients' examinations.

To facilitate dark adaptation, curtains are shown at the intersections of the technicians' and the patients' corridors. In addition to the illumination normally provided in the corridors, patients' toilet rooms, and dressing rooms, it is recommended that these areas be equipped with an independently controlled dim lighting system of red bulbs for dark adaptation.

## MISCELLANEOUS SERVICES
It is assumed that the central sterile supply department of the hospital will provide all such services required by the x-ray department.

The mobile x-ray unit should be stored in the radiology department where it will be under the supervision and control of the department and available when needed.

## OPTIONAL FACILITIES
*Intercommunication system.* Provision of a system within the department increases the efficiency of the staff and speeds up service. Outlets are shown at the desk of the secretary-receptionist, in the x-ray rooms and the darkroom, and in the technicians' corridor. It is recommended that a one-way intercommunication system, with a microphone in the control booth and a loudspeaker at the cassette changer, be installed so that the technician need not leave the control booth to give instructions to the patient at the far end of the x-ray room.

*Refrigerator.* Some items used in the x-ray department, such as barium suspensions for fluoroscopic examinations of the upper gastrointestinal tract, cream for a gall bladder series, and carbonated beverages for carbon dioxide distention of the stomach, require refrigeration. The space under one end of the barium counter at the sink (No. 75) in the technicians' corridor may be used for an under-counter type refrigerator.

*High-speed film dryer.* The plan provides sufficient space for an anhydrator, if desired, in lieu of the dryer shown (No. 31).

## FINISH MATERIALS
Materials used in this department are generally similar to those usually provided in hospitals. However, special attention should be given to some of the areas in the x-ray suite.

*Darkroom.* The cassette loading counter surface should be of a material which is static-free; wood or linoleum is often preferred. Vinyl or vinyl-asbestos tile, $\frac{1}{8}$ in. thick, appears to be a satisfactory material for floors in this size department. Experience indicates, however, that asphalt tile and linoleum floors do not stand up well under the effects of spilled solutions. A pattern of alternating dark and light tiles improves visibility when working under a safe light.

*X-ray rooms.* No special finishes are required for the x-ray rooms. Asphalt tile floors are satisfactory and a pattern of alternating dark and light tiles is also desirable here. Plaster walls and ceilings are acceptable, but acoustical tile ceilings are preferred since they aid in reducing reverberation.

*Toilets.* Tile floors and wainscot are highly desirable for easy cleaning.

*Doctors' viewing room.* Acoustical treatment is recommended to lessen the possibility of doctors' conversations being overheard by nearby waiting patients.

## ELECTRICAL INSTALLATIONS
Voltage supplied to the x-ray unit should be constant so that fluoroscopic images and radiographs will be uniform. An independent feeder with sufficient capacity to prevent a voltage drop greater than 3 per cent is recommended. To minimize voltage fluctuations, a separate transformer for the x-ray feeder is required for most installations.

## ILLUMINATION
Illumination intensities in the various areas of the suite should comply with recommendations given in the Lighting Handbook, 3rd Edition (1959), published by the Illuminating Engineering Society. Briefly, the general illumination should be not less than 10 footcandles in corridors and in rooms where reading is not required. The waiting room should have 15 footcandles, with supplemental lighting for reading. Offices and areas where clerical work is performed should have at least 50 footcandles, preferably 70 footcandles.

Indirect or cove lighting fixtures are recommended for the x-ray rooms so that patients need not be inconvenienced by glare when lying face upward during radiographic examinations.

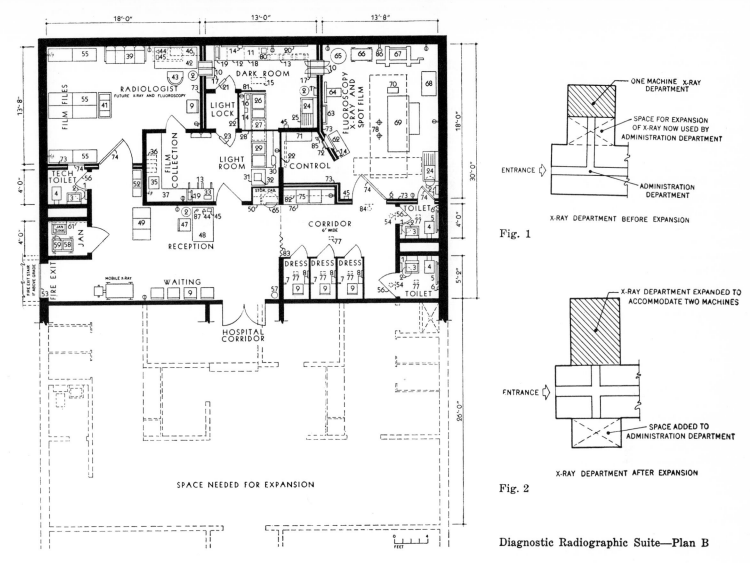

**Fig. 1**

ONE MACHINE X-RAY DEPARTMENT

SPACE FOR EXPANSION OF X-RAY NOW USED BY ADMINISTRATION DEPARTMENT

ENTRANCE ⇨

ADMINISTRATION DEPARTMENT

X-RAY DEPARTMENT BEFORE EXPANSION

**Fig. 2**

X-RAY DEPARTMENT EXPANDED TO ACCOMMODATE TWO MACHINES

ENTRANCE ⇨

SPACE ADDED TO ADMINISTRATION DEPARTMENT

X-RAY DEPARTMENT AFTER EXPANSION

Diagnostic Radiographic Suite—Plan B

## RADIATION PROTECTION

Protection against ionizing radiations in excess of a tolerable amount is necessary. Methods for determining protective barriers are given in Handbook 60, as amended, "X-ray Protection," issued by the National Bureau of Standards.

The barrier design should be checked by a qualified expert before the construction plans are approved and the completed installation should be surveyed with radiation detecting devices before the facility is used. A resurvey should be made after any alteration or structural change which might permit increased radiation into an occupied area.

For the protection of the staff and persons in adjacent areas from radiation, barriers of lead or equivalent materials should be provided to attenuate the radiation so that no one will receive radiation in excess of the "maximum permissible dose." (Refer to Handbook 60, as amended.) Adequate protection of the darkroom from radiation, to minimize fogging of unprocessed films, should be provided.

Primary barriers should be provided on all surfaces of the x-ray rooms which are exposed, or which may be exposed, to the useful beam between the x-ray tube and occupied areas. Secondary barriers should be provided on all other room surfaces where protection is needed. In determining secondary barriers, consideration should be given to direct or leakage radiation which passes through the tube housing, and also to the secondary or scattered radiation emitted from objects being irradiated by either the useful beam, leakage radiation, or other scattered radiation.

## PLAN B—DESIGN FOR EXPANSION

This one-machine department, designed to handle a daily average of about 20 patient examinations, could satisfactorily serve a hospital of 50 to 100 beds, depending upon the extent of outpatient services provided. As in Plan A, its volume of examinations can be increased, depending on the staffing pattern and other factors, discussed previously.

The staff usually required for this workload includes: 1 part-time radiologist, 1 technician, 1 secretary-receptionist-technician, 1 orderly (as needed).

This plan will result in a functional unit. It has another important advantage in that it may be expanded to include all the features of Plan A. Such expansion is usually indicated when the hospital is served by a full-time radiologist, when the average daily load approaches 30 examinations per day, and when the proportion of time-consuming examinations becomes high.

Expansion problems frequently occur in a hospital of 100 beds or less, where there is only one x-ray machine and a part-time radiologist. As the volume of work increases, the radiologist spends more time at the hospital, and a second machine is installed. Unfortunately, in most of these cases, the lack of planning for a future expansion program and expansion area results in an inefficient layout. This limits the usefulness of the equipment and the efficiency of the staff. Examples of such limitations are: poor location of the darkroom in relation to the new x-ray room, inadequate size of the darkroom, insufficient number of toilet facilities and dressing rooms, lack of office and waiting areas, and limited film filing space.

Remodeling an x-ray department is more expensive than remodeling other areas of a hospital because of the shielding, wiring, and plumbing. Expansion of the x-ray department should be incorporated in the original plan. Roughing in the plumbing and building in the shielding and electrical conduits in the expansion space will result in future savings and an efficient x-ray suite.

Minimum alterations to Plan B necessary to duplicate the facilities of Plan A would be the remodeling of the film collection area to accommodate a new control booth, the elimination of the partition between the lightroom and reception space, the elimination of the dressing rooms and the partition behind them.

Until the need for remodeling becomes apparent, part of the administration offices of the hospital may temporarily be situated in the expansion space. When enlarging the x-ray department, other space may then be added to the administration department. The dotted lines on Plan B and Figures 1 and 2 illustrate how this expansion may be designed.

## AIR CONDITIONING

Air conditioning with positive ventilation and a well-defined pattern of air movement within the department is necessary to provide an acceptable environment. In order to prevent the spread of odors from the radiographic and fluoroscopic rooms, darkroom, toilets, and janitor's closets, the ventilation system should be designed so that a negative air pressure relative to the adjoining corridors will be maintained in these rooms. This can be done by exhausting more air from these rooms than is supplied to them, and by reversing this procedure in the corridors. Doors to the toilets and the janitor's closet should be undercut or louvered so that air from the corridors may flow into these areas and be exhausted without recirculation.

Because of the odor problem, the air from the fluoroscopic and x-ray rooms should not be recirculated during the time these rooms are in use, unless adequate odor removal equipment is incorporated in the ventilation system. For economical operation, where odor control equipment is not used, the exhaust system should be provided with motor-operated dampers, switched from within the room, which will direct the air to the outdoors when the rooms are being used, or recirculate the air during idle periods.

As the darkroom will be used for longer periods than the x-ray rooms, an independent system to exhaust the air to the outdoors should be provided. The exhaust from the darkroom should be controlled from a switch in the room and the system should be dampered to regulate the amount of air handled. The exhaust from the film dryer in the lightroom should be connected into the darkroom exhaust system.

The following conditions are recommended for the comfort of patients and personnel:

*Administration and waiting areas.* A temperature of 72 deg F with a relative humidity of 50 per cent and a ventilation rate of 1-1½ air changes per hour.

*Patients' and technicians' corridors.* A temperature of 75 deg F to 80 deg F with relative humidity of 50 per cent and a ventilation rate of 2 air changes per hour.

*Fluoroscopic and x-ray rooms.* A temperature of 75 deg F to 80 deg F with relative humidity of 50 per cent and a ventilation rate of 6 air changes per hour.

*Darkroom.* A temperature of 72 deg F with relative humidity of 50 per cent and a ventilation rate of 10 air changes per hour.

## FIRE SAFETY

To provide an adequate measure of fire safety for the patients and the staff in this department, consideration must be given to factors of design and construction relating to fire prevention and fire protection. The basic structure should be built with fire resistive materials and incombustible finishes and provided with approved equipment.

Closed metal files are recommended for storage of x-ray films. If open shelves are used instead, an automatic sprinkler system should be installed over this storage area to neutralize the hazard of the large volume of combustible materials which would be exposed to possible fire.

Fire extinguishers (carbon dioxide type preferred) should be provided, as located on the plans, to assist in controlling fire.

In accordance with good fire safety practice, two means of egress are provided in the plan: one at the entrance to the department and an emergency exit located off the patient's corridor (door No. 53). The emergency fire exit should lead directly to the ground level outside the building, through an appropriate exit stairway.

## ACKNOWLEDGMENTS

"These plans are the product of extensive studies by the staff of the Division of Hospital and Medical Facilities in co-operation with the Division of Radiological Health, Public Service, and hospital architects, radiologists, administrators, engineers, and manufacturers throughout the country. Without their generous assistance, the work would not have been possible."

*Jack C. Haldeman, Chief, Division of Hospital and Medical Facilities, Public Health Service*

"The authors gratefully acknowledge the valuable assistance received from the following: J. Robert Andrews, M. D., Chief, Radiation Branch, National Cancer Institute, Bethesda, Md.; Joe Lee Frank, Jr., M. D., Director, Department of Radiology, Roanoke-Chowan Hospital, Ahoskie, N. C.; Philip J. Hodes, M. D., Professor and Head, Department of Radiology, Jefferson Medical College, Philadelphia, Pa.; Ira Lewis, M. D., Chief, Radiology Service, U. S. Public Health Service Hospital, San Francisco, Calif.; Russell H. Morgan, M. D., Radiologist-in-Chief, The Johns Hopkins Hospital, Baltimore, Md.; Jacque B. Norman, Hospital Consultant, Greenville, S. C.; Wendell G. Scott, M. D. Associate Professor of Clinical Radiology, Washington University School of Medicine, St. Louis, Mo.; W. M. Sennott, M. D., Chief of Radiology Service, U. S. Public Health Service Hospital, Baltimore, Md.; George Shipman, M. D., Chief of Radiology, U. S. Public Health Service Hospital, Staten Island, N. Y.; Richard E. Zellmer, M. D., Chief, Radiology Department, U. S. Public Health Service Hospital, Chicago, Ill.; Picker X-ray Corporation, Washington, D. C., and White Plains, N. Y.; Westinghouse Electric Corp., X-ray Division, Washington, D. C.

*Diagnostic X-ray Suites*

*By the term teletherapy, we are restricting ourselves to the use of radiation at a distance; that is, the subject and source are separated by a distance of 50 centimeters or more. In particular, we are concerned with the use of the radioactive isotopes cobalt-60 and cesium-137 as sources of radiation in teletherapy units.*

*We have restricted our discussion to Co⁶⁰ and Cs¹³⁷, primarily because they are the more familiar of the isotopes suggested for use in teletherapy units. We are not including the use of radium and high energy X-rays, since some of the problems associated with these are quite different in their solution and nature.*

*The primary purpose of this article is to furnish architects anticipating a teletherapy unit, information on basic radiation protection ideas and techniques, and to serve as a guide in the solutions of certain architectural problems. We are by no means attempting to evaluate the advantages and disadvantages of Co⁶⁰ and Cs¹³⁷ units against other types of units.*

# Design of Teletherapy Units

*Radiation and Architectural Considerations for Cobalt 60 Units*

*by Wilbur R. Taylor, William A. Mills and James G. Terrill, Jr.\**

IN PLANNING A COBALT INSTALLATION, it should be understood that each type of machine and its location within the building will present a different problem which will require an individual solution. Consequently, no one type plan can be designed which will take care of the various shielding requirements presented by the different machines and installations. The architect is dependent upon other professionals for specific technical information he needs before he can intelligently design a building containing a cobalt teletherapy unit. The problems incurred may materially affect the orientation, location, and structural and functional design of the building. Therefore, during preliminary design stages, close cooperation between architect, radiologist and radiation physicist is necessary to develop an efficient and economical layout.

It should be noted that the Atomic Energy Commission places responsibility upon the applicant for conditions of installation and use of the facility. Since the use of a facility is largely dependent upon the conditions of installation, it is to the applicant's advantage to secure the services of a radiation physicist at the inception of a project. His function is to advise the applicant and architect on radiation requirements, assume responsibility for the final design as to shielding provided and furnish the supporting information required in Application Form AEC-313 relative to exposure rates in areas surrounding the teletherapy room and occupancy factors assigned.

Fundamental decisions as to: (1) the type of machine, (2) strength of the source, (3) desired location, and (4) the shielding required for floor, walls and ceiling must be made before the building's structural system can be designed. During the early design, it may be determined that the structural system cannot support the weight of the shielding, or perhaps soil conditions will not permit sufficient excavation for a subgrade installation. It may then be necessary to change or alter one or more of the following: the machine or its operation, the source strength or the location of the room.

To those not familiar with such shielding problems, the included plans have been developed to illustrate the shielding necessary for three types of machines in specific locations. However, before considering the detailed plans, it may be desirable to discuss some of the general requirements of such facilities.

### Location

The cobalt suite should adjoin the X-ray therapy department. This location permits the joint use of waiting, dressing, toilet, examination, work and consultation rooms. In addition, it offers the important advantage of having the staff concentrated in one area, thereby eliminating the considerable

*\*Wilbur R. Taylor is a Hospital Architect in the Division of Hospital and Medical Facilities, Bureau of Medical Service, Public Health Service, Department of Health, Education, and Welfare; and William A. Mills and James G. Terrill, Jr. are respectively Radiation Physicist and Chief of Radiological Health Program, Division of Sanitary Engineering Services, Bureau of State Services, Public Health Service.*

loss of time involved in traveling to a remote location. This is an important consideration and justifies the cost of any additional shielding that may be necessary to achieve it.

A location below grade, unoccupied above and below, will require less shielding. However, if such a location separates the cobalt and the X-ray therapy department, it may be more costly in both loss of staff time and efficiency than the cost of concrete shielding amortized over several years. If, for example, twenty-five minutes per day are lost in traveling to a remote location, one additional patient could be treated in this time each day — or 240 patients per year. Assuming a staff salary of $20,000 per year, this loss of twenty-five minutes per day results in an indirect salary loss of $1032 per year, which would soon equal the cost of shielding in a new facility.

A corner location for the cobalt room is usually desirable since through traffic is eliminated, only two interior walls require shielding, distance to the property line utilizes the inverse square law to reduce shielding and the structural requirements are more easily solved.

### Teletherapy Room Details

*Size.* The room size may vary to suit different manufacturers' equipment. A room approximately 15 ft by 18 ft by 9 ft-6 in. plus the necessary entrance maze, will accommodate most of the machines commercially available with the exception of the largest rotating models. For reasons of cost, the room should be as compact as possible after allowing space to install the equipment and to position the treatment table.

*Shielding.* The shielding necessary for a room must not only be considered in terms of floor, ceiling and wall shielding, but also such things as doors, windows, ventilation and heating ducts, and safety locks. Radiation that might escape through such possibilities could result in overexposure to personnel, if proper precautions are not taken.

*Entrance.* The primary purpose of specific entrance construction is to protect personnel. It should also provide sufficient space to admit a stretcher and the largest crated piece of equipment. In some cases, a considerable savings in cost of assembling equipment may be had by making the door and maze large enough to admit the crated assembled machine. For this purpose, some manufacturers specify a door opening of 4 by 7 ft and a minimum distance of 6 ft at the end of the maze.

Rather than add large amounts of lead to doors, the shielding problem may be solved to some degree by having the door to the teletherapy room open into a maze. This maze should be built so that no primary radiation could fall directly on the door. In designing doors for such a room, a good practice is to have a door of wood with a layer of lead. This lead can either be on the inside surface, or between layers of wood. Commercially available x-ray doors serve well for this purpose. The space between the door and floor can usually be shielded by using a lead strip under the door or by making a slight rise in the floor containing lead, on the outer side of the door. Lead shielding at the jamb and head between the frame and buck may be eliminated by the use of a combination frame and buck set in concrete.

For safety precautions, the door lock should be such that the door can be readily opened from inside the cobalt room.

*Control View Window.* It is standard practice to locate this window at a height which will permit the operator to be seated during the treatment period, 4 ft-0 in. from the floor to the center of the window being an optimum distance. In plan, the window should be located in the area of minimum radiation and for convenient observation of the patient. This position, for a rotational machine, would be along the axis of rotation, and for a fixed beam unit, 90° to the plane of tilt.

From the control view window the entire room should be in full view, using mirrors when necessary. The glass should contain lead or other materials in amounts which would provide shielding equivalent to the surrounding concrete. The frame is usually packed with lead wool and should be designed to offset the shielding loss of the reduced concrete thickness at beveled areas. The cost of such special glass and frame increases rapidly with size and an 8 by 8 in. window is considered an optimum size.

*Heating and Air Conditioning.* The only problem in relation to heating and air conditioning not encountered in other buildings is that of providing shielding where walls are pierced with supply and return ducts. The usual solution is to locate ducts and openings in walls which are least subject to radiation and offset the path of ducts through the wall, lead or other high density material being added, where necessary, to maintain the shielding value of the wall displaced by ducts.

*Electrical.* Electrical service required for the machine, will vary with each manufacturer's equipment. Voltage will vary from 110-single phase to 220-three phase for large machines.

Room lighting should assure good over-all illumination, preferably from cove lighting or an indirect type of fixture. It is essential that the operator be able to observe any movement of the patient during treatment and shadows produced by a rotating machine interfere with observation.

In providing a safety lock for the door, it has been found of great value to interlock the machine control with the door, so that opening the door automatically shuts off the machine.

Conduits should be provided for power and control wiring.

*Environment.* The general effect to be created in this department should be one of cheerfulness and restfulness. Use of color and even murals have been used effectively on the walls of the cobalt room.

The usual hospital finishes such as acoustical ceiling tile and resilient flooring are desirable in this area.

*Remodeling.* Unless previously designed for super voltage X-ray, remodeling an existing building can be expensive. It is often impossible to build in sufficient shielding which makes it necessary to control nearby occupancy and restrict direction of the beam, thereby handicapping the usefulness of the machine. Other problems such as relocating plumbing, heating, electrical services and disturbing the normal operation of the building during remodeling must be considered.

In new construction, concrete shielding is relatively cheap, but in remodeling the cost is high. For this reason the use of masonry units may be preferable since no form work is necessary and the work can be performed intermittently. Good workmanship, of course, is necessary to prevent voids in mortar joints.

In some cases it might be better to add to the building, rather than to remodel an existing portion. Normal hospital operation would not be interfered with, costs may be lower and a more efficient layout would probably result.

SPECIAL FACILITIES

THIS ARTICLE WAS DEVELOPED at the request of the Committee on use of Radioisotopes in Hospitals of the American Hospital Association and as a result of many requests from architects and hospitals for information on the design of such facilities.

## ACKNOWLEDGMENTS

The authors gratefully acknowledge the valuable assistance received on the text and plans from the following:

Alexander H. Bacci, Architect, firm of Schmidt, Garden and Erikson
Architects and Engineers
Chicago 3, Illinois

Richard P. Gaulin
Mechanical Engineer
Architectural and Engineering Branch
Division of Hospital and Medical Facilities
Public Health Service

Noyce L. Griffin
Electrical Engineer
Architectural and Engineering Branch
Division of Hospital and Medical Facilities
Public Health Service

August F. Hoenack
Chief, Architectural and Engineering Branch
Division of Hospital and Medical Facilities
Public Health Service

Frank E. Hoecker,
Chief, Architectural and Engineering Branch
Division of Hospital and Medical Facilities
Public Health Service

Frank E. Hoecker, Ph. D.
Radiological Physicist
University of Kansas

George Ivanick
Assistant Chief
Architectural and Engineering Branch
Division of Hospital and Medical Facilities
Public Health Service

Clinton C. Powell, M. D.
Chief, Radiological Health Medical Program
Division of Special Health Services
Public Health Service

Julian Smariga, Structural Engineer
Architectural and Engineering Branch
Division of Hospital and Medical Facilities
Public Health Services

Edwin G. Williams, M.D.
Chief, Radiological Protection Branch
Division of Hospital and Medical Facilities
Public Health Service

# FUNDAMENTALS OF RADIATION PROTECTION

In considering a teletherapy unit, architects are immediately thrown into a world of new definitions, concepts and terms.

Listed in the Glossary are some of the more frequent occurring definitions that turn up during the course of a discussion on teletherapy units.

In addition to definitions and terms, one must become acquainted with new technical fundamentals having to do with the decay of radioactive isotopes, and the passage of the radiation through matter.

A very important law having to do with radioactive decay is stated simply by the equation:

$$N = N_0 e^{-\lambda t} \qquad (1)$$

Where,

$N$ = the number of atoms of the isotope present after a time = $t$,

$N_0$ = the initial number of atoms present at a time equal to zero,

$e$ = the base of the natural log = 2.718,

$\lambda$ = the decay constant for the isotope.

This is usually written in the form of the given half-life for the isotope, and appears as:

$$N = N_0 e^{-\frac{0.693}{T}} \quad \text{Where, } T = \frac{0.693}{\lambda}$$

For our purpose we will not speak of the number of atoms decaying in terms of N, but we will use the more familiar term of *curie*. Where, as defined,

1 curie = $3.7 \times 10^{10}$ disintegrations/sec. This is approximately the disintegrating rate of 1 gm of natural radium atoms. In speaking of $Co^{60}$, we must keep in mind that each disintegrating atom results in the emission of two gamma rays, and each disintegrating atom $Cs^{137}$ results in one gamma ray. We will discuss this in greater detail later in this paper.

Another important fundamental to which one becomes exposed is that pertaining to the intensity of radiation, and is expressed as:

$$I = \frac{I_0 B}{D^2} e^{-\mu x} \qquad (2)$$

Where,

$I$ = The intensity in mr/hr at a distance of D cm from the source

$I_0$ = The intensity at 1 cm from the source

$D$ = Distance between source and subject in cm

$B$ = Buildup factor in the shielding material

$\mu$ = Total absorption coefficient of the shielding material in cm$^{-1}$.

$X$ = Thickness of shielding material in cm.

In utilizing such an equation as (2), one neglects the attenuation due to the air present between the subject and source. We will apply essentially this idea in designing of shields for personnel protection, in latter parts of this article.

Perhaps before one becomes involved in a situation of using either $Co^{60}$ or $Cs^{137}$ in a teletherapy unit, he should understand some of the basic characteristics of each of these isotopes.

First of all, we will look at the $Co^{60}$ isotope. This isotope is produced in nuclear reactors, by subjecting naturally occurring cobalt ($Co^{59}$) to intense neutron bombardment. Naturally occurring $Co^{59}$ is not radioactive, but by adding a neutron to its nucleus, it becomes the highly radioactive $Co^{60}$. This isotope has a half-life of 5.2 years and emits two gamma rays of 1.17 and 1.33 Mev. A close approximation of the dose rate delivered by $Co^{60}$ is

R = $1.35 \times 10^4$ Roentgens per hour at a distance of 1 cm from
1 curie source of $Co^{60}$.

When considering the use of $Cs^{137}$, one has a different source of radiation in that the half-life of the material is greater, but the radiation emitted per curie is not as large as for $Co^{60}$. $Cs^{137}$ is one of the fission products produced in the process of operating a nuclear reactor, and this is one of the primary reasons it serves as a good source for teletherapy units. Of course, the expense involved in this material, is in separating it from the many other materials produced in the reactor fuel elements. However, the supply is increasing steadily. $Cs^{137}$ has a half-life of 30 years and results in the emission of a 0.662 Mev gamma ray. The radiation produced from a curie quantity of $Cs^{137}$ is

R = $0.39 \times 10^4$ r/hr at 1 cm.

## SHIELDING

Now we would like to discuss the shielding necessary for personnel protection. In thinking about shielding, one is conscious of a statement made by Dr. K. Z. Morgan of the Oak Ridge National Laboratory, "radiation need not be feared, only appreciated." This is a good basic idea to keep in mind when thinking about the shielding of dangerous quantities of radioactive material.

There are many different materials used in shielding of radiation, but perhaps the more useful ones are earth, lead and concrete. Such materials as water, steel and marble can make suitable shields depending on the type of radiation and the architectural circumstances. A rough rule of thumb in comparing different materials is that $\frac{3}{4}$ in. of lead, $1\frac{1}{2}$ in. of steel, $4\frac{1}{2}$ in. of concrete, $7\frac{1}{2}$ in. of earth and $10\frac{1}{2}$ in. of water are equivalent for shielding. In this paper, we will only explore the usefulness of concrete in the attenuation of radiation from sources of $Co^{60}$.

Perhaps before going further, we should examine the process of attenuation of gamma rays in shielding material. Gamma rays are electromagnetic waves, highly energetic, and can result in heat development. Thus, gamma rays in passing through a material lose their energy by various processes, but basically all result in an increase in heat of the material. However, the heat generated is insignificant.

In designing shielding for radiation, one is concerned with two types of shielding, primary and secondary. Primary shielding is that needed to attenuate the direct radiation from the unit, and secondary shielding is that which is needed to attenuate the scattered radiation from the patient, primary barrier, etc.

What are the maximum values that we are "shooting" for in designing shielding?

According to a proposed revision of the National Bureau of Standards Handbook 59, "Permissible Dose from External Sources of Ionizing Radiation," for design purposes occupational exposures should not exceed 100 milliroentgens (mr) per week, and non-occupational exposures not over 10 milliroentgens per week. These are total body or critical organ exposures.

In this discussion we will allow the occupational exposure to be given over a work week of 48 hours.

In designing shielding for any teletherapy unit, there are many variables which one must consider. Such things as degree of occupancy, type of machine being considered, the source strength and actual running time of the machine will affect the amount of shielding necessary to give proper protection. Two basic equations for primary and secondary radiation that consider some of these variables are

$$B = \frac{(MPD)D^2}{WT} \text{ (3) and } B_s = \frac{(MPD)S^2}{0.001\ WT} \text{ (4)}$$

Where,

$B$ = permissible transmission for the primary beam

$B_s$ = permissible transmission for the secondary beam (scattered radiation at angles equal to or greater than 90°)

$MPD$ = maximum permissible weekly exposure for occupational or non-occupational

$D$ = distance from source to position in question

$S$ = distance from scatterer to position in question

$W$ = total weekly exposure for the primary beam at 1 meter from the source (obtained by multiplying the roentgens per hour at 1 meter by 48 hours of weekly operation)

$T$ = the occupancy factor.

Graphs showing the permissible transmission values $B$ and $B_s$ versus the thickness of concrete required for protection are given in Figures 1 and 2.

# GLOSSARY*

*Absorption Coefficient:* Fractional decrease in the intensity of a beam of radiation per unit thickness (linear absorption coefficient), per unit mass (mass absorption coefficient), or per atom (atomic absorption coefficient) of absorber.

*Attenuation:* The reduction of intensity of radiation due to an interposed medium (particle attenuation, energy attenuation).

*Backscattering:* The deflection of radiation by scattering processes through angles greater than 90 degrees with respect to the original direction of motion.

*Build Up Factor:* The ratio of the intensity of X- or gamma radiation (both primary and scattered) at a point in an absorbing medium to the intensity of only the primary radiation. This factor has particular application for "broad beam" attenuation. "Intensity" may refer to energy flux, dose, or energy absorption.

*Curie:* That quantity of a radioactive material having associated with it $3.7 \times 10^{10}$ disintegrations per second.

*Decay Radioactive:* Disintegration of the nucleus of an unstable element by the spontaneous emission of charged particles and/or photons.

*Decay Constant:* The fraction of the number of atoms of a radioactive isotope which decay in unit time. Symbol: $\lambda$.

* All definitions are from the *Radiologic Health Handbook.*

*Depth Dose:* The radiation dose delivered at a particular depth beneath the surface of the body. It is usually expressed as a percentage of surface dose or as a percentage of air dose.

*Direct Radiation:* All radiation coming from one source, except the useful beam.

*Dose (Dosage):* According to current usage, the radiation delivered to a specified area or volume as to the whole body. Units for dose specification are roentgens for X- or gamma rays, reps or equivalent roentgens for beta rays. In radiology the dose may be specified in air, on the skin, or at some depth beneath the surface; no statement of dose is complete without specifications of location. The entire question of radiation dosage units is under consideration by the International Congress of Radiology. (See Rad).

*Dose Rate (Dosage Rate):* Radiation dose delivered per unit time.

*Dosimeter:* Instrument used to detect and measure an accumulated dosage of radiation; in common usage it is a pencil size ionization chamber with a built-in self-reading electrometer; used for personnel monitoring.

*Electron Volt:* A unit of energy equivalent to the amount of energy gained by an electron in passing through a potential difference of one volt. Larger multiple units of the electron volt are frequently used, viz: *Kev,* for thousand or kilo electron volts; *Mev.* for *million electron volts*

and *Bev.* for *billion electron volts.* Abbreviation: ev.

*External Radiation:* Exposure to ionizing radiation when the radiation source is located outside the body.

*Film Badge:* A pack of photographic film used for approximate measurement of radiation exposure for personnel monitoring purposes. The badge may contain two or three films of differing sensitivity, and it may contain a filter which shields part of the film from certain types of radiation.

*Gamma Ray:* Short wavelength electromagnetic radiation of nuclear origin with a range of wave lengths from $10^{-9}$ to $10^{-12}$ cm, emitted from the nucleus.

*Geiger-Mueller (G-M) Counter:* Highly sensitive gas-filled radiation-measuring device which operates at voltages sufficiently high to produce avalanche ionization.

*Health Physics:* A term in common use for that branch of radiological science dealing with the protection of personnel from harmful effects of ionizing radiation.

*Ionization Chamber:* An instrument designed to measure quantity of ionizing radiation in terms of the charge of electricity associated with ions produced within a defined volume.

*Ionizing Radiation:* Any electromagnetic or particulate radiation capable of producing ions, directly or indirectly, in its passage through matter.

*Isotope:* One of several different nuclides having the same number of protons in

SPECIAL FACILITIES

their nuclei, and hence having the same atomic number, but differing in the number of neutrons, and therefore in the mass number. Almost identical chemical properties exist between isotopes of a particular element.

*Lead Equivalent:* The thickness of lead affording the same reduction in radiation dose rate under specific conditions as the material in question.

*Leakage (or Direct) Radiation:* The radiation which escapes through the protecting shielding of an X-ray tube or teletherapy unit.

*Linear Absorption Coefficient:* A factor expressing the fraction of a beam of radiation absorbed in unit thickness of material. In the expression $I = I_0 e^{-ux}$, $I_0$ is the initial intensity, I the intensity after passage through a thickness of the material, x, u is the linear absorption coefficient.

*Mass Absorption Coefficient:* The linear absorption coefficient per cm divided by the density of the absorber in grams per cu cm. It is frequently expressed as u/p, where u is the linear absorption coefficient and p the absorber density.

*Maximum Permissible Dose (MPD):* The dose of ionizing radiation that, in the light of present knowledge, is not expected to cause detectable bodily injury to a person at any time during his lifetime.

*Milliroentgen (mr):* The submultiple of the roentgen equal to one thousandth (1/1000) of a roentgen. (See Roentgen.)

*Primary Protective Barriers:* Barriers sufficient to reduce the useful beam to the permissible dose rate.

*Protective Barriers:* Barriers of radiation-absorbing material, such as lead, concrete and plaster, that are used to reduce radiation hazards.

*Rad:* The unit of absorbed dose, which is 100 ergs/g. The rad is a measure of the energy imparted to matter by ionizing particles per unit mass of irradiated material at the place of interest. It is a unit that was recommended and adopted by the International Commission on Radiological Units at the Seventh International Congress of Radiology, Copenhagen, July 1953.

*Radiation:* 1. The emission and propagation of energy through space or through a material medium in the form of waves; for instance, the emission and propagation of electromagnetic waves or of sound and elastic waves. 2. The term radiation, or radiant energy, when unqualified, usually refers to electromagnetic radiation; such radiation commonly is classified, according to frequency, as Hertzian, infrared, visible (light), ultraviolet, X-ray, and gamma ray. 3. By extension, corpuscular emissions, such as alpha and beta radiation, or rays of mixed or unknown type, as cosmic radiation.

*Radiological Health:* The art and science of protecting human beings from injury by radiation.

*Radiological Survey:* Evaluation of the radiation hazards incident to the production, use or existence of radioactive materials or other sources of radiation under a specific set of conditions. Such evaluation customarily includes a physical survey of the disposition of materials and equipment, measurements or estimates of the levels of radiation that may be involved and a sufficient knowledge of processes using or affecting these materials to predict hazards resulting from expected or possible changes in materials or equipment.

*Roentgen:* The quantity of x- or gamma radiation such that the associated corpuscular emission per 0.001293 grams of air produces, in air, ions carrying 1 electrostatic unit of quantity of electricity of either sign.

*Roentgen Equivalent Man (Rem):* That quantity of any type ionizing radiation which when absorbed by man produces an effect equivalent to the absorption by man of one roentgen of x- or gamma-radiation (400 KV).

*Roentgen Equivalent Physical (Rep):* The amount of ionizing radiation which will result in the absorption in tissue of 83 ergs per gram. (Recent authors have suggested the value 93 ergs per gram.)

*Rotation Therapy:* Radiation therapy during which either the patient is rotated before the source of radiation or the source is revolved around the patient's body.

*Scattered Radiation:* Radiation which, during its passage through a substance, has been deviated in direction. It may also have been modified by an increase in wavelength. It is one form of *secondary radiation.*

*Scattering:* Change of direction of subatomic particle or photon as a result of a collision or interaction.

*Scintillation Counter:* The combination of phosphor photo-multiplier tube and associated circuits for counting light emissions produced in the phosphers.

*Secondary Protective Barriers:* Barriers sufficient to reduce the stray radiation to the permissible dose rate.

*Secondary Radiation:* Radiation originating as the result of absorption of other radiation in matter. It may be either electromagnetic or particulate in nature.

*Stray Radiation:* Radiation not serving any useful purpose. It includes direct radiation and secondary radiation from irradiated objects.

*Teletherapy:* A method of using a radioisotope as a radiation source in which the radioelement is shielded on all sides except one, thus giving a directional beam of radiation which is directed at the area to be treated.

*Useful Beam (In radiology):* That part of the primary radiation which passes through the aperture, cone, or other collimator.

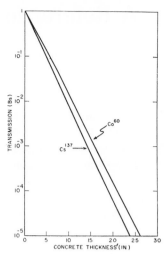

**Figure 1**

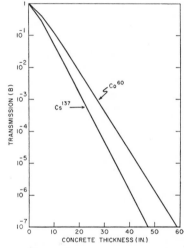

**Figure 2**

The curves shown above were extrapolated from National Bureau of Standards Handbook 54

*Teletherapy Units*

# A Reference Guide to Hospital Electrical Facilities

*by Noyce L. Griffin, Electrical Engineer, Architectural and Engineering Branch, Division of Hospital and Medical Facilities, Public Health Service*

*It is essential that the electrical supply for hospitals be adequate and dependable. Blood banks, refrigerators, respirators, surgical lightings, as well as other vital equipments, cannot be without electrical power for even short periods.*

*The demand on electrical energy is usually higher than for most building types. For this reason, the quality of materials and equipment must be high and future maintenance must be considered during the course of the design.*

## ELECTRICAL SERVICE
### MAIN ELECTRIC SERVICE

The electric service brought into the building may be primary or secondary depending upon the load demands and other local conditions. An underground service usually costs four to eight times that of a conventional overhead service but is generally preferred for hospitals because of landscaping and reduction of the probability of service interruption due to storms, ice loads, or other overhead disturbances.

TRANSFORMERS. If the service brought into the hospital is primary or high voltage, several types of step-down transformers may be used. A nonflammable, nonsludging, insulating, liquid-filled transformer offers high impulse strength and low maintenance. However, air-cooled and gas-cooled transformers of high quality are available.

The open dry-type transformer has less impulse strength than the liquid-filled type. Frequent cleaning is required and it is suitable for indoor use only. The sealed dry-type transformer has many advantages of the liquid and the open dry types, and it has the same impulse strength limitations as the open dry-type transformer; but in addition it is dust-tight and weatherproof. It can be installed at lower cost and requires less space than the liquid type.

CIRCUIT BREAKERS for switching of main secondary circuits are usually the drawout type in larger hospitals, or the molded case type in smaller hospitals. The drawout type is more expensive to install but provides a higher degree of protection, reliability, and ease of maintenance.

DISTRIBUTION. Three-phase, 4-wire 208y/120 volt distribution systems are generally preferred for small hospitals because of economy and convenience in providing for both 3-phase and single phase connections

at the distribution panels. A higher voltage system such as the 3-phase, 4-wire 480y/277 volt system, using dry-type transformers for 120-volt service may be more economical for large hospitals which operate several large motors. The nominal voltage of any distribution system should be that of an industry standard conforming to American Standards Association Publication 84.1, "Preferred Voltage Ratings for A-C Systems and Equipment."

The simplest and cheapest scheme of distribution is the "simple radial system." Improvement in flexibility and dependability may be obtained at additional cost by one of several variations of this system. Many schemes of distribution are workable, and general information may be obtained from handbooks on electrical facilities for hospitals.

## EMERGENCY POWER

A reliable source of emergency power for lighting and for operation of essential equipment is necessary. The three sources of power which have been used are storage battery, second utility line, and generator. A generator on the hospital site is preferable to either a storage battery or a second utility line for the following reasons: (a) storage batteries have a limited capacity and the direct current for services such as operation of motorized equipment or fluorescent lighting; (b) a second utility line is usually subjected to the same factors contributing to power interruption as those of the main utility service.

When a second utility line is used as the only source of emergency power, it should be from a generating plant separate from the source of main power and should be routed and connected so that any fault on the main feeder would not be transmitted to, or likely to cause an outage of the emergency feeder.

Generators on the hospital site may be driven by any suitable prime mover such as gasoline, gas, or diesel oil internal combustion engines or steam turbines. The selection of the type of generating unit is usually influenced by the dependability of fuel supply or whether the emergency power will be used frequently to carry a part of the load during normal operation. Generally, the internal combustion engine generating units are intended as a standby service only, while the steam turbine units are sometimes operated during periods of maximum demands daily, and where such operation may result in a more favorable power rate from the utility company.

A switch-over gas and gasoline fuel supply for small and medium sized internal combustion engines offers greater flexibility

of operation in case of scarcity or depletion of either fuel. Starting gasoline engines on bottled gas and then switching to gasoline has been suggested as a more positive assurance of avoiding failure of automatic starting.

An arrangement of feeders so that a planned selection of loads may be connected or dropped from the emergency service is desirable, to more fully utilize the available capacity of the emergency service and also to prevent overloading to the point of trip-out of the entire service. Such a design is a particularly important convenience when adding fixed or mobile emergency capacity to an existing system and also for minimizing a trip-out of service to a highly important area. The switching of emergency power for critical areas should be automatic. Pickup or dropout of other circuits should be selective and may be either manual or automatic. In some hospitals designed for treatment of poliomyelitis patients, circuit feeders are divided into three groups designated as "critical," "semicritical," and "noncritical."

TELEPHONE SERVICE should be brought into the building underground, where practicable, and should be kept well separated from electric power service. Telephone cables should be routed to avoid locations where they would be subject to mechanical injury, excessive heat, or chemical erosion.

## PANELBOARDS AND SWITCHBOARDS

All panelboards and switchboards should be of the dead front type, enclosed in metal cabinets with hinged doors and latches, and with the connection schedule under a transparent protective material. Where locked cabinets are provided, all locks should be keyed alike.

Suitable working space at panelboards and switchboards should be provided and maintained as required by the National Electrical Code, Section 1116.

Switchboards which have thermal trip overload devices should be located in a well ventilated space to prevent trip-out at less than the preset current rating due to excessive ambient temperature.

Distribution panelboards should be located in corridors rather than in confined spaces such as linen or janitor's closets. Panelboards serving lighting circuits should be located on the same floor as the respective lighting outlets and should be spaced so that the length of the branch circuits will not exceed approximately 100 ft.

## SWITCHES

Automatic circuit breakers for power and light feeders and for the lighting and receptacle branch circuits, while more expensive than fused switches for the initial installation, are preferred.

The general types of automatic circuit breakers usually employed are thermal or magnetic, or a combination of both. The thermal type will permit a long delay before tripping on light overloads or a short delay on heavy overloads. The magnetic type will permit instantaneous tripping on heavy overloads or short circuits. A combination thermal and magnetic tripping action for the circuit breaker has wide applications and is preferred for protection of small wires and flexible cords used on lighting and appliance branch circuits.

Local and wall switches of the silent type are recommended in all patient areas to reduce noise. Wall-mounted switches are preferred to pull switches to reduce maintenance. Where lights are installed in small closets, door-operated switches are recommended. Switches installed or operated within a location defined as hazardous because of use or storage of combustible anesthetic agents should be approved for use in Class 1, Group C hazardous atmospheres. Switches controlling the ungrounded circuits in anesthetizing locations such as operating and delivery rooms must have a disconnecting pole in each conductor.

Switching of lighting circuits by means of a low voltage control system is applicable to hospitals, particularly in large areas such as auditoriums, assembly halls, or laboratories.

## WIRE

All feeders and branch circuits should have high grade insulation as required or permitted by the National Electrical Code to assure optimum life and dependability of the electrical system. High temperature wire is required at range hoods, boilers, etc. Lead sheath or waterproof wire should be used underground and where condensation may form, as in outdoor conduits, refrigerator boxes, roof slabs, and connections to outside lights. The Code should be consulted for special conditions.

## CONDUIT

All hospital wiring should be in conduit to facilitate alterations and repairs. Wiring for the patient-nurse call system should be in conduit of ample size to permit a reasonable amount of change in the system with a minimum amount of labor and structural changes.

Where only one set of service conductors is brought into the building underground, spare conduit facilities should be provided to expedite restoration of service in case of a failure in the service conductors between the building and the street or main service connection.

Underground conduit should be nonmetallic and encased in concrete. Explosion-proof wiring must be in rigid conduit. Spare conduits or conduit sleeves through walls or floors are advisable where future service is planned or contemplated.

## LIGHTING

Lighting in all areas of the hospital should be designed for comfortable seeing. Luminaires should be durable, a standard type, neat, attractively designed, easily cleaned and relamped.

WORK SPACES should be relatively free from shadows and have sufficient illumination on work areas to eliminate the need for portable units with extension cords on floor or work area.

GENERAL AREAS. The lighting of offices, corridors, assembly halls, shops, boiler and machine rooms, kitchens, and storage spaces can be treated as in other types of buildings. The Illuminating Engineering Society Handbook should be consulted.

PATIENTS' ROOMS should have installed lighting for three distinct services: (1) general illumination for the room, (2) a reading light for each patient, and (3) a night light in the room. A fourth service, a doctor's examining light, may be an installed unit or a feature incorporated into the patient's reading light, or the light may be supplied by a portable lamp with an extension cord. This examining light should produce approximately 100 foot-candles over a limited area. A fixed ceiling-mounted examining light arranged to illuminate the entire bed area might be uncomfortably glaring for the patient, but it need not be left on longer than required for the examination. Such an arrangement is preferred to hand-held or portable examining lights.

NIGHT LIGHTS can be included as an added feature to the reading light or other units, but the flush wall-mounted type is generally preferred. Wall-mounted night lights should be about 18 in. above the floor, located so that they are not likely to be covered by furniture or drapes. Night lights should be switched at the door.

RECOVERY ROOMS and intensive care rooms of Progressive Patient Care units should have about 30 foot-candles of general illumination.

Patients frequently complain about the radiation of heat from a nearby reading light. A unit with an output intensity sufficient to permit adequate lighting when the unit is located a greater distance from the patient will reduce the objectionable heat. Where two or more beds are located in one room, the reading lights should be of a type that can be installed or adjusted so as not to shine in other patients' eyes. Each reading light should have a switch control accessible to the patient.

OPERATING AND DELIVERY ROOMS should have general illumination of about 100 foot-candles for the room area and special, separately controlled lights for the tables.

The major operating light should provide a multibeam of larger area for directing a minimum of 2500 foot-candles in the center of a 10-in. diameter circular area on the operating table, and tapering to not less than 500 foot-candles at the edge of that circle.

DELIVERY ROOMS require about the same general illumination as operating rooms. If the room is used for all deliveries, including Caesarean section and others which require extensive surgery, lighting at the table should be equal to that recommended for operating rooms. Where it is contemplated that the room will be used only for normal deliveries and for those which require only minor surgery, the light at the table may be somewhat less than that required for operating rooms.

MINOR SURGERY, EMERGENCY ROOMS, CYSTOSCOPIC ROOMS, AND AUTOPSY ROOMS should have about 100 foot-candles general illumination. These rooms should have supplemental lighting either by ceiling-mounted adjustable luminaires or portable units which will provide spot intensities of 2000 to 2500 foot-candles.

FRACTURE ROOMS need about 90 foot-candles general illumination with supplemental lighting for the table of about 200 ft-c.

LABORATORIES require about 50 to 100 foot-candles, depending upon the seeing task. Currently recommended foot-candles listed in the IES Lighting Handbook, Third Edition, 1959, should be consulted.

Where critical observation of color is required, as in surgery, laboratories, and autopsy rooms, color correction of the light may be necessary to provide a color effect as nearly as possible to that by which tests or specimens are ordinarily viewed. Daylight and incandescent filament lamp lighting have in the past been the most commonly accepted sources of illumination for critical seeing involving color determination.

*(Minimum on the task at all times)*

| | |
|---|---|
| Anesthetising and preparation | |
|   room | 30 |
| Auditorium | |
|   Assembly | 15 |
|   Exhibition | 30 |
| Autopsy and morgue | |
|   Autopsy room | 100 |
|   Autopsy table | 2500 |
|   Morgue, general | 20 |
| Central sterile supply | |
|   General | 30 |
|   Needle sharpening | 150 |
| Corridor | |
|   General | 10 |
|   Operating and delivery | |
|     suites and laboratories | 20 |
| Cystoscopic room | |
|   General | 100 |
|   Cystoscopic table | 2500 |
| Dental suite | |
|   Waiting room | |
|     General | 15 |
|     Reading | 30 |
|   Operatory, general | 70 |
|   Instrument cabinet | 70 |
|   Dental chair | 1000 |
|   Laboratory, bench | 100 |
|   Recovery room | 5 |
| Dining areas | 20 |
| Encephalographic suite | |
|   Office | 100 |
|   Workroom | 30 |
|   Patients' room | 30 |
| Emergency room | |
|   General | 100 |
|   Local | 2000 |
| EKG, BMR and Specimen room | |
|   General | 20 |
|   Specimen table (supplementary) | 50 |

| | |
|---|---|
| Examination and treatment room | |
|   General | 50 |
|   Examining table | 100 |
| Eye, ear, nose and throat suite | |
|   Dark room | 10 |
|   Eye examination and | |
|     treatment room | 50 |
|   Ear, nose and throat room | 50 |
| Exits, at floor | 5 |
| Flower room | 10 |
| Formula room | 30 |
| Fracture room | |
|   General | 50 |
|   Fracture table | 200 |
| Kitchen | |
|   Central | 70 |
|   Floor, kitchen and pantry | 70 |
|   Dishwashing | 30 |
| Laboratories | |
|   Assay rooms | 30 |
|   Work tables | 50 |
|   Close work | 100 |
| Laundry | 70 |
|   General | 30 |
|   Pressers and ironers | 70 |
|   Sorting | 70 |
| Libraries | 70 |
| Linen closet | 10 |
| Locker rooms | 20 |
| Lobby | 30 |
| Lounge rooms | 30 |
| Maintenance shop | |
|   General | 30 |
|   Work benches | 100 |
|   Paint storage | 10 |
| Medical records room | 100 |
| Nurses' station | |
|   General | 20 |
|   Desk and charts | 50 |
|   Medicine room counter | 100 |

| | |
|---|---|
| Nurses' workroom | 30 |
| Nurseries | |
|   General | 10 |
|   Examination table | 70 |
|   Play room, pediatric | 30 |
| Obstetrical | |
|   Cleanup room | 30 |
|   Scrubup room | 30 |
|   Labor room | 20 |
|   Delivery room, general | 100 |
|   Delivery table | 2500 |
| Offices | |
|   General | 100 |
|   Bookkeeping and fine work | 150 |
|   Conference and | |
|     consultation room | 30 |
|   Information and switchboard | 30 |
|   Retiring room | 10 |
|   Waiting room | 20 |
| Parking lot | 5 |
| Power plant | |
|   Boiler room | 10 |
|   Machine room | 20 |
|   Switchboard room | 30 |
|   Transformer room | 10 |
| Pharmacy | |
|   General | 30 |
|   Work table | 100 |
|   Active storage | 30 |
|   Alcohol vault | 10 |
| Private rooms and wards | |
|   General | 10 |
|   Reading | 30 |
| Psychiatric disturbed | |
|   patients' areas | 10 |
| Radioisotope facilities | |
|   Radiochemical laboratory | 30 |
|   Uptake measuring room | 20 |
|   Examination table | 50 |
| Retiring room | 10 |
| Sewing room | |
|   General | 20 |
|   Work area | 100 |
| Solariums | 20 |
| Stairways | 20 |
| Storage, central | |
|   General | 15 |
| Office | 70 |
| Surgery | |
|   Instrument and sterile | |
|     supply room | 30 |
|   Cleanup room (instruments) | 100 |
|   Scrubup room | 30 |
|   Operating room, general | 100 |
|   Operating table | 2500 |
|   Recovery room | 30 |
| Therapy | |
|   Physical | 20 |
|   Occupational | 30 |
| Toilets | 10 |
| Utility room | 20 |
| Waiting room | |
|   General | 15 |
|   Reading | 30 |
| X-ray room and facilities | |
|   Radiography and fluoroscopy | 10 |
|   Deep and superficial therapy | 10 |
|   Dark room | 10 |
|   Waiting room, general | 15 |
|   Waiting room, reading | 30 |
|   Viewing room | 30 |
|   Filing room, developed films | 30 |
|   Storage, undeveloped films | 10 |

EMERGENCY LIGHTING should be provided for safety of patients, staff, and protection of plant. As a minimum in any case, emergency lighting should be provided for operating and delivery rooms, exits, stairs, corridors, switchboard, and boiler rooms. Additional emergency lighting will be needed where hospitals may be without the normal service for days or weeks due to disasters and where care is to be provided for a large number of casualties.

Exit, stair, and corridor lighting should conform to local and State codes, or if such codes are not in effect, the "Building Exits Code" of the National Fire Protection Association.

Illuminated signs may be required in areas where there is much visitor traffic, such as at the information desk, cashier's office, and outpatient department. Where such lighting is likely to be required, plug-in receptacles should be conveniently located.

An X-ray film illuminator is required in each operating room. It is also desirable that one be installed in the doctors' locker room of the obstetrical suite.

### RECEPTACLES

Convenience outlets should be installed in all places where plug-in service is likely to be required. Duplex receptacles are generally preferred, except for heavy duty service or other specific requirements. Grounding type receptacles should be installed in kitchens, pantries, utility rooms, laundries, laboratories, boiler rooms, and other work areas likely to have wet floors.

Each operating and delivery room should be provided with not less than three receptacles of the lock-in type suitable for interchangeable type plugs as described in NFPA No. 56 of The National Fire Protection Association.

Patients' bedrooms should have at least three duplex outlets for single-patient rooms, with two outlets near the head of the bed. Rooms for more than one patient should have a similar arrangement of outlets. Preferably, there should be two duplex outlets at the head of each bed, or at least three outlets on the head wall for each two beds side-by-side.

Each bed in recovery rooms and in intensive care nursing rooms should have two duplex receptacles near the head of the bed. Intensive care nursing rooms should, in addition, have two 3-phase, 4-pole outlets, 30 amperes or larger, as required, for motorized equipment and mobile X-ray. The recently introduced 30 ma mobile X-ray re-

quires 60-ampere, 230-volt receptacles. Corridors should have grounding type outlets, rated at 20 or 30-amperes, as required for use of mobile X-ray and cleaning machines. In corridors of patient areas, outlets should be spaced on 40-ft.

## HAZARDOUS LOCATIONS

Anesthetic storage rooms within the surgical suites are considered hazardous throughout. Rooms for bulk storage of unopened containers of anesthetic agents in a relatively remote area are generally not considered hazardous locations.

The extent of the hazardous location of an anesthetizing space for administering flammable anesthetics or disinfectants is considered to include the entire floor area of the room, and to a height of 5 ft above the floor. All hazardous locations require special attention to construction, equipment, and operation as precautions against ignition of these agents which cause fires and explosions. All equipment used in these areas should be approved for use in Class 1, Group C hazardous atmospheres. For specific requirements, see NFPA No. 56.

All hazardous locations require conductive floors for electrically intercoupling all people and equipment in the room to prevent electro-static sparks which might ignite flammable gasses or vapors.

Operating and delivery rooms require ungrounded electrical distribution systems for all wiring, except for fixed nonadjustable lighting fixtures located more than 8 ft above the floor for the purpose of minimizing the hazard of electric shock and sparks from the electric system.

A ground detector system is required for the purpose of warning of accidental or fault ground on the ungrounded system. Wiring and equipment installed above hazardous location, more than 5 ft above the floor, should be enclosed or guarded to prevent sparks or hot particles from falling into the hazardous location. All furniture and mobile equipment should be conductive and in electrical contact with the conductive floor.

Controlled humidity of at least 50 per cent is considered an important factor in the control of static electricity.

## COMMUNICATION SYSTEMS

### NURSES' CALL SYSTEMS

Call systems for nursing service vary from the simplest type of a signal system to two-way voice communication. An important feature common to all systems is that the switch provided for patients' use will register the call at the nurses' station. This feature may be varied to fit any practicable situation by the various types of switches for actuating calls and the various points and means of registering calls. Cord operated switches are preferable for isolation or contagious areas because these cords are inexpensive

and may be removed and incinerated. A new cord can then be installed for each new patient.

Registration of calls should include a signal light in the corridor over the door of the room where the call originates. A selection of lights, buzzers, bells, chimes, and annunciators are available for registering calls at the nurses' station, floor pantries, utility rooms, or other duty stations.

Emergency calls, actuating distinctive signals, are usually installed in patients' toilets and sometimes incorporated into the regular call station at the patient's bed for use by the nurse when she needs assistance. Call stations should be provided for nurses' use in nurseries, children's wards, operating, and delivery rooms.

Two-way voice communication is a feature which may be added to the signal system described. Where it is planned for economy reasons to first install a signal system and later add the voice feature, conduits large enough to accommodate the wiring of the final installation should be included in the original installation.

### PAGING SYSTEMS

Paging systems for doctors and staff may be the wired or radio type. The wired paging system usually includes a microphone and/or a sending station for calling or signaling to one or a combination of the following: loud speakers, coded chimes, illuminated numerals, bell taps, or annunciator drops.

### DOCTOR'S IN-AND-OUT REGISTER

Usually these registers include boards containing staff doctors' names at all entrances normally used by doctors and at the telephone switchboard. All boards are electrically connected to register the same signal simultaneously. A recall feature may be included which consists of a flasher unit having a motor driven interrupter which actuates a flashing light at the doctor's name on all register boards. The control for this unit is located at the telephone switchboard. The recall feature assures the doctor's attention upon entering or leaving the hospital.

### CALL-BACK SYSTEM

Call-back systems provide a relatively inexpensive means of "wake-up" or calling service for interns and nurses. Calls originating in the office or at the switchboard actuate a bell or buzzer in the quarters. An answer switch is provided for acknowledgement that the call has been received. Wiring

may be arranged for individual calls or, if desired, it can be connected so that one button may call several rooms or stations simultaneously.

### TELEPHONES

Interconnecting telephones should be provided for all department heads, assistants, operation and delivery suites, nurses' stations, offices, housekeeper, maintenance supervisor, doctors' rooms, record rooms, and diet kitchens. These may be connected on a dial system which will permit interior communication through the hospital switchboard without the assistance of an operator. At all private and semi-private beds, telephone jacks should be installed so that a telephone can be plugged in at any time, with a minimum rental charge to the hospital. This arrangement is efficient and satisfactory.

Conduit should be provided for all telephone wiring. Installation and connection of wiring is usually done by the telephone company. Provision should be made for public telephones at convenient locations for visitors and others requiring the use of pay stations.

### INTERCOMMUNICATION SYSTEMS

Telautograph transcribers which transmit written messages from one department to another are being used successfully in some hospitals. These systems leave a written record of the mesage at the sending and receiving stations. Where installation of this equipment is contemplated, conduit should be installed for the necessary wiring. This equipment may be obtained on a rental or purchase agreement.

Audible speaker systems are frequently used for communication between departments and within specific branches. These systems may be arranged for individual as well as collective announcements.

Loud speaker systems which include microphone, amplifier, and loud speakers are often required for extending the voice range, as in auditoriums, outdoor assembly, parking lot, or to issue general instructions as in the case of fire or any other type of disaster.

### CARRIER TUBE SYSTEMS

Pneumatic tube systems are extremely useful to carry records, prescriptions, or orders from one department to another. The carriers of these systems are propelled by electrically operated vacuum systems or vacuum-pressure combinations.

Nonpowered gravity drops with hand-operated lifts are sometimes useful between one floor and another directly above or below.

## ELEVATORS

Size and shape of the elevator car and its door opening are related to the needs of vehicle traffic. The length and width of patients' beds are determining factors in car depth and door width.

Hospital elevators are usually limited to three sizes, as standardized by the industry and the National Elevator Manufacturers' Institute. These sizes comply with the requirements of the American Standard Safety Code for Elevators, A17.1-1955 and in respect to rated load capacity in pounds and the outside dimensions of the car platform the sizes are as follows: 3500 lb, 5 ft 4 in. by 8 ft; 4000 lb, 5 ft by 8 ft 4 in.; and 5000 lb, 7 ft by 8 ft 4 in.

Small and medium size hospitals, where comparatively few elevators are needed, use these hospital-size cars almost exclusively because of the economic advantage of their "all-purpose" characteristics. Automatic operation without an attendant, except during peak service demands, visiting periods, and vehicle transportation, is common practice in most of the small and medium size hospitals. Larger hospitals sometimes employ a few "office building-size" cars for passenger service only. Automatically operated elevators should be provided with a keyed switch which permits an attendant to bypass any calls and travel directly to any station. This feature is needed for hospital-type elevators as it is not desirable to combine passenger traffic with vehicle traffic such as bed or stretcher patients or food carts.

It is desirable that the electric service to elevators be arranged so that at least one of the hospital-type elevators may be operated on the emergency system. Switching should be arranged to permit connection of the emergency power to bring any elevator to a landing in case it has been trapped between floors by interruption of the normal power.

## FIRE ALARMS

Fire alarms are required in every hospital. Alarms as required by the "Building Exits Code" apply except where they may be modified by additional requirements of local or state codes.

Devices used in the alarm system should be listed by Underwriters Laboratories, Inc., or Factory Mutual Laboratories, or certified to comply with the requirements of the listed devices. In all cases the system should be electrically supervised, preferably the code signal type and should comply with NFPA No. 72, "Proprietary Signaling Systems." To minimize panic among patients when a fire alarm is sounded, a pre-signal feature is generally recommended, designed so that the initial signals will sound only in department offices, engine rooms, fire brigade stations, nurses' stations, and other central locations. Chimes or lighted signal gongs are recommended in nursing areas.

## CLOCKS

An electric clock system, rather than individual clocks, should be provided with clocks in all offices, nurses' stations, main lobby, waiting rooms, telephone switchboard, kitchen, dining room, laundry, boiler room, operating and delivery rooms. The clocks should be of the recessed type, preferably with a narrow frame. Clocks in operating and delivery rooms should have sweep second hands. The need for elapsed time indicators in operating and delivery rooms is controversial.

Two types of clock systems are available: the wired and the electronic. The wired system requires wiring from the individual clocks to the master control clock. The electronic system requires no wiring connection between the individual clocks and the master clock. Control is by means of electrical impulses sent out by the master control clock and picked up by a radio-type receiver in each clock which is operated from any convenience outlet.

## X-RAY

Voltage supplied to the X-ray unit should be nearly constant so that images and pictures will be uniform. An independent feeder with capacity sufficient to prevent a voltage drop greater than 3 per cent is recommended. A separate transformer for the X-ray feeder is desirable and is a requirement for most installations.

## REFERENCES

1. U. S. Department of Commerce, National Bureau of Standards, *National Electrical Safety Code, Handbook H30,* U. S. Government Printing Office, Washington 25, D. C., 1949, 408 pp.

2. National Fire Protection Association, *National Electrical Code,* NFPA No. 70, National Fire Protection Association, Boston, Mass., 1956, 491 pp.

3. Illuminating Engineering Society, *Lighting Handbook, 3rd Edition,* Illuminating Engineering Society, New York, N. Y., 1959, 1100 pp.

4. National Fire Protection Association, *Building Exits Code, 15th Edition,* NFPA No. 101, National Fire Protection Association, Boston, Mass., 1958, 256 pp.

5. National Fire Protection Association, *Recommended Safe Practice for Hospital Operating Rooms,* NFPA No. 56, National Fire Protection Association, Boston, Mass., 1956, 48 pp.

6. American Society of Mechanical Engineers, *Safety Code for Elevators, Dumbwaiters and Escalators,* A17.1-1955, The American Society of Mechanical Engineers, New York, N. Y., 1955, 290 pp.

7. Underwriters Laboratories, Inc., 207 East Ohio Street, Chicago 11, Ill.

8. Factory Mutual Laboratories, 1151 Boston-Providence Turnpike, Norwood, Mass.

9. National Fire Protection Association, *Proprietary, Auxiliary, Remote Station and Local Protective Signaling Systems,* NFPA No. 72, National Fire Protection Association, Boston, Mass., 1958, 29 pp.

10. American Standards Association, *Preferred Voltage Ratings for A-C Systems and Equipment. ASA 84.1* (EEI R-6; NEMA 117), American Standards Association, 1954.

11. General Electric Company, *Hospital Handbook for Architects and Engineers,* General Electric Company, Schenectady, N. Y., 1949.

12. Westinghouse Electric Corporation, *Hospital Electrical Planning for Architects and Engineers,* Westinghouse Electric Corporation, East Pittsburgh, Penna., 1951, 238 pp.

13. Griffin, N. L., *Emergency Power for Hospitals,* (AIEE Conference Paper No. Cp 56-278), American Institute of Electrical Engineers, New York, N. Y., Jan. 30-Feb. 3, 1956.

14. Griffin, N. L., "Telephone Systems for Hospitals," *Architectural Record,* Vol. III, No. 6, pp. 221-225, June 1952.

15. Griffin, N. L., "Recomended Lighting Practices—Put the Hospital in its Best Light," *Modern Hospital,* Vol. 84, No. 3, pp. 84-87, March 1955.

16. Griffin, N. L. "Electrical Safety in Hospital Operating Rooms," (AIEE Conference Paper No. 58-579), American Institute of Electrical Engineers, New York, N. Y., April 30, 1958. Published in *Power Apparatus and Systems,* No. 38, pp. 698-702, Oct. 1958.

17. Kusters, N. L., "The Ground Detector Problem in Hospital Operating Rooms," *Transactions,* Vol. 2, No. 1, Engineering Institute of Canada, Ottawa, Canada, 1958.

18. McKinley, D. W. R., "An Electronic Ground Detector," *Transactions,* Vol. 2, No. 1, Engineering Institute of Canada, Ottawa, Canada, 1958, 44 pp.

# REHABILITATION CENTERS

# Rehabilitation Facilities for Multiple Disability

*Preliminary Type Plan by*
*U. S. Public Health Service,*
*Thomas Galbraith, Architect*

REHABILITATION is a big word in the country's new health program. Society realizes that civilization has progressed beyond the "survival of the fittest." Handicapped persons are not to be sloughed off as discards, to be tucked away some place with mere custodial care. So — rehabilitation, for continued usefulness, and a reasonable chance for rewarding activity.

Medical science of rehabilitation made rapid strides during the war. And the benefits of wartime techniques and training programs are now available for peacetime development. The need now is for the necessary physical facilities.

The plan here shown — a preliminary concept by the Public Health Service — is for rehabilitation facilities, for multiple disability, as part of a medical center. The rehabilitation facility might also be conceived as a separate center, for both in-patients and out-patients, again for multiple disability. Or there might be a facility for just out-patients. A fourth concept would be a rehabilitation unit for a single disability — blindness, cerebral palsy, retarded children, alcoholism, etc.

Under the program, priority is given to rehabilitation facilities providing multiple disability service, located in medical centers, medical schools or universities. Reasoning here is that a wide variety of medical specialists is usually required by a patient, especially in the early stages of rehabilitation. There is also a need for developing new techniques, and for training new personnel. Also, it is believed, such concentration of newly financed facilities would give the program the best start.

In official language, a rehabilitation service is defined as: "a facility providing community service which is operated for the primary purpose of assisting in the rehabilitation of disabled persons through an integrated program of medical, psychological, social and vocational evaluation and services under competent professional supervision. The major portion of such evaluation and services must be furnished within the facility; and the facility must be operated either in connection with a hospital or as a facility in which all medical and related health services are prescribed by, or are under the general direction of, persons licensed to practice medicine or surgery in the State."

It is quite clear — from the plan, if not from the legalistic language — that rehabilitation here represents an all-out attack. The "multiple disability" phrase means that the facility might serve patients with many different types of infirmities: orthopedic cases, disabilities from injuries, arthritis, diseases of the heart or arteries, and neurological problems. With children there might be also post-polio, congenital malformations, and children's neurological problems. A consider-

able range of physical facilities is therefore required, yet many of those facilities would be useful to several classifications of patients. All-important is the availability of fairly complete medical services for such diverse patient groups.

As for planning the buildings, a considerable fund of data has been accumulated in the Public Health Service; for purposes of this preliminary presentation only general notes will be given.

Major elements of the rehabilitation unit include:
Administration Facilities
Evaluation and Treatment Facilities
1. Medical Facilities, including: Dental; Physical Therapy; Occupational Therapy; Teaching Activities of Daily Living; Speech and Hearing; Artificial Appliance Facilities; Nursing Units for Adults; Nursing Units for Children
2. Psychological Facilities
Social Service Facilities
Vocational Facilities

Wherever practicable, all of those elements should be located together within the department, for better coordination of the services and efficiency of operation. Some of the elements may already exist in a hospital,

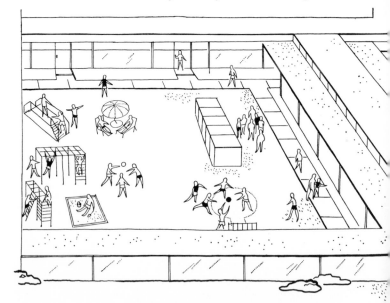

and would not necessarily have to be repeated. In addition to the services indicated, some patients might need additional facilities in the hospital, such as X-ray, laboratory, surgery, pharmacy, etc.

A ground floor location has several advantages. Access to outdoors and treatment areas without recourse to elevators is desirable, and out-patients would be well served.

The size of the facility will be based on the findings

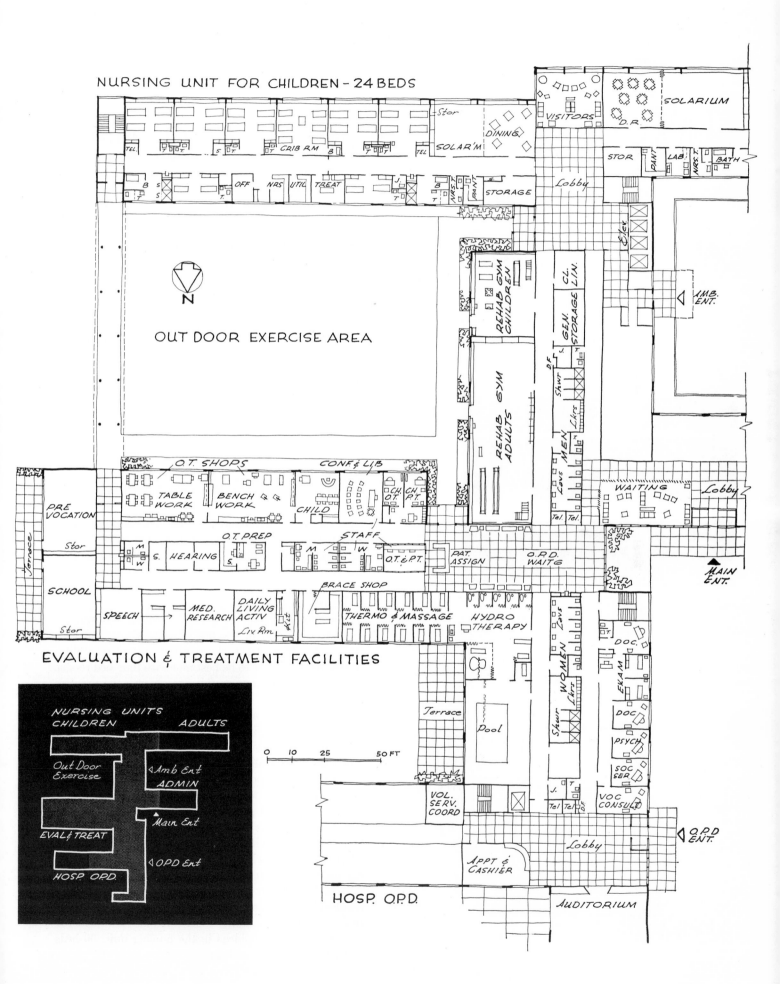

NURSING UNIT FOR CHILDREN — 24 BEDS

SOLARIUM

VISITORS

D.R.

DINING

SOLAR'M

STOR

PANT

LAB.

BATH

Lobby

STORAGE

N

OUT DOOR EXERCISE AREA

REHAB GYM CHILDREN

REHAB GYM ADULTS

GEN. STORAGE

CL. LIN.

MEN

AMB. ENT.

WAITING

Lobby

O.T. SHOPS

CONF & LIB

TABLE WORK

BENCH WORK

CHILD

PRE VOCATION

Stor

O.T. PREP

STAFF

HEARING

O.T. & P.T.

PAT. ASSIGN

O.P.D. WAIT'G

MAIN ENT.

SCHOOL

BRACE SHOP

SPEECH

MED. RESEARCH

DAILY LIVING ACTIV

Liv. Rm.

THERMO & MASSAGE

HYDRO THERAPY

Stor

EXAM

DOC.

DOC.

PSYCH

SOC SER

EVALUATION & TREATMENT FACILITIES

Terrace

Pool

WOMEN

VOC CONSULT

NURSING UNITS

CHILDREN      ADULTS

Out Door Exercise

Amb Ent

ADMIN

Main Ent

EVAL & TREAT

OPD Ent

HOSP. O.P.D.

0   10   25      50 FT

VOL. SERV. COORD

O.P.D ENT.

Lobby

APPT & CASHIER

HOSP. O.P.D.

AUDITORIUM

159

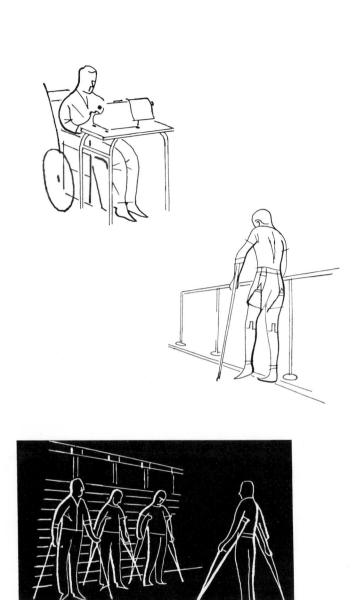

of the survey of needs of the region served. It should be remembered, in the study of size, that the out-patient load is usually much larger than the in-patient load. The service of the facility will probably extend beyond the boundaries of the local community, since a complete rehabilitation program is not feasible for most small hospitals.

The accompanying plans suggest an adult nursing unit of 38 beds and a unit for children of 24 beds and 6 cribs. Capacity of these units should not be considered a recommended ratio. It has been estimated that from 25 to 30 per cent of the total beds in the rehabilitation unit may be children's beds, with 14 years as the top age for children.

Grouping of disabled patients in a separate unit is psychologically advantageous. The morale of the individual is improved by knowing that admission to this unit indicates a good prognosis for recovery, and he tends to concentrate on showing maximum improvement. Grouping also facilitates more effective care. Moreover, requirements for housing such patients differ considerably from those of general hospital patients.

Many of the rehabilitation patients are up and active each day, getting around on crutches, wheel chairs and wheel stretchers. It should be recognized that such traffic requires greater clearances in bedrooms, day room, toilets, etc.

Although individual cases will vary widely, it is estimated that the length of stay will average approximately 60 days. The psychological needs of long-term patients should be considered in the general approach to design.

The number of beds in the adult unit may be greater than that usually recommended for medical and surgical units. Most patients will not need intensive bedside care and approximately 75 per cent may be ambulant or semi-ambulant. A capacity of 35 to 40 beds is recommended for economy and convenience in operation; 50 beds appears to be the maximum.

Need for flexibility in general medical and surgical units has resulted in the use of more single and two-bed rooms. In contrast, the requirements of rehabilitation patients appear to be best met with four-bed rooms. Social contact and opportunity to observe the progress of their roommates in bed exercises and other activities of daily living has a stimulating and therapeutic value. Competition arises in the group, and patients encourage and assist each other. Finally, the therapeutist's time is more efficiently utilized.

A few smaller rooms are desirable for the occasional use of a patient in need of a period of orientation, or one with a pronounced personality problem.

Accommodations for children in the rehabilitation facility of a hospital gives them access to essential medical services which often are not found in small specialized children's facilities, in no way impairs function, and results in better total service on a sound economical basis. It is essential to separate in-patient facilities from those for adults. Fourteen years is considered maximum age for children in the nursing unit; 30 beds including cribs is a good size.

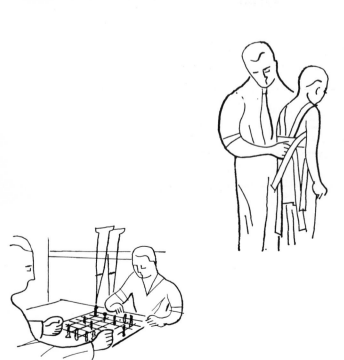

*Rehabilitation Facilities*

# Chronic Disease Hospital

*Preliminary Type Plan by*
*U. S. Public Health Service,*
*Peter Jensen, Architect*

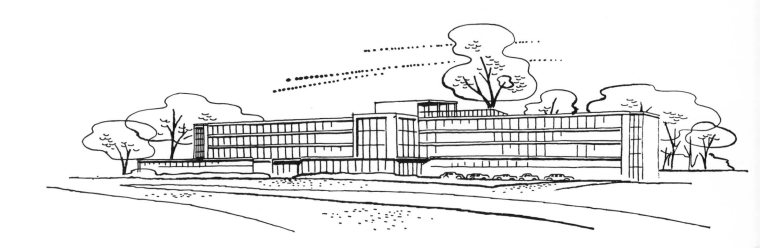

IN RECENT YEARS chronic disease hospitals have come in for new attention; in effect a new concept for such a hospital is being proposed. It has long been said that a high proportion of beds in most general hospitals are occupied by long-term patients, some of whom do not need such expensive quarters, such skilled medical attention, others of whom might require special services not available where they are. The broadening of the federal government's efforts in health facilities contemplate some sorting out of patients into chronic disease hospitals, rehabilitation centers, or nursing homes as new buildings can become available.

The Commission on Chronic Illness suggests that chronic patients should be treated and cared for at general hospitals or in special nursing units connected with general hospitals. However, many long-term patients are being treated and cared for in chronic disease hospitals.

Rehabilitation of long-term patients is a major part of this plan, whether in chronic disease hospitals or in separate rehabilitation centers. With the new skills in this area, it is said, many so-called chronic patients could be restored to active living, in some degree, and might not need hospital care at all.

These laudable objectives have led to serious study of the role of the chronic hospital, and perhaps some confusion. There is no difficulty, of course, in understanding the function of the specialized chronic hospital — for tuberculosis, for example, or heart cases. But the multiple disability type of chronic hospital, such as proposed now, has started some discussion as to medical facilities to be included, with an evident leaning toward the idea that very good medical facilities are required.

In federal regulations covering the state-aid program, the chronic disease hospital is defined: "a hospital for the treatment of chronic illness, including the degenerative diseases, in which treatment and care is administered by or under the direction of persons licensed to practice medicine or surgery in the State. The term does not include hospitals primarily for the care of the mentally ill or tuberculosis patients, nursing homes, and institutions the primary purpose of which is domicilliary care."

A chronic hospital provides services primarily to patients with non-acute illness for whom a prolonged period of hospitalization is anticipated, and whose principal care requirements are diagnosis, medication, nursing care, occupational therapy, medical social work, recreation and rehabilitation including some education and pre-vocational work.

The preliminary plan presented herewith illustrates space requirements and relationships of the various departments and services required in a 300-bed chronic disease hospital.

The first floor of this multi-story hospital contains complete rehabilitation facilities for in-patients and out-patients who can benefit most from these services. The rehabilitation portion shown closely follows the rehabilitation facility outlined for the medical center (page 159). It must be remembered that all chronic disease hospitals may not have such extensive facilities as shown in this plan.

This multi-story facility has two nursing units of 36 beds each on the first floor to accommodate those patients who can benefit most from the services provided on this floor, such as the departments of physical

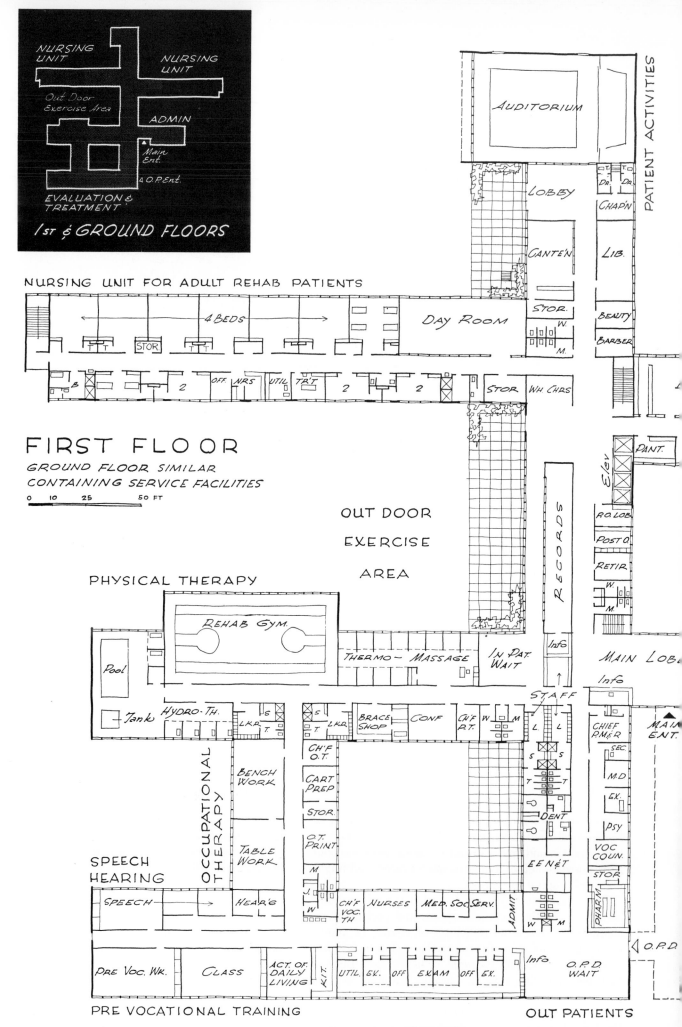

NURSING UNIT

NURSING UNIT

Out Door Exercise Area

ADMIN

Main Ent.

O.P. Ent.

EVALUATION & TREATMENT

## 1ST & GROUND FLOORS

NURSING UNIT FOR ADULT REHAB PATIENTS

4 BEDS

DAY ROOM

STOR.

STOR.

B · 2 · OFF. NRS UTIL TR'T 2 · 2 · STOR WH. CHRS

# FIRST FLOOR
### GROUND FLOOR SIMILAR
### CONTAINING SERVICE FACILITIES
0   10   25      50 FT

OUT DOOR

EXERCISE

AREA

PHYSICAL THERAPY

REHAB GYM.

Pool

Tank

HYDRO- TH.

THERMO ~ MASSAGE

In Pat. Wait

RECORDS

Info

STAFF

LKR.   S   S   LKR.   BRACE SHOP   CONF   CH'F P.T.   W   M   L   L

CH'F O.T.

CART PREP

STOR.

O.T. PRINT

BENCH WORK

TABLE WORK

SPEECH HEARING

OCCUPATIONAL THERAPY

SPEECH

HEAR'G

DENT

EE N&T

CH'F VOC. TH.

NURSES   MED. SOC. SERV.

PRE VOC. WK.   CLASS   ACT. OF DAILY LIVING   KIT.   UTIL. EX. OFF   EXAM   OFF EX.

PRE VOCATIONAL TRAINING

AUDITORIUM

PATIENT ACTIVITIES

LOBBY

Dr.   Dr.

CHAP'N

CANTE'N

LIB.

STOR.

W.

M.

BEAUTY

BARBER

Elev

PANT.

R.O. LOB.

POST O.

RETIR.

W.

M.

MAIN LOB.

Info

CHIEF PM&R

MAIN ENT.

SEC.

M.D.

EX.

PSY

VOC. COUN.

STOR.

PHARM

ADMIT

Info

O.P.D. WAIT

W   M

OUT PATIENTS

O.P.D.

# EVALUATION & TREATMENT FACILITIES

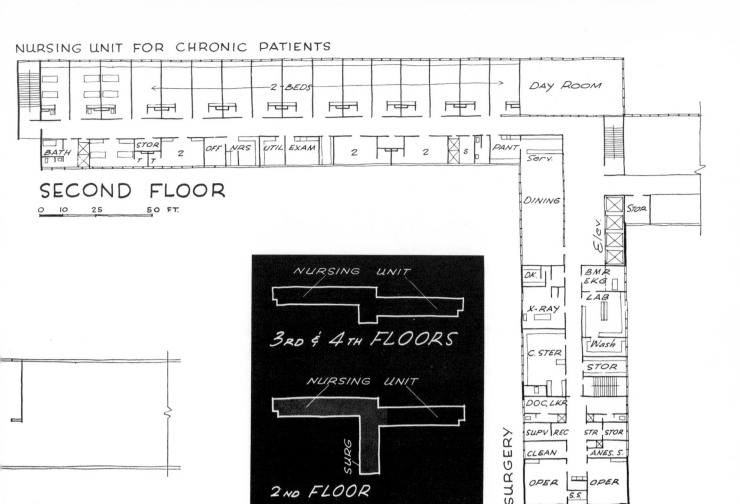

## SECOND FLOOR

0   10   25      50 FT.

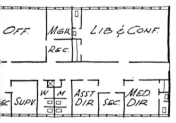

ADMINISTRATION

medicine, rehabilitation, occupational therapy and recreational facilities. About 75 per cent of the patients
on this service are ambulant or semi-ambulant.

The remaining six nursing units of 37 and 38 beds
each on the second, third and fourth floors would be
occupied by the more acute patients. Some 60 to 75 per
cent of these patients are ambulant or semi-ambulant
and can ambulate to and from the day rooms, dining
rooms and wash rooms provided on these floors. Diagnostic facilities, such as X-ray, laboratory, BMR and
EKG are located in a separate wing on the second floor
(available for out-patients) as are also the operating
suite and central sterilizing and supply rooms.

The out-patient department, pharmacy and the administration department are, as is customary, located on
the first floor. Dietary facilities, staff and help's dining
rooms, help's locker rooms, nurses' locker rooms, store
rooms, laundry, autopsy and morgue are on the ground
floor (not shown).

The major departments and facilities of a chronic
disease hospital are administration department, diagnostic and treatment facilities, nursing department,
surgical department, service dietary and out-patient
departments. Except for the rehabilitation nursing units
and the treatment facilities of the department of physical medicine the function and locations of the other departments are basically the same as in the general
hospital.

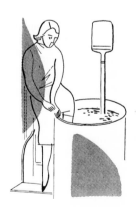

*Chronic Disease Hospital*

# Nursing Home Connected with a Hospital

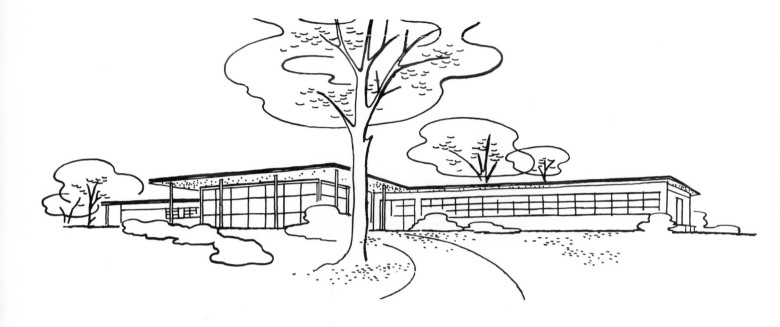

Nursing homes are a more or less familiar type of health facility now scheduled for some reexamination. They are included in types now eligible for federal aid, but there are a few provisos calculated to insure a high level of patient care.

Those conditions are stated in the official definition of a nursing home: "a facility which is operated in connection with a hospital, or in which nursing care and medical services are prescribed by or performed under the general direction of persons licensed to practice medicine or surgery in the State, for the accommodation of convalescents or other persons who are not acutely ill and not in need of hospital care, but who do require skilled nursing care and related medical services. The term 'nursing home' shall be restricted to those facilities, the purpose of which is to provide skilled nursing care and related medical services for a period of not less than 24 hours per day to individuals admitted because of illness, disease, or physical or mental infirmity and which provide a community service." They must also be operated by non-profit organizations.

The emphasis on medical care does not seriously strain the planning and equipping of the nursing home; it is not contemplated that the home have its own medical facilities. What is insisted upon is real medical supervision plus some tie-up with a hospital or other arrangement which would insure that medical attention was available on call. Implicit in that proviso are some factors influencing location of the home, and, of course, its organization.

Definitely the nursing home is for persons needing nursing care — not merely for somebody's Aunt Matilda who talks too much at home. Thus it is planned for the needs of partially sick people, and in a few respects this fact does affect its planning. It is not designed primarily for old people, but the common infirmities that come with age will bring many such patients to the home.

As a planning assignment the nursing home should appeal to the small architectural office. It is definitely not in the hospital category as to complications, though medical considerations do enter into the planning. Most important, it is a minimum facility, small in scale and domestic in character. It is a neighborhood affair, closely identified with the life and needs of a community, and designed as such. It should settle into the community, so that patients have no feeling of moving into a strange and institutional environment, so that friends and relatives can visit frequently and informally. More specifically, it should not have more than fifty beds, preferably about half that.

Clearly the site should be suitable for attractive landscaping, with space for some outdoor activity, if only sitting in the sunshine. Most important of all, however, it should not be isolated from community interests and activities. Patients should be able to observe the comings and goings of the community, to maintain a feeling of participation and to keep interests outside themselves or their fellow patients. Many of them will be there for a lengthy stay, and boredom will be a constant threat to health and morale.

It should be made as easy as possible for visitors to come, and for patients to go out to stores, churches, and so on, as they are able.

The plan on the opposite page suggests a generally satisfactory arrangement. A one-story building is usually

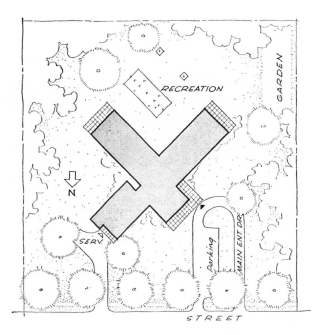

recommended, for obvious reasons. Here one wing takes all the services; wings for patients focus on the nurses' station as a control point. A large area combines for recreational and dining space, near the entrance, near the center of activities. It would be nice if the program afforded an additional solarium or lounge area, so that different groups or activities need not always be thrown together. Rooms are generally two-bed rooms, with each bed near the window. There are some single rooms, for the ill or poorly adjusted patients. There are scarcely any real medical facilities, but there are special toilets and baths designed to accommodate wheel chairs and arranged for the training of certain handicapped persons who must learn new methods of scrambling in and out of bathtubs.

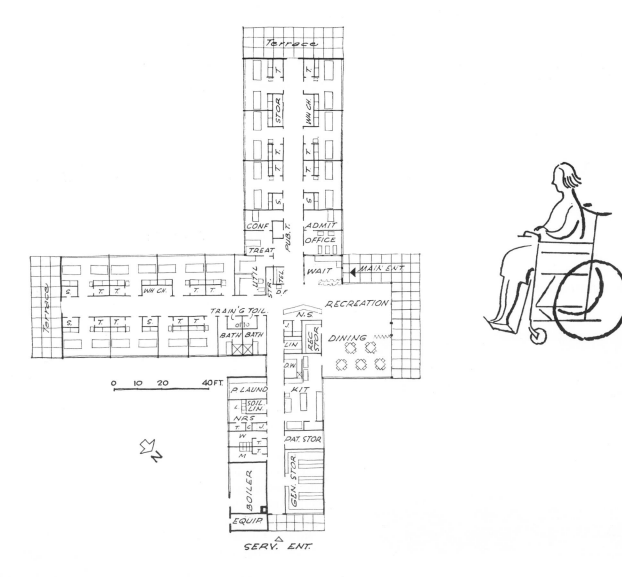

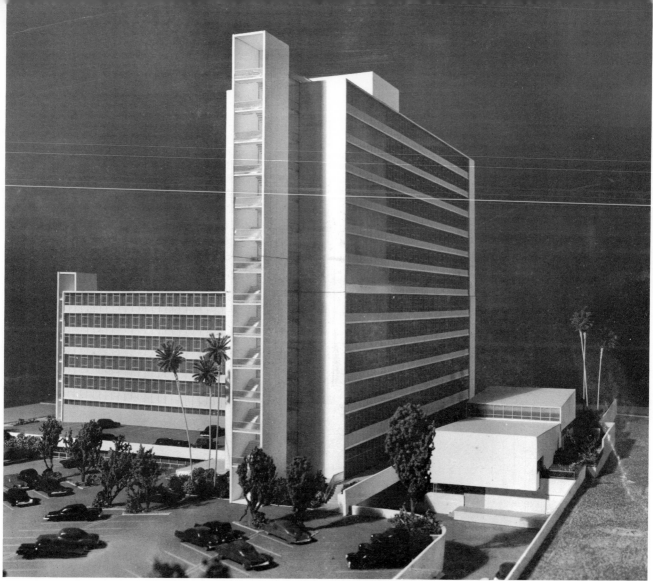

Douglas M. Simmonds

# Hospital with Emphasis on Chronic Cases

**New MT. SINAI HOSPITAL** , *Los Angeles, Cal.*

*Welton Becket & Associates; Palmer, Krisel & Lindsay; Architects and Engineers*

*W. J. Mezger, Hospital Consultant; Richard R. Bradshaw, Struct. Engineer; Ralph E. Phillips, Inc., Mech. and Elect. Engineers*

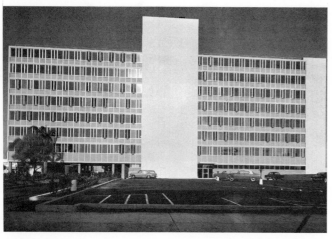

THE CONCERN of Mt. Sinai hospital for its chronically ill patients, also indigent cases, makes this an especially interesting hospital. The older Mt. Sinai Hospital, long established in Los Angeles, has always stressed this part of medical service; in planning its new building it kept this firmly in mind, not forgetting that modern medicine calls for all possible rehabilitative measures for such patients.

This new building, then, has especially comprehensive physical therapy and rehabilitation facilities (its second floor) and will have still more when its master plan is fully realized. The model photo above shows a six-story addition for the chronically ill, and five additional stories on the main portion; as now built, the hospital

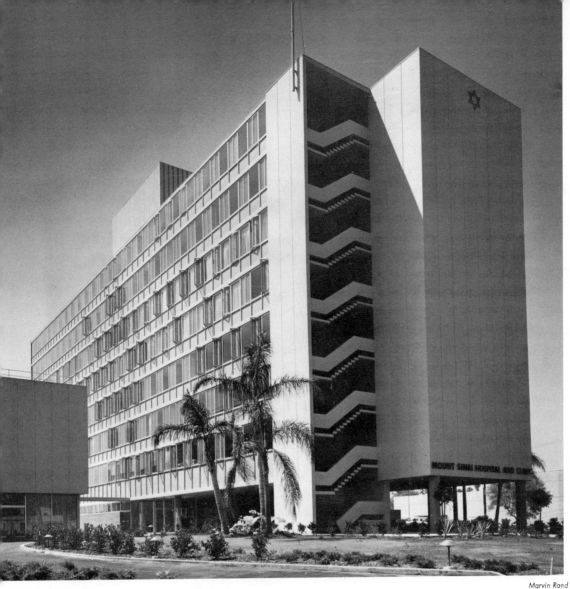

Marvin Rand

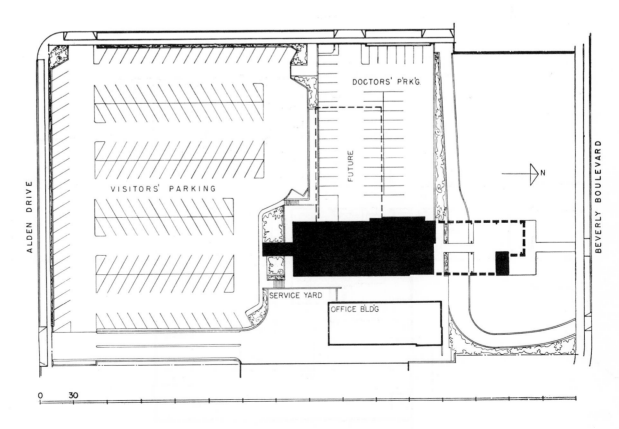

ALDEN DRIVE

VISITORS' PARKING

DOCTORS' P'RK'G.

FUTURE

SERVICE YARD

OFFICE BLD'G

BEVERLY BOULEVARD

N

0      30

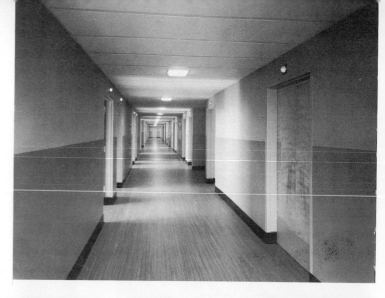

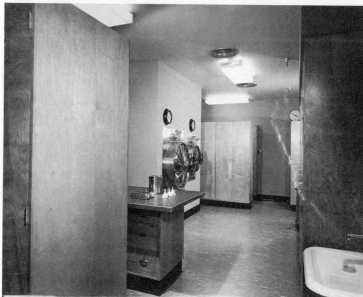

has eight stories in the main building. The existing hospital will continue to be operated largely for custodial cases.

In a sense, then, the present movement to do more for the chronically ill finds support in the program of this hospital. This concern, sharpened by the rapid strides since the war in rehabilitation, has led to a great deal of discussion of the proper place for the chronically ill patient, with a considerable body of sentiment in favor of the general hospital as the place. Whether by intention or not, this Mt. Sinai hospital becomes a case in point. In any case, the Los Angeles area has more than its normal share of persons who are, or soon will be, more or less chronic invalids, and a consequent need for facilities.

The new building has approximately 252 beds, about half of which are considered for indigent patients, half for private patients at full rate. Thus some of the floors have most of the 40 beds in semi-private rooms, others most of them in four-bed wards.

Arrangement of nursing stations on these floors is particularly interesting. The station itself is quite large, and has clustered around it utility rooms, diet kitchen, visitors' rooms, and bathrooms. The station is in the center of the nursing unit, immediately opposite the elevators. The handling of these 40-bed units involves a floor secretary, seated at the front of the nurses' station, to relieve the nurses of much of the non-medical work. This job is staffed from 8 A.M. to 10 P.M.

The second floor devoted to physical therapy and re-

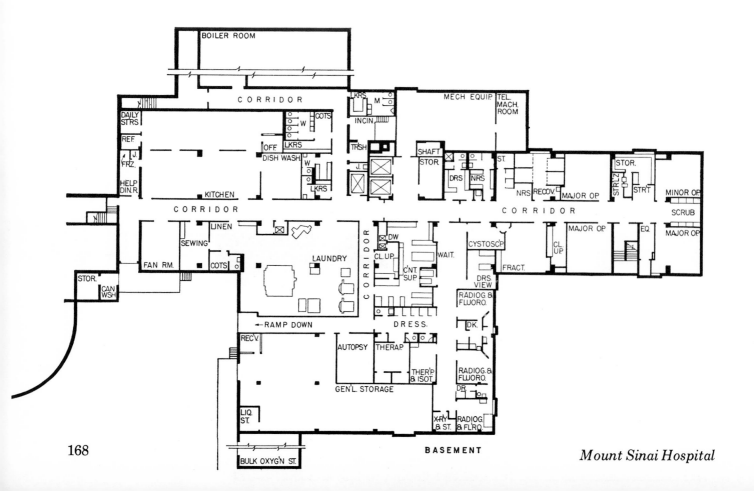

BASEMENT

*Mount Sinai Hospital*

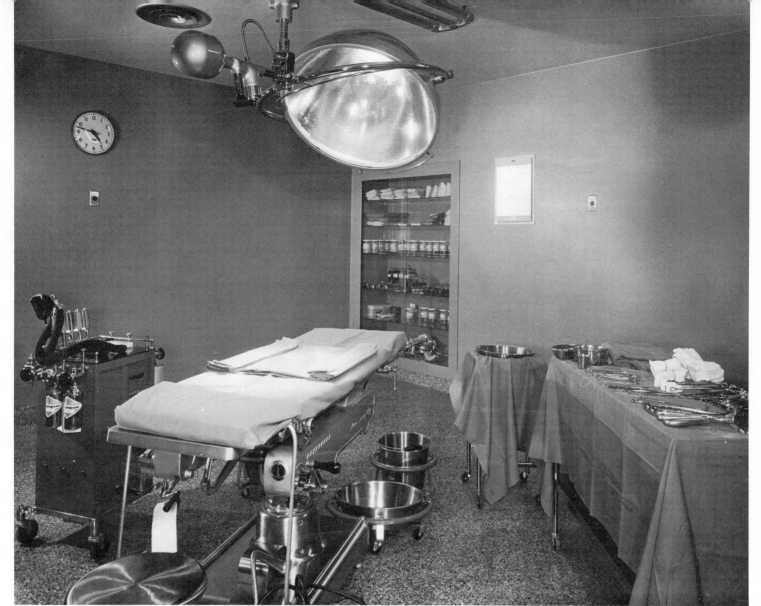

Marvin Rand

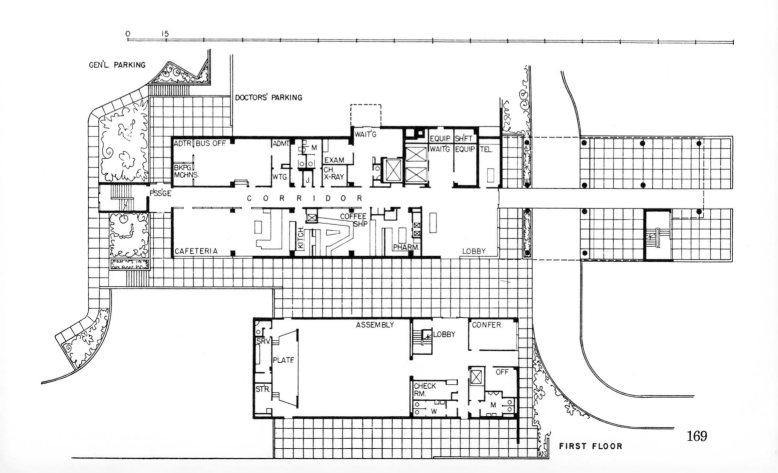

GEN'L. PARKING

DOCTORS' PARKING

ADTR | BUS.OFF | ADMT | M | WAIT'G | EQUIP | SHFT
BKPG MCHNS. | WTG | J | EXAM CH. X-RAY | WAIT'G | EQUIP | TEL.
PSS'GE

C O R R I D O R

CAFETERIA | KITCH | COFFEE SHP | PHARM. | LOBBY

ASSEMBLY | LOBBY | CONFER.
SRV
PLATF
STR | CHECK RM. | W | OFF | M

FIRST FLOOR

169

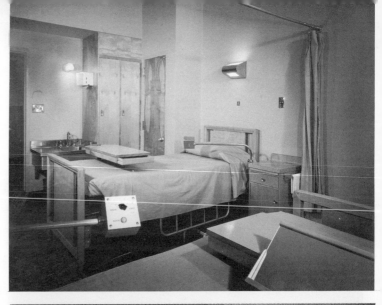

habilitation is especially noteworthy. It probably sets a new high for a general hospital in the lavishness of the equipment. This section is in charge of a doctor, over the physical therapists; notice that there are consultation rooms and examining rooms where patients may have individual attention, even private exercise booths for cases needing psychological help with their exercises. There is space on this floor for a dayroom with special dining facilities; in general, rehabilitation patients profit from contact with each other and from a spirit of competition in their struggles to improve.

Unusual in hospital design is the three-story separate building housing auditorium and office space. Fundraising is important to a hospital so definitely charitable as this one, and will be handled from separate offices here. The auditorium will be used for a wide variety of social and charitable activities.

Completion of the proposed six-story wing and the added stories atop the main building will bring the bed capacity up to around 450. This will call for some additions also to various departments, which may result in some horizontal extension of lower floors.

The site, containing something over three acres, will eventually introduce some problems, especially in the matter of parking. The vertical concept of the building was of course dictated by the limitations of the plot, but this idea is not so readily available for the automobile problem. The master plan leaves this item for future consideration, with the recommendation that more land be acquired when the additions go forward.

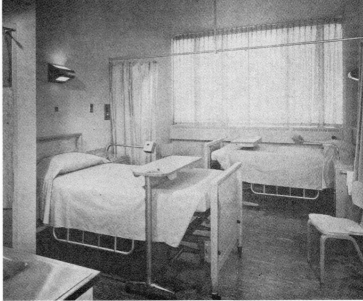

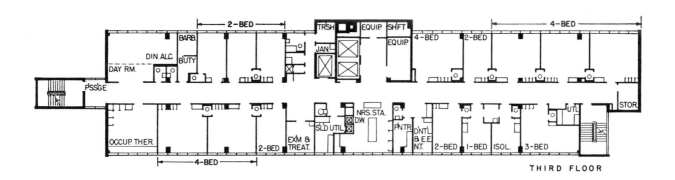

THIRD FLOOR

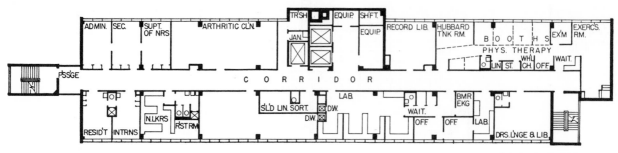

SECOND FLOOR

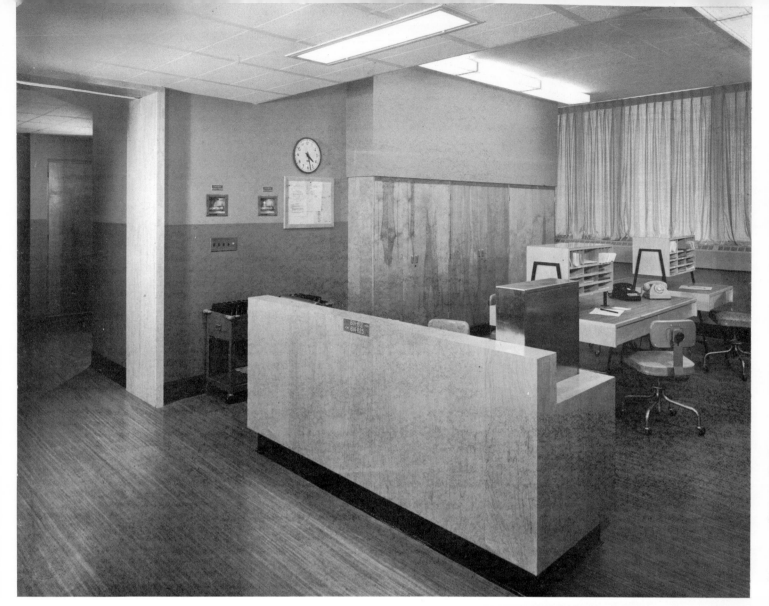

Marvin Rand

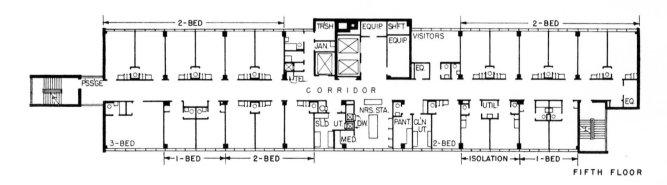

FIFTH FLOOR

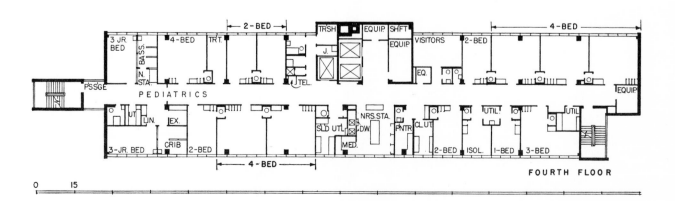

FOURTH FLOOR

0    15

*Mount Sinai Hospital*

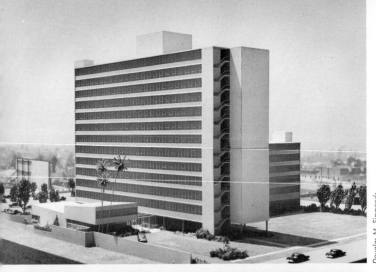

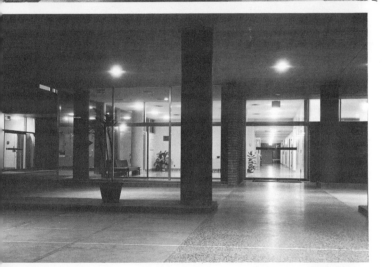

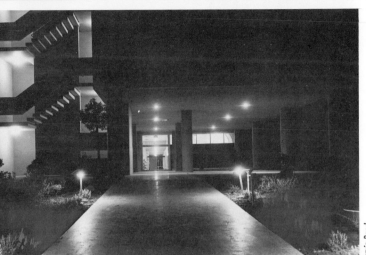

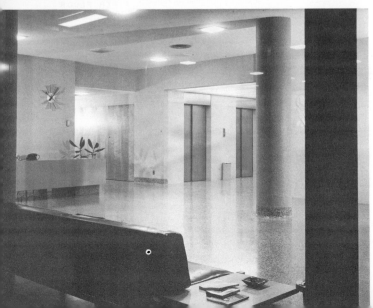

## STATEMENT OF APPROXIMATE FINAL COST
## MT. SINAI HOSPITAL AND AUDITORIUM

*Hospital Building and Auditorium*

| | |
|---|---:|
| Building Structure Cost | $1,792,877 |
| Added Costs due to sub-surface water problem | 56,400 |
| Elevators and Dumbwaiter | 152,175 |
| Plumbing | 280,000 |
| Sprinklers | 10,000 |
| Heating and Ventilating | 160,000 |
| Air Conditioning (Surgeries only) | 100,000 |
| Kitchen equipment | 45,000 |
| Sterilizers and O.P. Lts. | 15,000 |
| Paging System & Intercom System | 39,000 |
| | $2,651,052 |
| Builder's Fee | 95,723 |
| **TOTAL COST** | **$2,746,775** |

| | |
|---|---:|
| Cost of Auditorium (3 floors) | $ 200,000 |
| Cost of Hospital Bldg. Proper | 2,546,775 |
| Approx. Total Constr. Cost | $2,746,775 |

| | Floor Area | Bldg. Cube |
|---|---:|---:|
| Hospital | 114,965 | 1,262,760 |
| Auditorium | 9,160 | 111,310 |
| | 124,125 | 1,374,070 |

| | Cost per sq ft | Cost per Bed |
|---|---|---|
| Auditorium | $21.48 | |
| Hospital | 22.16 | (252 Beds) @ $10,106 |

*Mount Sinai Hospital*

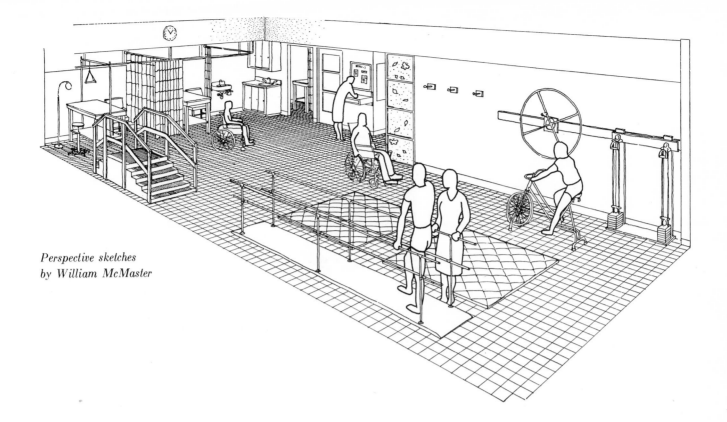

*Perspective sketches
by William McMaster*

This chapter, "Suitable Environment," is from the manual "Physical Therapy Essentials of a Hospital Department" prepared by the Joint Committee of the American Hospital Association and the American Physical Therapy Association.

Planning is by Thomas P. Galbraith and Peter N. Jensen, Hospital Architects of the Architectural and Engineering Branch, Division of Hospital and Medical Facilities, Public Health Service.

# Planning the Physical Therapy Department

Of the many environmental factors which condition the effectiveness of physical therapy service to patients, the most important are space, location and work areas. Ventilation, lighting, interior finish and related considerations also contribute toward providing a suitable environment. The keynote is function.

### Location

Location is closely related to function. The area selected for physical therapy should be centrally located to minimize problems of transporting patients and to facilitate giving bedside treatment when necessary. At least half of the patients treated in a general hospital physical therapy department are likely to be out-patients. With this in mind, special attention should be given to accessibility, and to having as few steps as possible to climb, as few long corridors and heavy doors to negotiate. A ground floor location, convenient for both in- and out-patients and for access to an outdoor exercise area, is recommended.

Availability of daylight and fresh air should also be considered in selecting a location.

In new hospitals, physical therapy is frequently placed in an area which includes other out-patient services, social service, occupational therapy, recreation. It is particularly important that physical and occupational therapy be in close proximity.

### Amount of Space

The amount of space needed depends on the number of patients treated, the kinds of disabilities and the treatments required. Also to be considered is the fact that some space-consuming equipment — such as a whirlpool bath, treatment tables, parallel bars, etc. — are minimum essentials for even a one therapist department. These pieces of equipment will not be multiplied in direct proportion to increases in staff and patient load.

Efforts to correlate bed capacity and physical therapy space requirements are not satisfactory. Hospitals with 50–100 beds may serve large numbers of out-patients. The amount of space given over to physical therapy in a small hospital is, justifiably, out of proportion to the bed capacity.

No absolute standard can be recommended as the amount of space needed for physical therapy in a general hospital. The most that can be said is that, if possible, it is desirable to plan for at least a thousand square feet of floor space, free of structural obstructions. About half of that should be exercise area.

This does not mean that a hospital cannot begin an effective physical therapy service in smaller quarters. Many have done so successfully, using to full advantage whatever space resources they had. But crowded quarters do subject the staff to strain and call for more than ordinary ingenuity and good

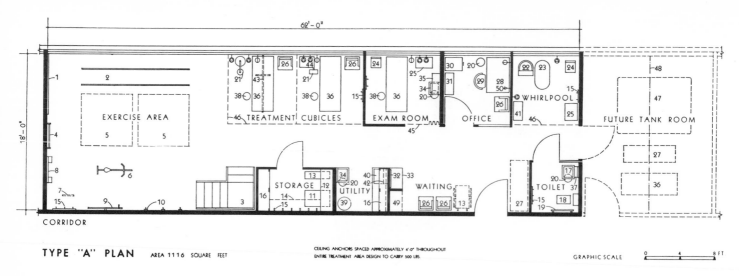

62'-0"

18'-0"

EXERCISE AREA

TREATMENT CUBICLES    EXAM ROOM    OFFICE    WHIRLPOOL    FUTURE TANK ROOM

STORAGE    UTILITY    WAITING    TOILET

CORRIDOR

TYPE "A" PLAN    AREA 1116 SQUARE FEET

CEILING ANCHORS SPACED APPROXIMATELY 4'-0" THROUGHOUT
ENTIRE TREATMENT AREA DESIGN TO CARRY 500 LBS.

GRAPHIC SCALE    0    4    8 FT

NOTE: MAJOR PIECES OF EQUIPMENT RECOMMENDED FOR ONE
PHYSICAL THERAPIST AND AID INDICATED ON TYPE PLANS

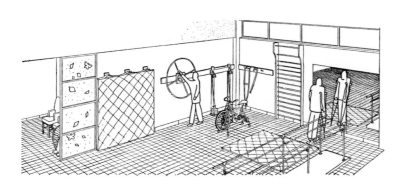

humor in order to make it possible for patients to obtain maximum benefit from treatment.

### Work Space Components

Whatever the eventual size of a physical therapy department, from the very beginning plans must be made to provide certain kinds of work space. These essential components can be expanded, multiplied or refined as the physical therapy department grows but the fundamental requirements are the same for a small or large department. They include: (1) reception area, (2) staff space, (3) examining room, (4) treatment areas, (5) toilet facilities, (6) storage.

Experienced physical therapists have many suggestions for increasing the efficiency of physical therapy departments by giving attention to details of planning and arranging these component work areas. For example:

Reception area — accommodations for in-patients and out-patients, if possible. Adequate space for stretcher and wheelchair patients.

Staff space — private. Office space suitable for interviewing patients, attending to administrative and clerical duties, housing files, etc. Writing facilities for the staff adequate for dictation, record keeping. There should be space for staff lockers and dressing rooms separate from the patient area,

either within the department or near to it.

Examining room — floor to ceiling partitions for privacy. Arranged so that necessary examining equipment can remain in the room permanently. Possible to use this space for special tests and measurements or for treatment when privacy is desirable.

Treatment area — there are three types of treatment areas: cubicle (dry), underwater exercise (wet) and exercise (open). Each is designed to meet the particular requirements of the special equipment used for different kinds of treatment.

Cubicle — each unit large enough for the physical therapist to work on either side of the table without having to move equipment belonging in the cubicle. Preferably cubicles divided by curtains for easier access for wheelchair and stretcher cases, for expansion of useable floor area for gait analysis, group activity or teaching purposes.

Curtain tracks should be flush with the ceiling and curtains should have open panels at the top for ventilation when drawn. Both curtains and tracks should be sturdy. In or near the cubicles, out-patients need a place or locker for their outer clothing.

Underwater exercise area — all equipment requiring special plumbing and water supply concentrated in one section of the department but accessible and adjacent to other treatment areas. Should include a treatment table, especially in the room

174

1. Posture Mirror
2. Parallel Bars
3. Steps
4. Stall Bars
5. Gym Mat
6. Stationary Bicycle
7. Sayer Head Sling Attached to Ceiling
8. Pulley Weights
9. Shoulder Wheel
10. Gym Mat Hooks
11. Cart with Open Shelves
12. Open Shelves
13. Wheel Chair
14. Shelf
15. Wall Hooks
16. Wall Cabinet
17. Lavatory, Gooseneck Spout
18. Water Closet
19. Hand Rail
20. Waste Paper Receptacle
21. Portable Equipment
22. Adjustable Chair
23. Whirlpool
24. Chair
25. Table
26. Chair, preferable with arms
27. Wheel Stretcher
28. Desk
29. Swivel Chair
30. File Cabinet
31. Bookcase
32. Bulletin Board
33. Wall Desk (counter, shelf below)
34. Lavatory, Gooseneck Spout and Foot Control
35. Wall Cabinet with Lock
36. Treatment Table, Storage below
37. Mirror and Glass Shelf over Lavatory
38. Adjustable Stool
39. Laundry Hamper
40. Sink with Drainboard
41. Paraffin Bath
42. Glass Shelf over Sink
43. Overbed Trapeze
44. Three Single Outlets on separate branch circuits. 1 outlet 2-pole, 2 outlets 3-pole
45. Folding Door
46. Cubicle Curtain
47. Under Water Exercise Equipment
48. Overhead Lift
49. Coat Rack
50. Telephone Outlet

TYPE "B" PLAN    AREA 1350 SQUARE FEET

CEILING ANCHORS SPACED APPROXIMATELY 4'-0" THROUGHOUT ENTIRE TREATMENT AREA DESIGNED TO CARRY 500 LBS.

NOTE:
MAJOR PIECES OF EQUIPMENT RECOMMENDED FOR ONE PHYSICAL THERAPIST AND AID INDICATED ON TYPE PLANS

GRAPHIC SCALE

with a tank or exercise pool. Fixed overhead lifts are absolutely essential for the efficient use of tanks and failure to provide lifts severely limits the usefulness of this valuable equipment. Plumbing and other installation requirements, humidity and noise from motors call for special care and attention. Electrical and metal equipment in other treatment areas may suffer damage unless the underwater exercise area is carefully planned.

Exercise area — very flexible open space planned to accommodate patients engaged in diverse individual or group exercise activities. Used extensively by people in wheelchairs, on crutches or canes, or with other disabilities which limit their motion and agility. At least one wall should be reinforced for the installation of stall bars and similar equipment.

Toilet facilities — separate toilet facilities for patients and staff, if possible. Patient facilities should be designed to accommodate wheelchair patients. If the department serves small children, seat adaptors with foot rests should be provided.

Storage — designed to meet special needs in and near work areas. Should also be storage space on the wards for equipment and supplies usually needed for bedside treatments. For wheelchairs, stretchers, etc., it is best to plan "carport" space, not closets. All storage space should be accessible, simple, well lighted.

*Special Considerations*

Ventilation: Adequate, controlled ventilation is of extreme importance in a physical therapy department. Many of the treatment procedures require the use of dry or moist heat, or active exercise, which raise body temperatures. A continuous, reliable flow of fresh air is essential to the comfort of patients and staff. This includes protection from drafts.

Air conditioning, desirable for the entire department, will be a necessity for certain areas of the physical therapy department, in most sections of the country. The reduction of humidity for comfort, protection of equipment and reduction of the hazard of slippery floors makes air conditioning vital in the underwater exercise area. It has been demonstrated as desirable in the exercise area and in treatment cubicles, especially where heat producing equipment is used. Air conditioning engineers should be consulted before ventilation equipment is installed.

Sinks: Hospital hand washing lavatories with hot and cold water mixing outlets, preferably foot operated, should be located at the proper height in convenient places. At least one sink should be of sufficient width and depth to accommodate the care of wet packs and other special washing needs.

Interior finishes: The activity of patients in wheelchairs, on stretchers and crutches subject floors and walls to heavy wear. Materials which will stand up under such rough usage, remain

*Physical Therapy Department*

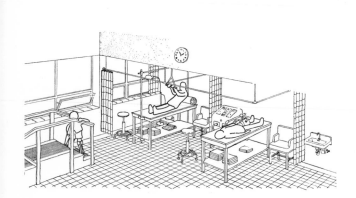

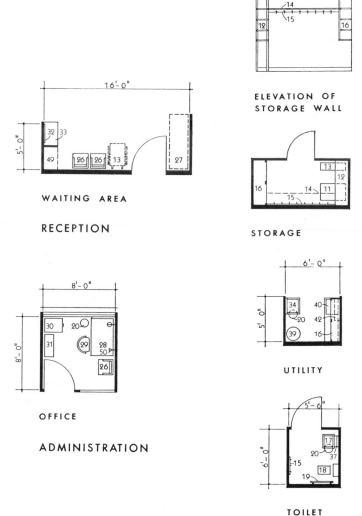

ELEVATION OF
STORAGE WALL

WAITING AREA

RECEPTION

STORAGE

OFFICE

ADMINISTRATION

UTILITY

TOILET

attractive and require a minimum of maintenance should be specified despite higher costs.

All interior wall surfaces of the department should have a durable and attractive wainscot to protect them against damage by wheelchairs, stretchers and carts. Ceramic wall tile or glazed structural units will serve the purpose but they emphasize the institutional character of the hospital. In patient areas this should be minimized as much as possible. In the last several years vinyl wall covering has gained in popularity as a wainscoting material, and to some extent for the entire wall. Two weights of the material are available; the heavier weight for areas subjected to severe abuse, the lighter weight for other parts of the wall.

The use of decorative colors for interior finishes and equipment is, of course, highly desirable in this department as it is in other parts of the hospital. Research in "color therapy" for hospitals adds to decorators' ideas the therapeutic value of combinations of pastel colors. "Cool" pastels — green, blue, violet and their many derivatives — are considered mildly restful. Some light colors in general are stimulating and may be of advantage in the exercise area.

Doors: For accommodation of stretcher and wheelchair traffic, doors within the department should be at least 40 inches wide. Raised thresholds should be eliminated.

Ceiling moorings: These moorings, strategically located in the ceiling in treatment areas, have been found useful for attaching overhead equipment such as hoists, pulleys, bars, counter balancing equipment, etc. They should be constructed and attached to joists in such a manner that each supports at least 500 pounds.

*Layout*

It is impossible to anticipate all of the practical problems of layout in a particular building or to say in advance that one plan or another is the right one. A few guidelines, however, may be useful in making decisions about layout.

Expect to expand and plan for it from the beginning. It is impossible to overestimate the value of the exercise area. Give it as many square feet of appropriate space as possible.

Note the need to have the underwater exercise equipment grouped in one area, separate but adjacent and accessible to the other treatment areas.

When deciding which units to place next to each other or group together, consider how they are used by patients, especially the flow of traffic from one unit to another. Try to avoid needless traffic. Try to conserve the energies of staff.

Visit other physical therapy departments and find out what the physical therapists like or would like to change in the layouts of their own departments.

176

1. Posture Mirror
2. Parallel Bars
3. Steps
4. Stall Bars
5. Gym Mat
6. Stationary Bicycle
7. Sayer Head Sling Attached to Ceiling
8. Pulley Weights
9. Shoulder Wheel
10. Gym Mat Hooks
11. Cart with Open Shelves
12. Open Shelves
13. Wheel Chair
14. Shelf
15. Wall Hooks
16. Wall Cabinet
17. Lavatory, Gooseneck Spout
18. Water Closet
19. Hand Rail
20. Waste Paper Receptacle
21. Portable Equipment
22. Adjustable Chair
23. Whirlpool
24. Chair
25. Table
26. Chair, preferable with arms
27. Wheel Stretcher
28. Desk
29. Swivel Chair
30. File Cabinet
31. Bookcase
32. Bulletin Board
33. Wall Desk (counter, shelf below)
34. Lavatory, Gooseneck Spout and Foot Control
35. Wall Cabinet with Lock
36. Treatment Table, Storage below
37. Mirror and Glass Shelf over Lavatory
38. Adjustable Stool
39. Laundry Hamper
40. Sink with Drainboard
41. Paraffin Bath
42. Glass Shelf over Sink
43. Overbed Trapeze
44. Three Single Outlets on separate branch circuits. 1 outlet 2-pole, 2 outlets 3-pole
45. Folding Door
46. Cubicle Curtain
47. Under Water Exercise Equipment
48. Overhead Lift
49. Coat Rack
50. Telephone Outlet

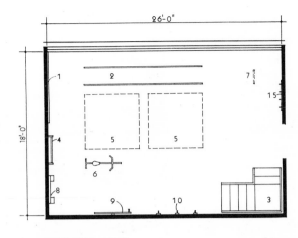

EXERCISE AREA

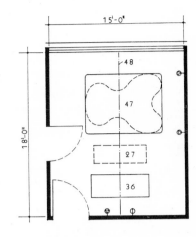

TANK ROOM

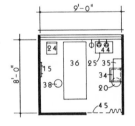

EXAMINATION ROOM

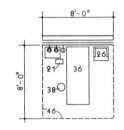

TREATMENT CUBICLE

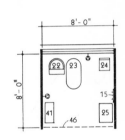

WHIRLPOOL

EXAMINATION AND TREATMENT

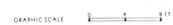

GRAPHIC SCALE     0     4     8 FT

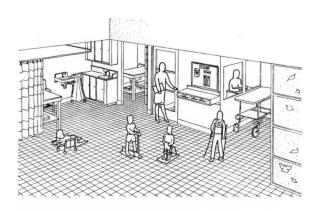

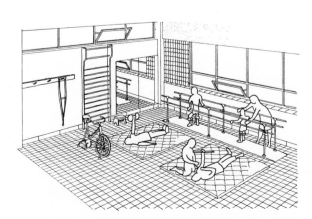

*Physical Therapy Department*

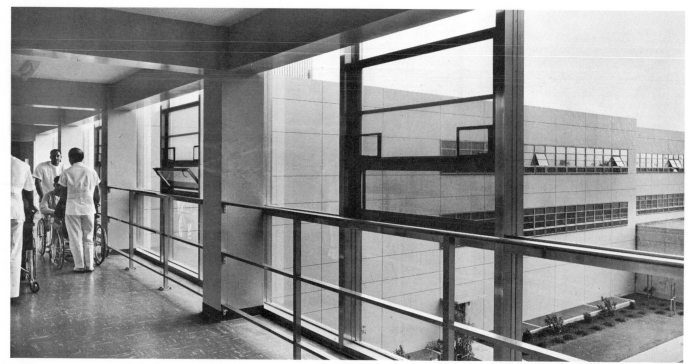

# First Complete Facilities for Paraplegics

*Addition to Long Beach Veterans Administration Hospital, Long Beach, Cal. Welton Becket and Associates, Architects; Murray Erick and Associates, Structural Engineers; Ruth Shellhorn, Landscape Architect; Gust K. Newberg, General Contractor*

With the completion of a new addition, the huge Long Beach Veteran's Administration Hospital has the first specially-planned facilities for paraplegics ever built in this country. Five wings extend from a broad, central spine, which, with four floors, have a total of 296,000 sq ft with a capacity of 561 beds, 205 of which are used for paraplegic veterans. The facilities are also planned to care for an out-patient load measured at 980 cases.

According to Dr. Ernest Bors, chief of spinal cord injury service at the hospital, two important considerations of location led to the selection of the Los Angeles area for this facility: mild weather and proximity to a large metropolitan center. A further dividend is the willingness of aircraft companies in this area to hire paralytics.

Each new injury case to enter the center is diagnosed by Dr. Bors and his assistants and a specific method of treatment scheduled. There is no general or normal course of treatment. Patients are about equally divided between paraplegics and quadruplegics and no two cases are exactly the same. Treatment involves medical rehabilitation, physical rehabilitation, and vocational-industrial rehabilitation and the center provides facilities for each.

Specific facilities include a gymnasium, physical therapy and occupational therapy areas, a cystoscopy clinic, central bathtub and enema room, swimming pool, and therapeutic pools and brine tanks. The central nursing area, with bathtubs and enema room, is one of the center's features. It is the most economical and efficient method of handling some fifty per cent of patients who are completely helpless. Instead of costly individual facilities for each quadruplegic, the central rooms require less nursing personnel and can handle more patients.

Doctors' and specialists' offices are located on one side of the first floor corridor in the central spine, with treatment facilities and consultation rooms directly across the hall from each office. Private rooms and ward areas are located in the five wings of the first floor.

Physical and vocational rehabilitation areas are in the lower level. These areas, some of which are used by general hospital patients as well as spinal cord injury patients, include a machine shop, carpentry, photography, weaving, jewelry making, metal work, lapidary, and radio repair facilities. In the swimming pool and gymnasium, patients learn to use new muscles or tone up old muscles for walking, swimming, and other normal activities.

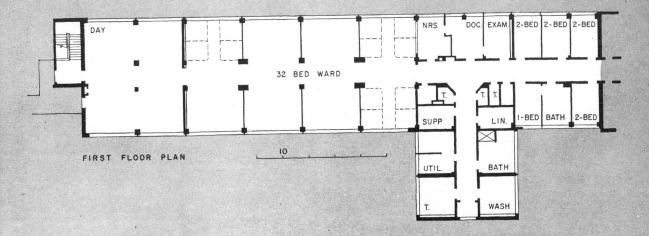

**FIRST FLOOR PLAN**

10

Plan above is typical of nursing wings for paraplegic inpatients. Most of the patients are in four-bed open wards, with head-high partitions separating one ward from another, and all open to the corridor. Bays are rather spacious, because of all of the paraphernalia necessary. There are, as the plan shows, one single and a few double rooms, for the occasional patients who need more privacy than is possible in the wards

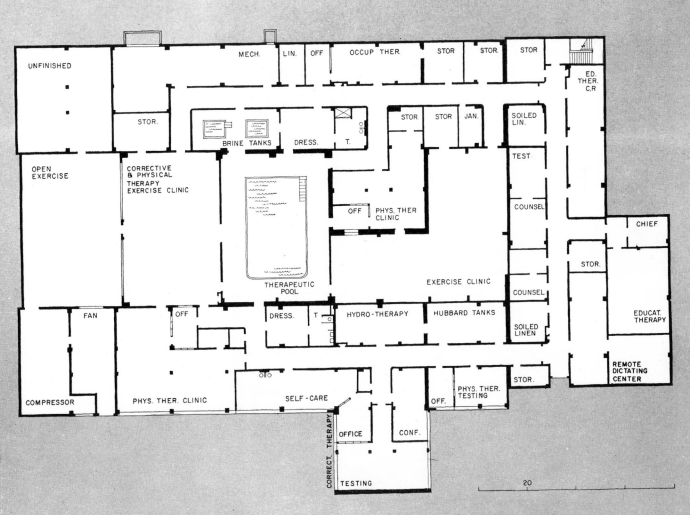

20

This plan shows what is said to be the most extensive layout of facilities for rehabilitation of paraplegics. Hydrotherapy is most important in the retaining of old muscles and the development of new ones, hence the pool, Hubbard tanks, brine tanks, and so on. Exercise of all types is of course important, so there are extensive areas for it both indoors and outdoors. There is also (plan not shown) a wing devoted to occupational therapy shops

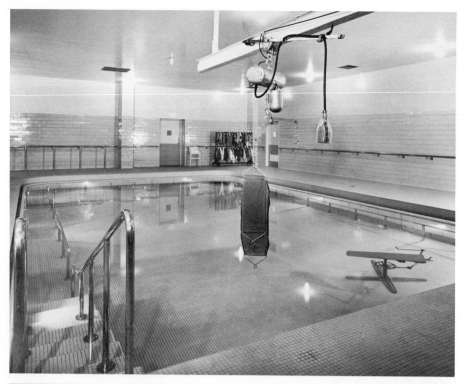

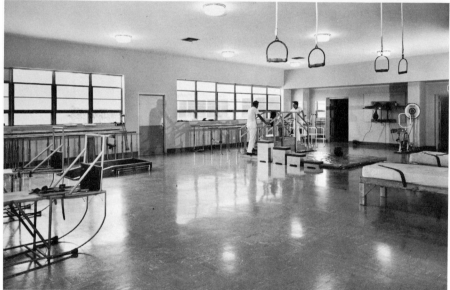

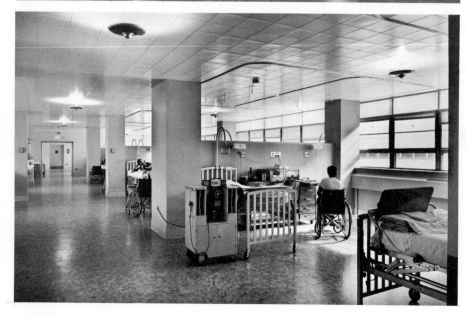

Swimming is an especially good exercise for paraplegics, helping them to develop new muscles and tone up old ones. Note the suspended harness, the submerged table and railings. The gymnasium also has a wide variety of exercising devices; it can be used by both bed patients and outpatients. Most of the beds are in wards, but rather spacious wards, because of all of the paraphernalia that goes with the treatment and rehabilitation of patients

*Facilities for Paraplegics*

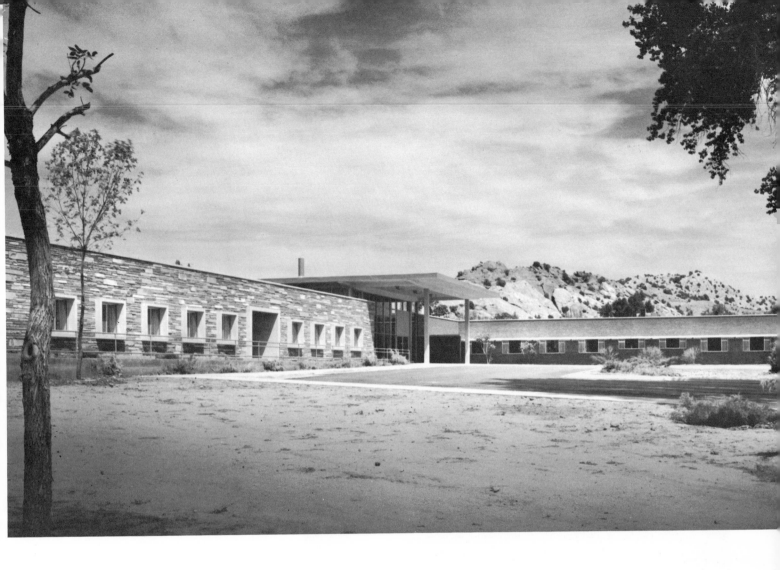

# General Hospital Combined with Rehabilitation Center

GOTTSCHE
REHABILITATION CENTER
AND HOT SPRINGS
MEMORIAL HOSPITAL,
THERMOPOLIS, WYOMING

ARCHITECTS:
*Fisher and Davis*

STRUCTURAL ENGINEERS:
*Ken R. White Engineers*

MECHANICAL ENGINEERS:
*Marshall and Johnson*

ELECTRICAL ENGINEERS:
*Swanson and Rink*

CONTRACTOR:
*J. C. Boespflug*

In this unusual building, a 51-bed general hospital is combined with rehabilitation facilities for children and adults. Officially, there are two institutions here—the county hospital (built with the aid of Hill-Burton funds) and the rehabilitation center (built by a private foundation). By combining their efforts and sharing certain facilities, the two institutions have been able to achieve improved services and economies not possible if each had been built separately.

The new buildings are near an existing home for the aged. The rehabilitation center is equipped for the treatment of patients with polio, multiple sclerosis, cerebral palsy and other crippling diseases. The hospital beds are subdivided as follows: general acute—27 beds, maternity—8 beds, and rehabilitation—16 beds. The rehabilitation beds are in addition to those for children in the cottages and are intended primarily for occupancy by adult patients from outside the county. They are supported by the rehabilitation foundation.

The foundations of the buildings are concrete on wood piling. The frame is steel with a concrete slab floor and gypsum roof deck. Exterior walls are brick and native sandstone with aluminum sliding windows. Interior partitions are plaster on steel studs; plaster or acoustical suspended ceilings are used.

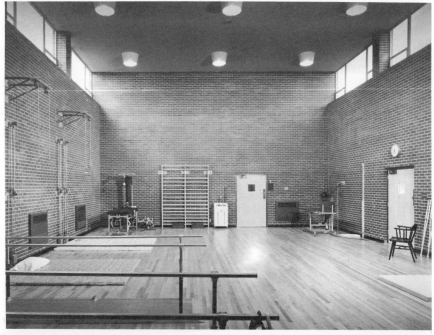

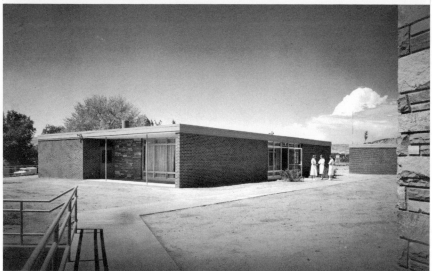

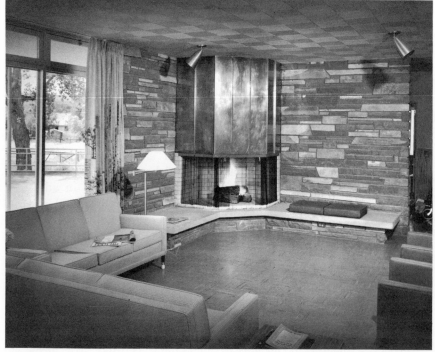

If the need should arise, a portion of the basement of the rehab center may be used for a kitchen for the center, separate from that of the hospital. Also, the storage area of the hospital, adjacent to the present kitchen, was designed for possible use as a future hospital cafeteria. At present, a single dietary service is used for both facilities. However, separate dish storage and washing areas for the two facilities are now provided. Left, above: view of the adult gymnasium. A separate gym is provided for children. Left, center: view of one of the children's cottages of the rehabilitation center. Left, bottom: view of a living room in one of the children's cottages

*Warren Reynolds, Infinity, Inc. photos*

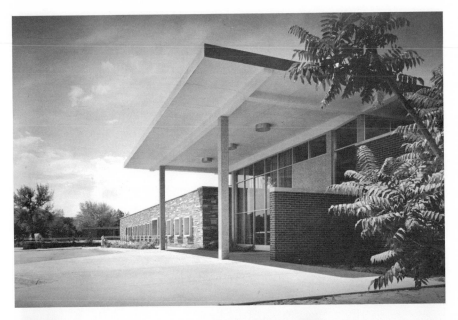

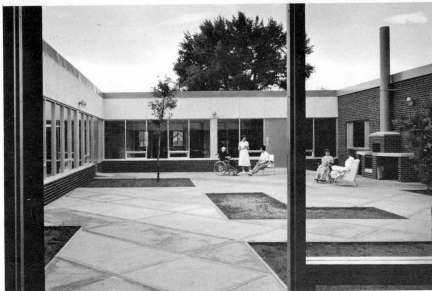

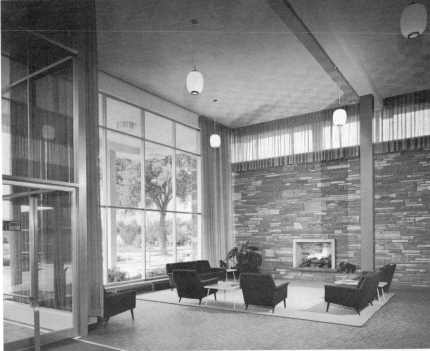

Right top: main entrance with the rehab center in background. Emergency entrance is located on the right side of the building. Right, center: view of the central court of the rehabilitation center. This area is used for recreational activities for the patients. On the right is the barbecue pit, in the background, the cafeteria. Right, bottom: the main lobby, between the hospital and the rehab center, serves both areas. The rehabilitation center also has a public entrance

*Gottsche Rehabilitation Center and Hot Springs Memorial Hospital*

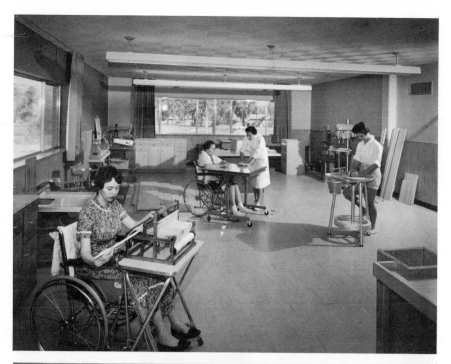

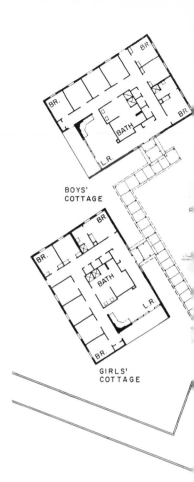

BOYS' COTTAGE

GIRLS' COTTAGE

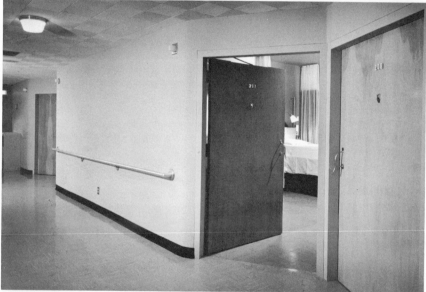

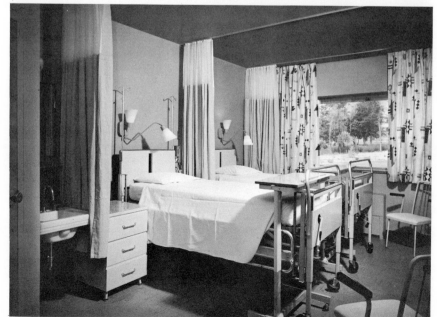

General-acute beds are located in the hospital wing projecting toward the front; the rear wing contains beds for adult rehabilitation patients; maternity and obstetrics are located in the front portion of the main hospital and are segregated from other facilities. The kitchen, laundry, and other service areas are located in the basement. The rehabilitation center facilities are grouped around a central court. In each of the two detached children's cottages six two-patient bedrooms, a living room, bath, and supervisor's room are provided. The unfinished basement area will eventually be used for a swimming pool and expanded therapy areas. <u>Left, top</u>: view of the occupational therapy area. <u>Left, center</u>: the rehab section of the main hospital was planned for specialized needs of these patients. <u>Left, bottom</u>: each of the patient rooms in the hospital is planned for two beds

REHABILITATION

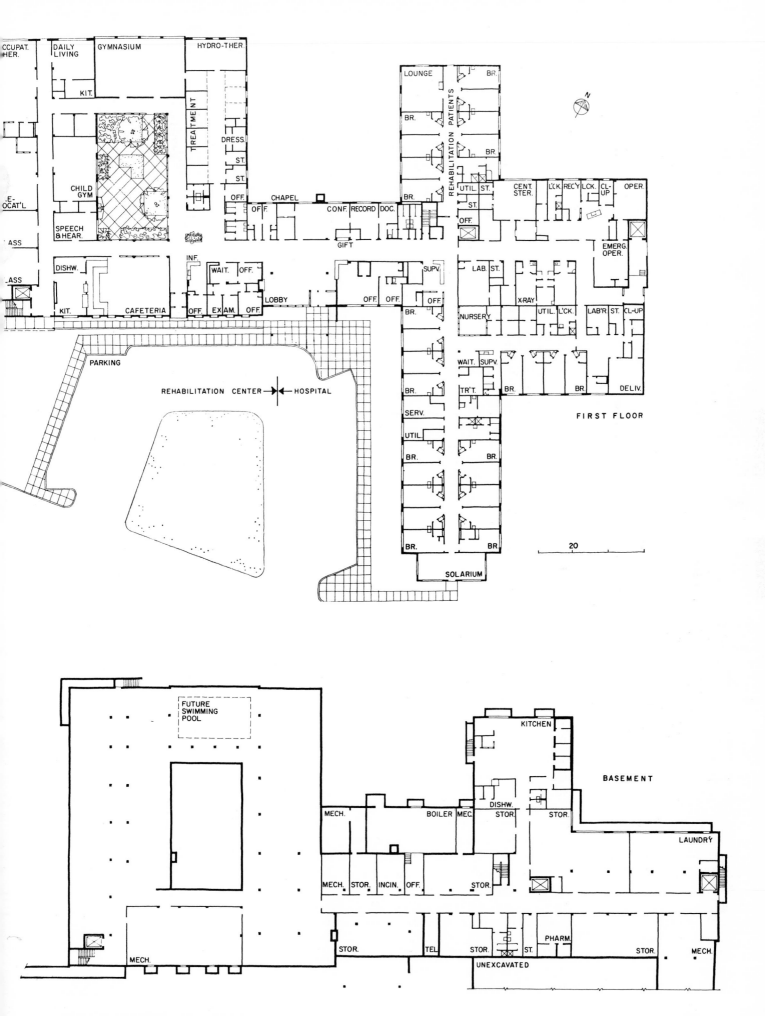

*Gottsche Rehabilitation Center*

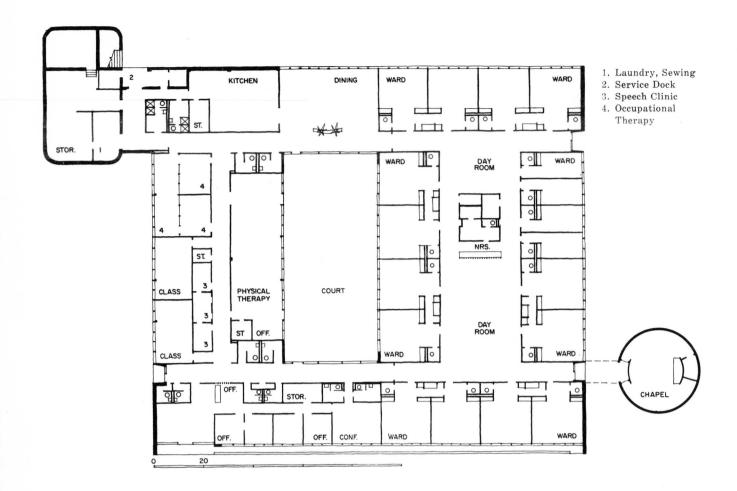

# Rehabilitation Hospital School for Children

A specialty among medical facilities, this cerebral palsy hospital school represents the consolidation, in a new building of its own, of a development which began years ago. For several years the State Department of Education operated a school of about 40 beds capacity housed in rebuilt army surplus buildings. Necessity of removing the old building, to make way for the University Medical School and Teaching Hospital, forced a move, and the need to continue the work was obvious. Perhaps a more accurate description of the facility would be a "children's rehabilitation hospital school." Treatment of a case frequently extends over several years, and prognosis as to treatment time is difficult, though the present hospital is planned for treatment of other types of children's illnesses, such as polio or orthopedic cases. As the plan indicates, children are housed largely in wards, as children need company and profit from the example and stimulus provided by others. While there are some classrooms, the bulk of the space in the school portion is devoted to physical and occupational therapy.

*Mississippi Hospital School for Cerebral Palsy Jackson, Miss.*

*Architects and Engineers: Biggs, Weir & Chandler*

*Structural Engineers: Post and Witty*

*Frank Lotz Miller photos*

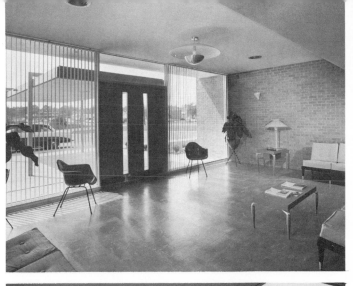

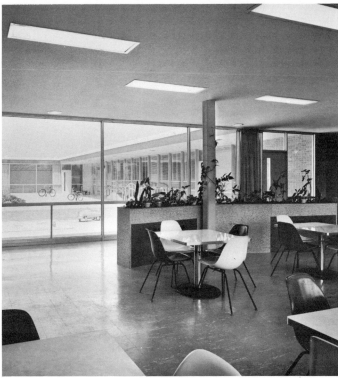

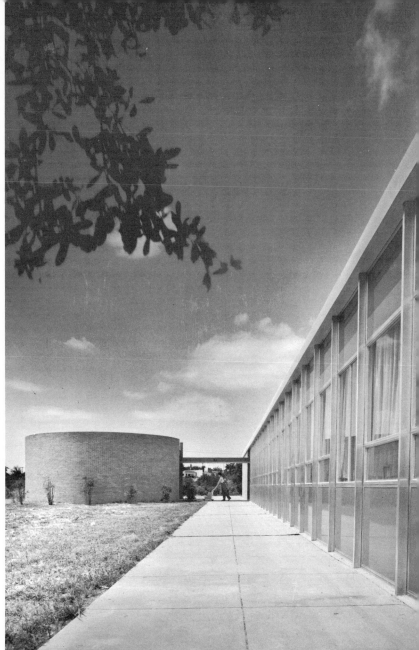

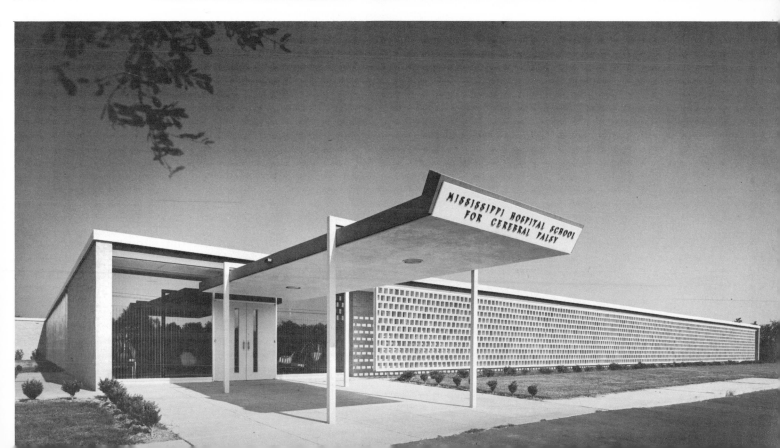

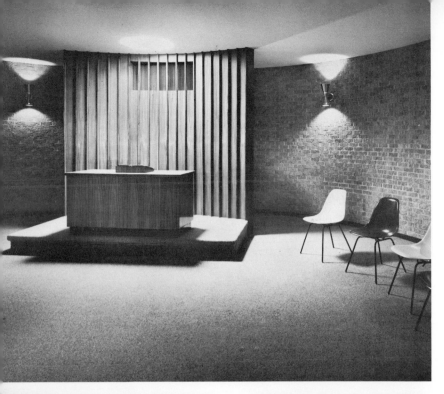

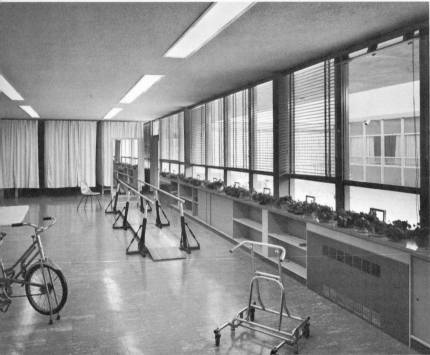

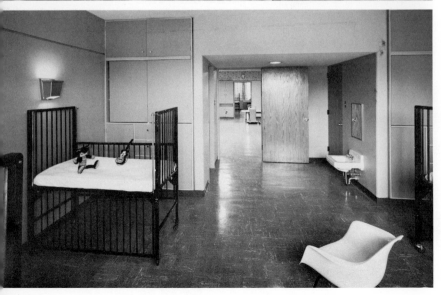

In both ward section and school and therapy rooms the building is kept scaled to children, though in general areas are quite large. The influence of the group is quite important, and children are encouraged to retrain their bodies by watching others. The scheme puts great stress on the enclosed courtyard for play of a therapeutic nature

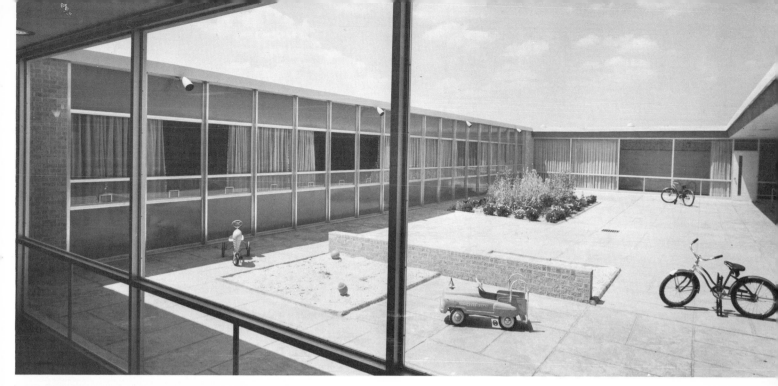

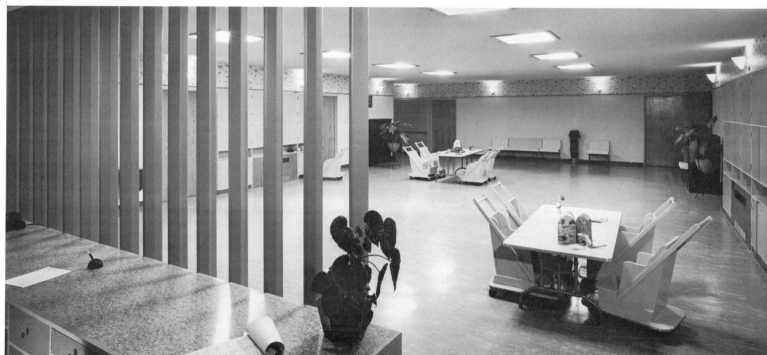

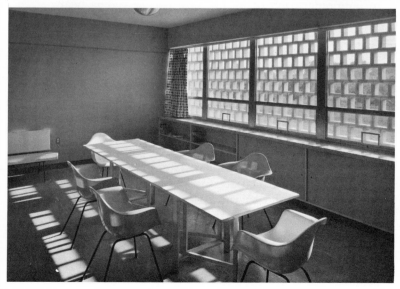

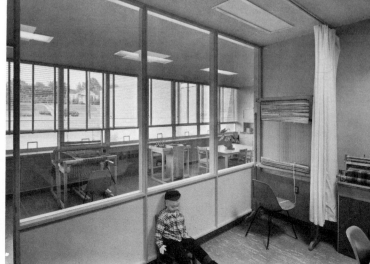

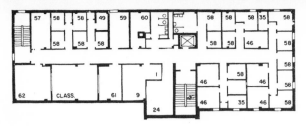

THIRD FLOOR PLAN

| | | |
|---|---|---|
| 1. Control | 22. Otol. Exam. | 43. Artic. & Psychom. |
| 2. P & C Research | 23. E.N.T. Dr's. Off. | 44. Artic. Testing |
| 3. Physical Acoust. Research | 24. Waiting | 45. Artic. & Audio. Test. |
| 4. Elec. Equip. Test. | 25. Psychologist | 46. Clinician |
| 5. Test Chamber | 26. Psyco. Test. | 47. Staffing |
| 6. Research Dir. Off | 27. Play Therapy | 48. Speech Direct. |
| 7. Elect. Engr. Off. | 28. Game Storage | 49. Recording |
| 8. Animal Surgery | 29. Clin. Voc. Rehab. | 50. Reception |
| 9. Secretaries | 30. Repair | 51. Business Manag. |
| 10. Med. Director | 31. Kitchen | 52. Director |
| 11. Staff Seminar | 32. Projection | 53. Dir. Stud. Train. |
| 12. Acoust. Super. | 33. Upper Physical Acoustic Research | 54. Grad. Stud. Work |
| 13. P.G. Skin Respon. | 34. Cerebral Palsy Nursery | 55. Stud. Coat Room |
| 14. Audiom'c Test | 35. Observation | 56. Central Files |
| 15. Clinical Audio Logist | 36. Recovery & Rest | 57. Group Therapy Speech |
| 16. Psy'tic & Test | 37. Teacher | 58. Stud. Therapy |
| 17. Audio Lab. | 38. Special Therapy | 59. Air Conditioning |
| 18. Interview | 39. Social Worker | 60. Clinician Lounge |
| 19. Pediat'c Exam. | 40. Playroom | 61. Demonstration |
| 20. Dental Operat. | 41. Audit. Training | 62. Group Therapy Hearing |
| 21. Dental Lab. | 42. Articulat. Test. | |

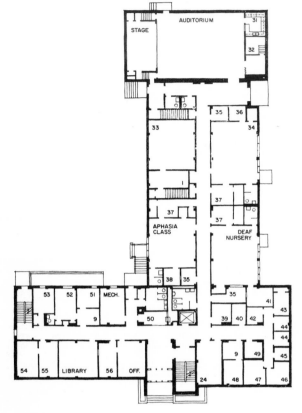

SECOND FLOOR PLAN

# Hearing and Speech Center

*Bill Wilkerson Hearing and Speech Center, Nashville, Tenn. Owner: State of Tennessee. Architects: Brush, Hutchinson & Gwinn. Structural Engineers: Barge, Waggoner & Sumner. Consulting Structural Engineers: Severud-Elstad-Kreuger. Mechanical Engineers: Lindstrom, McLendon & Holbrook, Inc. Electrical Engineers: Bush-May & Associates. Acoustical Consultant: Robert W. Benson. Interior Designers: Ken White Associates. Sculptor: Julian Harris.*

An interesting medical specialty, this building is hurriedly included in this group, though it is too early for adequate presentation. Functionally it is an agglomeration of highly interesting rooms bearing such titles as anechoic chamber, audiologic laboratory, sound room, speech research chamber, electronics shop, psychogalvanic skin response chamber, and so on, all devoted to speech and hearing problems. The building itself is interesting in its provisions for acoustical isolation. There are double masonry walls in some places to insulate against outside noises, sand-floated floor slabs, heavy partitions, and a great variety of measures to prevent transmission of sound through air conditioning ducts. Medically the building includes a great range of facilities for diagnostic and therapeutic work in the fields of audiology and speech pathology. Preschool training plays a large part in the work, in the hope that the deaf, cerebral palsied and aphasics can be prepared to enter the special education facilities in the public schools.

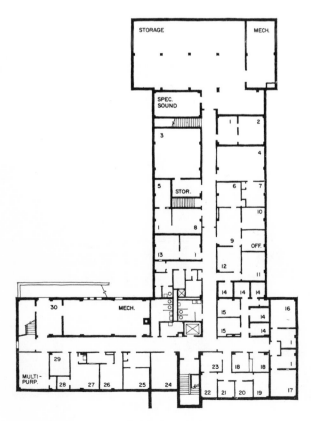

FIRST FLOOR PLAN

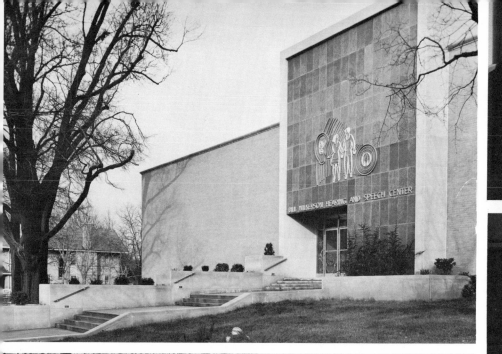

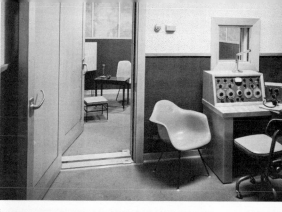

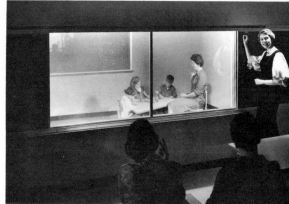

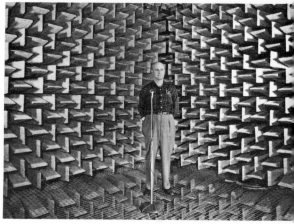

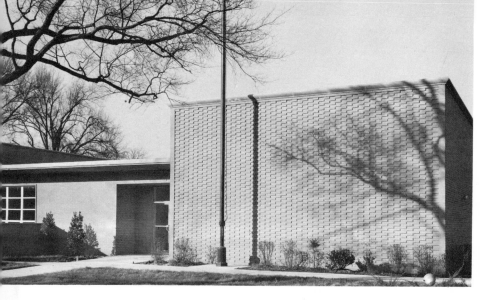

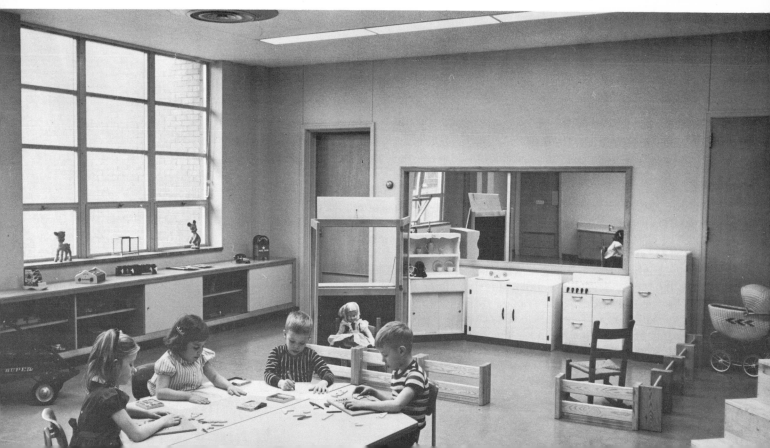

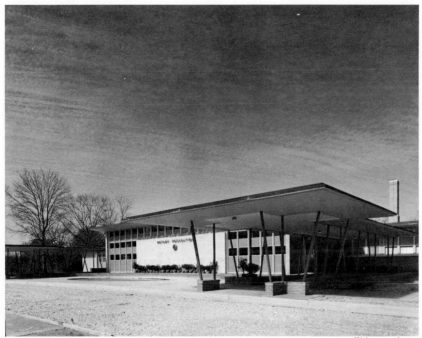

# Comprehensive Rehabilitation Center

For some years now medical authorities have hoped for the establishment of rehabilitation centers; since the doctrine of effective rehabilitation has spread so widely, facilities are necessary for carrying on the work. Who was to sponsor and finance such facilities was not as obvious as the need. This is just such a facility as was envisioned; the sponsors in this case comprise a considerable group of voluntary organizations starting with Rotary Clubs and continuing the Alabama Society for Crippled Children and Adults. Many other organizations participated in the study as well as in financing plans.

The building will house both in-patient and out-patient departments. Principal medical services will include physical and medical evaluation, physical therapy, occupational therapy, speech therapy, audiological services, prosthetic appliances, psychiatric services, and dentistry. Out-patient clinics will be operated for: orthopedic clinic; cerebral palsy clinic; cleft palate clinic; eye clinic; hearing clinic; epileptic clinic; muscular dystrophy clinic; amputee clinic; plastic clinic.

The center is located within reasonable distance of four hospitals, so that other medical services, such as x-ray and laboratory, will be available close by. There will also be vocational counseling, psychological service, and social evaluation along with the medical.

As for the building, it is poured-in-place concrete frame resting on spread footing foundation. The twenty-year built-up roof has copper gutters and downspouts. The exterior walls are a combination of pink face brick, limestone and porcelain enamel panel walls. All public areas in the interior are structural glazed tile with structural

*Rotary Foundation Clinic
and Rehabilitation Center
Mobile, Ala.*

*Architects:
Platt Roberts & Company*

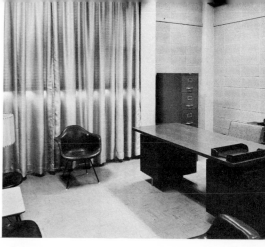

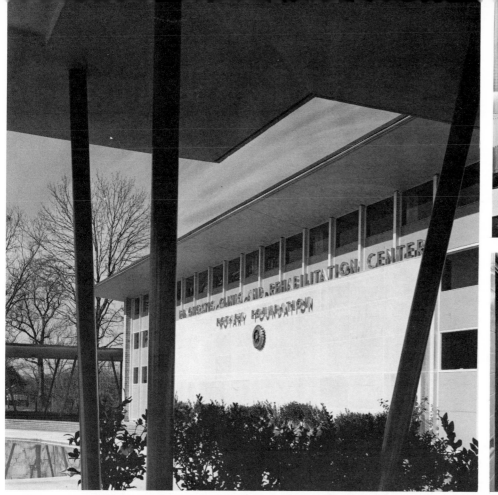

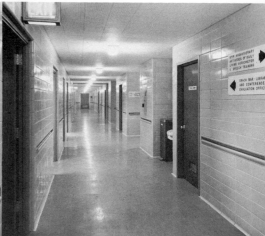

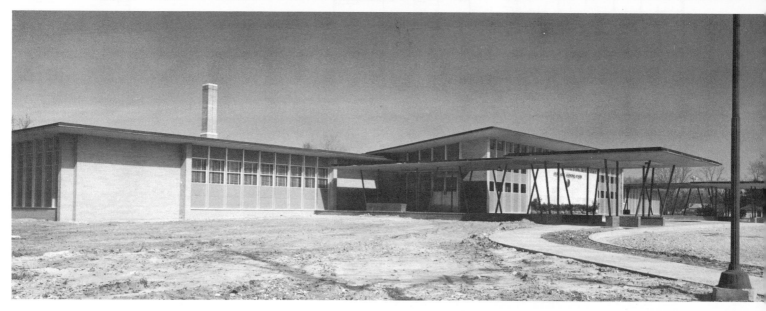

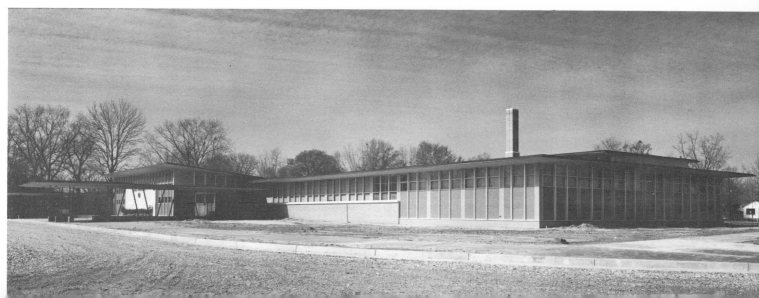

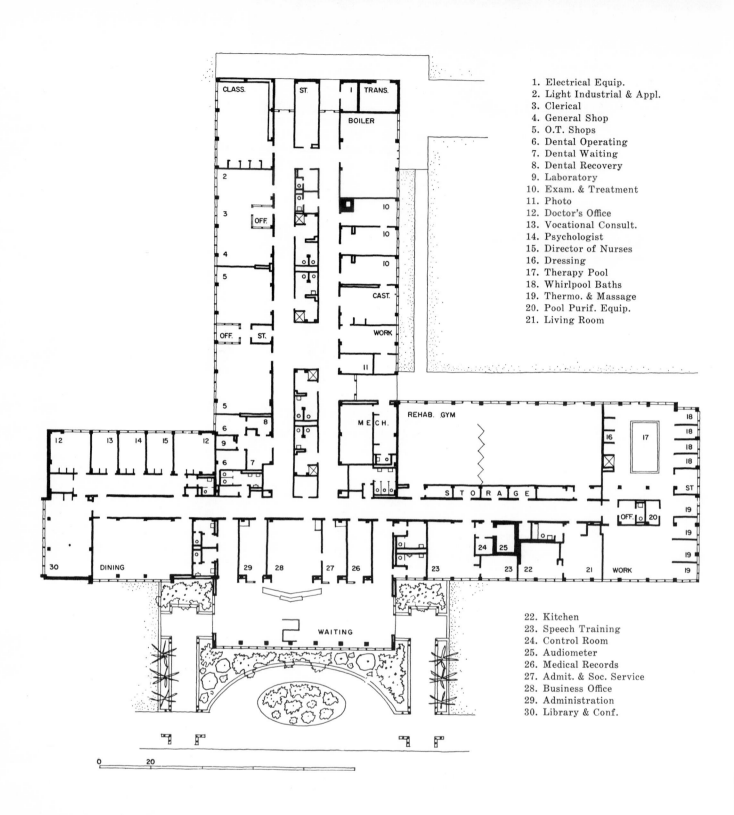

1. Electrical Equip.
2. Light Industrial & Appl.
3. Clerical
4. General Shop
5. O.T. Shops
6. Dental Operating
7. Dental Waiting
8. Dental Recovery
9. Laboratory
10. Exam. & Treatment
11. Photo
12. Doctor's Office
13. Vocational Consult.
14. Psychologist
15. Director of Nurses
16. Dressing
17. Therapy Pool
18. Whirlpool Baths
19. Thermo. & Massage
20. Pool Purif. Equip.
21. Living Room

22. Kitchen
23. Speech Training
24. Control Room
25. Audiometer
26. Medical Records
27. Admit. & Soc. Service
28. Business Office
29. Administration
30. Library & Conf.

glazed tile hand-rails for handicapped persons; except the lobby: it is marble, metal panel and aluminum frame. All ceilings are acoustically treated with 12 by 12 perforated acoustical tile hung by suspension system. All floors, except for the lobby, are vinyl tile; the lobby floor is terrazzo. All doors are hollow-core formica covered, 3 ft 10 in. in width to allow for wheel chairs and stretchers. The hydrotherapy room is tile throughout. The gymnasium is concrete block, painted. The building is air conditioned throughout.

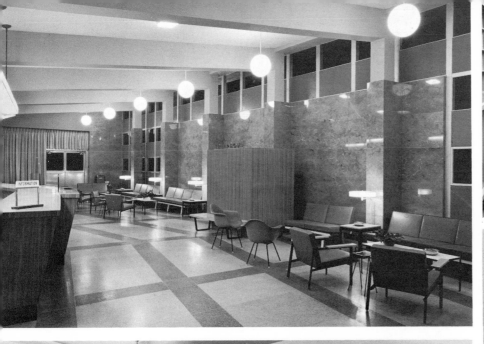
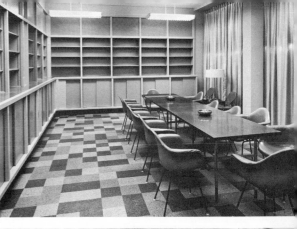
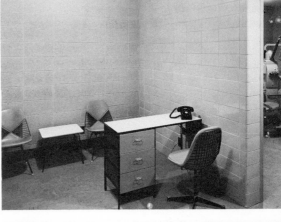
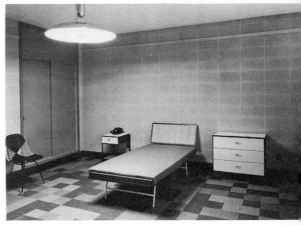
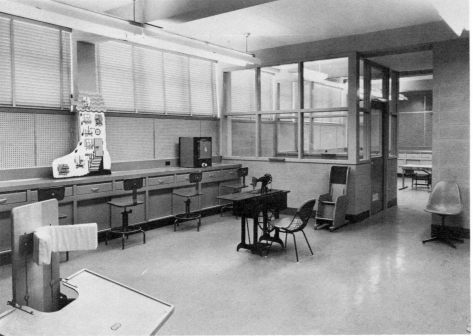
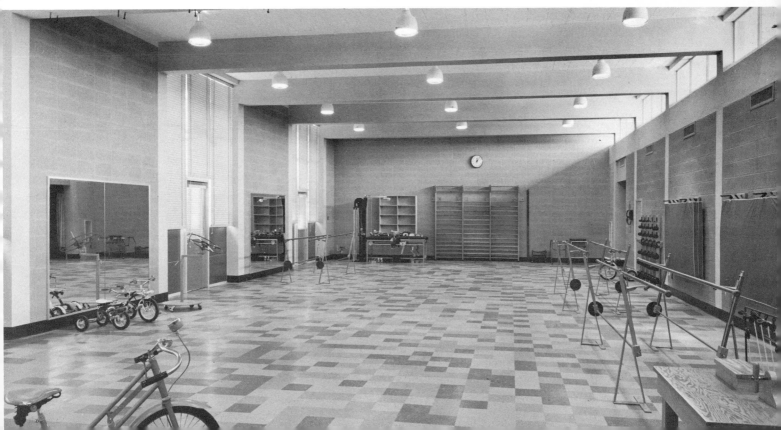

# Rehabilitation Center with Research Facilities

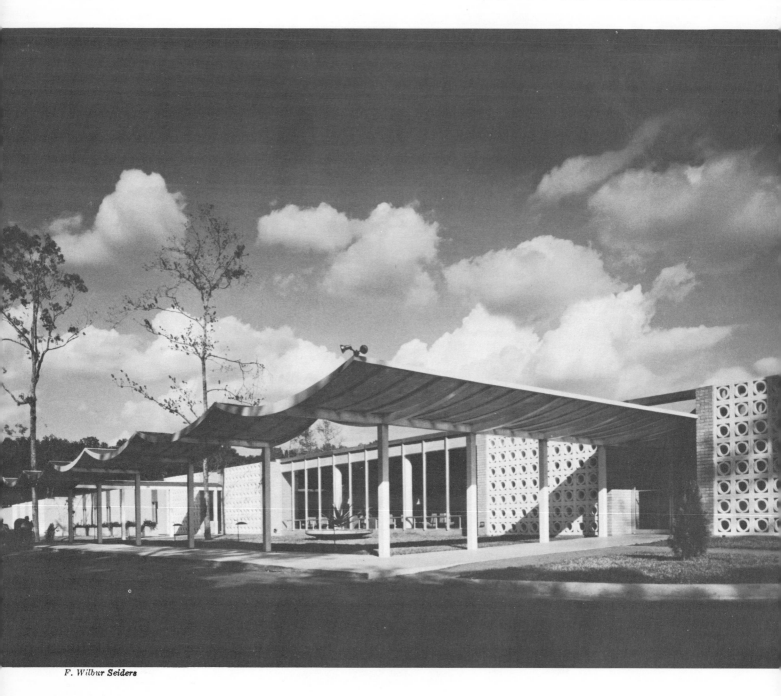

F. Wilbur *Seiders*

TEXAS INSTITUTE FOR REHABILITATION AND RESEARCH

LOCATION: *Houston, Texas*

ARCHITECTS: *Wilson, Morris, Crain and Anderson*

STRUCTURAL ENGINEER: *Walter P. Moore*

CONSULTING ENGINEERS: *Dale S. Cooper and Associates*

CONTRACTOR: *Knutson Construction Company*

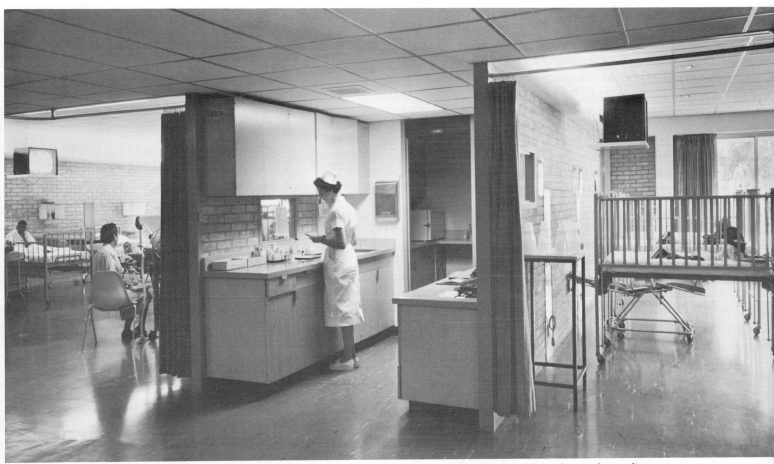

A nurse's station is located in the center of each nursing unit. Here it subdivides the children's nursing unit

F. Wilbur Seiders

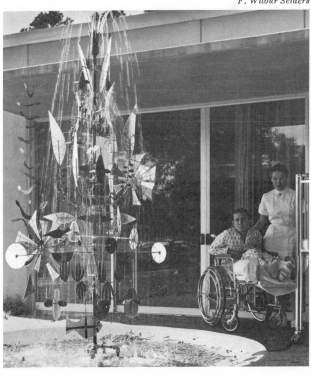

In recent years government financial aid has encouraged the construction of rehabilitation centers for the survivors of catastrophic disease. These people, rendered tragic and desperate by their disabilities, through comprehensive treatment and training can learn to enjoy their lives, take care of themselves, and play their role in society. The Texas Institute for Rehabilitation and Research is a representative example of the new centers. A pilot project to demonstrate the value of a comprehensive medical program, it is a non-profit, charitable, scientific and educational enterprise. Physical medicine and physical therapy are the essentials of any complete rehabilitation service. This 54-bed unit for in-patients and out-patients with multiple disabilities of severe degree, provides intensive integrated services in the four basic areas of rehabilitation: medical, psychological, social and vocational. It also provides research and teaching facilities.

A playful fountain helps avoid a depressing institutional character

Total cost of the center was approximately $1,350,000. $676,000 of this came from Hill-Burton funds and the balance from local philanthropy. Hill-Burton, known officially as the Hospital Survey and Construction Program, provides Federal funds to match state and local tax funds or private contributions in the construction of both public and voluntary non-profit hospitals. Several years ago Hill-Burton was extended to include non-profit rehabilitation facilities for the disabled, and this Texas treatment center is among the first buildings completed under the extended program.

The site is a 4½-acre area located in Houston's Texas Medical Center. Rehabilitation units are best located in medical centers for several major reasons: 1. the many kinds of specialists required in the early stages of rehabilitation are available; 2. training programs exist or can be planned to relieve shortages of personnel; 3. specialists' assistance in the development of treatment techniques can be readily obtained; 4. rehabilitation can be begun as early as possible in conjunction with treatment provided patient in other parts of the center; 5. duplication of personnel and equipment is avoided.

The building is of concrete frame construction with a **suspended concrete floor** slab and pre-cast concrete joist roof framing. Interior walls are 4-in. brick, exterior walls are brick and stucco. Windows and doors are aluminum frame. Because of the great physical exertion involved in rehabilitation it has been recommended that every rehabilitation building be air conditioned. This one is provided with both summer and winter air conditioning.

The architects state that the building was modularly coordinated and that drafting and specification time was greatly reduced thereby. They maintained a low hospital budget with a construction cost of about $16.00 per sq ft which included much of the built-in cabinet work.

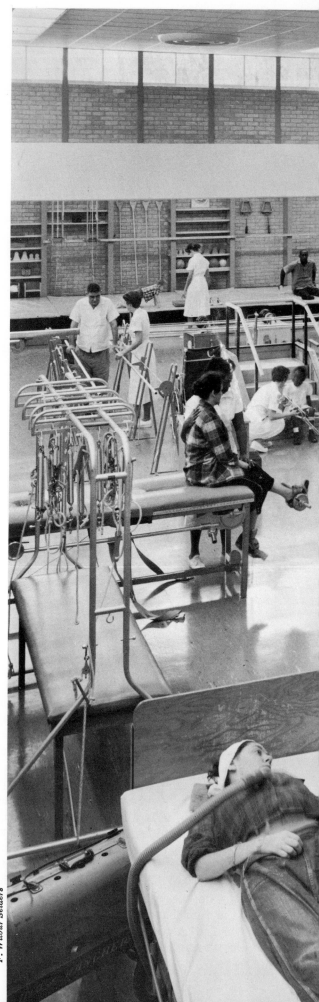

F. Wilbur Seiders

Most patients are paraplegics, quadriplegics or individuals with pulmonary or cardiovascular insufficiency. Non-functional, dependent, as a group they require every available service. A large open physical therapy room is recommended, not only for economy and ease of operation but for its value to patient morale. The patient takes comfort and encouragement in watching the constructive effort and improving skills of others. Note use of mezzanine for observation by professional staff

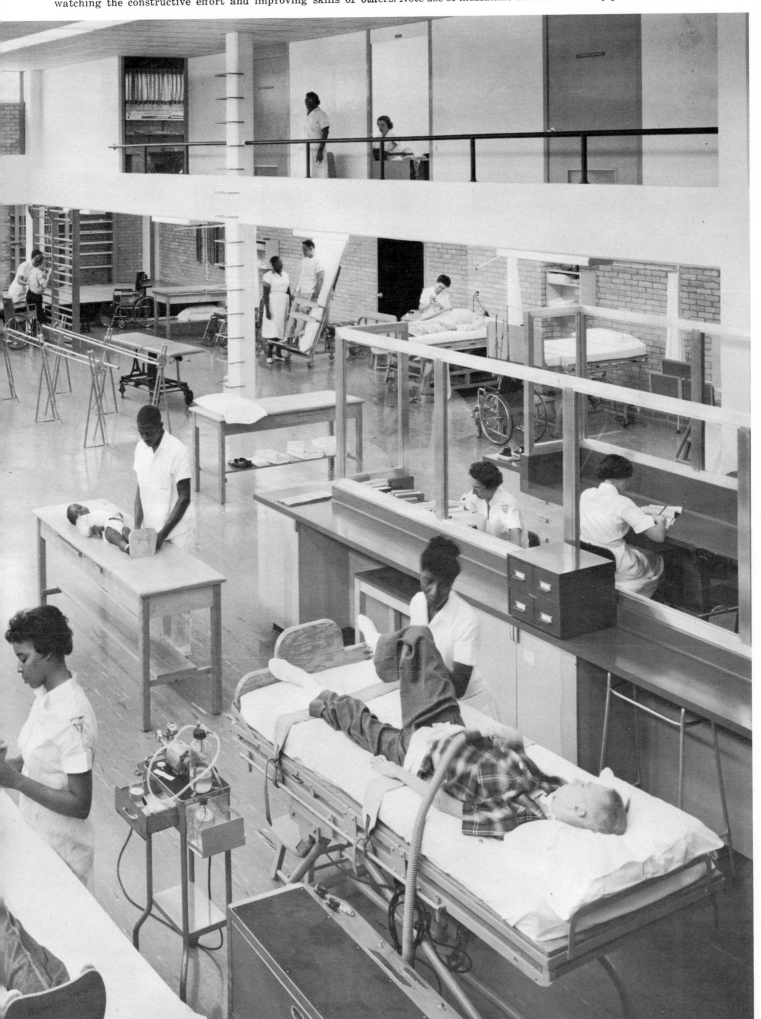

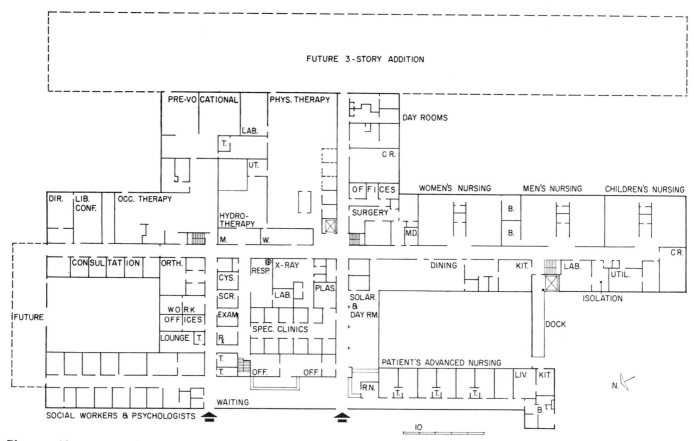

FUTURE 3-STORY ADDITION

Plan provides generous area for social workers and psychologists. In rehabilitation centers psychologists test, evaluate and counsel patients. They also counsel the staff about the reactions of the patients to their disabilities. Medical social workers are a link with the patient's family and community

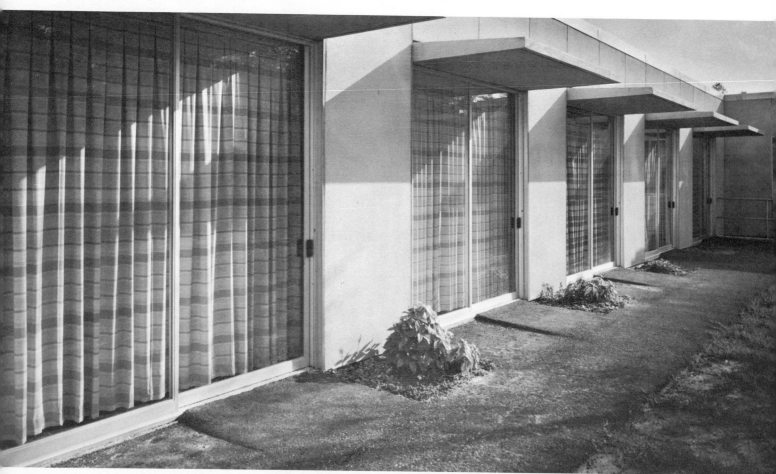

Sliding glass panels provide easy access to outdoors. Note gentle ramps for wheel chairs

*Texas Institute for Rehabilitation and Research*

# Rehabilitation Center for a Small Community

## CAROLYN ROSE STRAUSS REHABILITATION CENTER

OWNER: *Ouachita Parish Society for Crippled Children and Adults*

LOCATION: *Monroe, Louisiana*

ARCHITECTS: *Curtis and Davis, and Associated Architects and Engineers*

CONSULTING MECHANICAL AND ELECTRICAL ENGINEERS: *deLaureal and Moses*

CONTRACTOR: *F. C. Eason Construction Company*

In contrast to the preceding rehabilitation center, this one is very small in scope. It is restricted to children all of whom are ambulatory or wheel chair patients, and handles approximately fifteen of them per day. There are no in-patients. On two days each month general clinics are held and on these days 60 to 130 children accompanied by parents are accommodated. The center is in a small community and serves a large surrounding area in Northern Louisiana.

The waiting area could not economically be made large enough to take care of the twice monthly overflow crowds so a waiting patio and an outdoor canopied area have been provided. The patio admits sunlight to the waiting area. Built-in seating imposes an order on the crowds and conserves space. The examination and treatment areas are arranged in the sequence the patient travels and establish an orderly flow of traffic on clinic days. Office locations have been planned to help control and direct patients.

Three exterior walls face streets and are made of brick with no openings for the sake of privacy. Skylights are extensively used in the smaller rooms. The therapy rooms have been placed in the rear of the structure and overlook a fenced-in play yard which in the future will have a swimming pool. The rear wall is glass from floor to ceiling with doors providing access from the therapy rooms to the yard where other forms of therapy take place.

Certain rules for correct detailing in rehabilitation centers were followed. Heavy duty pre-polished vinyl flooring was used for its slip resistant quality and for its resistance to permanent indentation resulting from concentrated loads of equipment. Doors are oversized and furnished with special hardware, toilets are equipped with special grips and other devices, and drinking fountains project from the wall to facilitate use from wheelchair or crutches.

The entire building is air conditioned the year round. Built with the assistance of Hill-Burton funds, its cost was $124,770 including all construction, extras, built-in furniture and landscaping. Cost of land, other furniture, and architects' fee are not included in this figure.

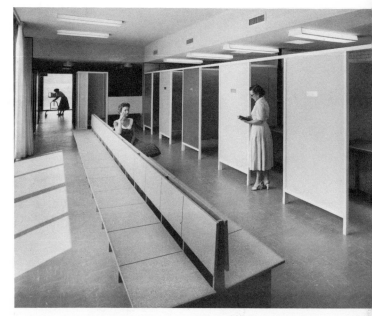

Waiting bench outside consultation and guidance booths

Entrance is without steps and protected by canopy. Seats are to help handle overflow on general clinic days

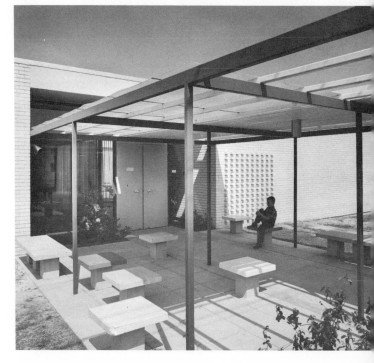

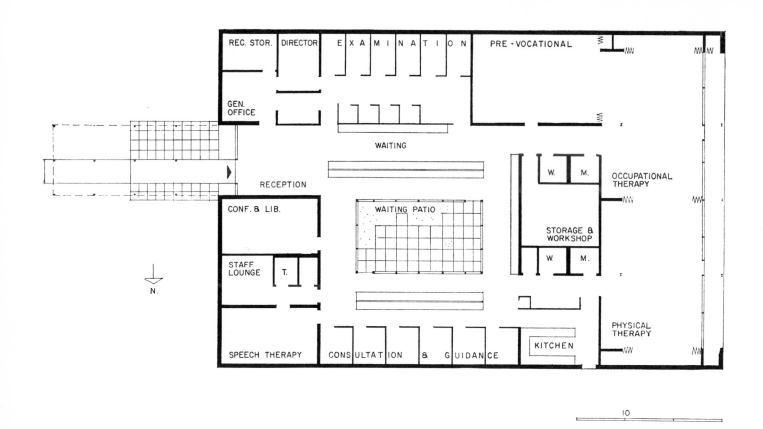

*Frank Lotz Miller*

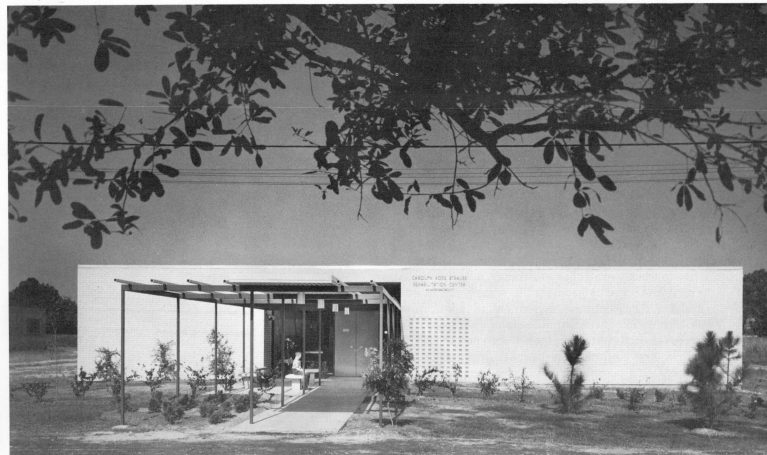

Because of need for privacy building is closed on three sides but opens onto a fenced play-yard at rear

# HEALTH CENTERS, CLINICS, and DOCTORS' OFFICES

# Planning the Public Health Center

HEALTH CENTERS under the Hill-Burton program, range in size from 1000 to 20,000 sq ft in area. The national median size is about 5000 sq ft, but the most common size is the health center with about 3000 sq ft. The latter is considered a small health center, capable of serving a rural area population of up to 35,000.

Desirable minimum or basic functions of a local health department include vital statistics, sanitation supervision, communicable disease control, laboratory services, maternal and child health, dental hygiene and health education. To these has recently been added control of chronic diseases, which promotes case finding and diagnostic services for arthritis, cancer, cardiac, or diabetes cases among others. Rehabilitation for these and other types of cases is very often available. Accident prevention, the hygiene of housing, industrial hygiene, school health services, and hospital and medical care are other areas of service which are being incorporated into many local health programs. Most state governments have established within their official health agencies consulting services which are prepared to assist in organizing these health services at the local level. Fitting the new service into the local health program must be carefully planned after thorough studies have been made. Such studies must aim at improving the whole field of public health.

Space requirements may be determined largely from the clinic schedule and the list of personnel. The clinic schedule is an arbitrary allotment of hours to accommodate estimated case loads for the several health services outlined in the program. Case loads are estimated from a study of local statistics, pertinent to each of the proposed health services. Type health center plans and schedules have been developed, using national averages and standards. It is suggested that these schedules be used only as patterns into which local statistics are substituted. Some services, such as dental hygiene, are quite variable in different areas and, as a result, solid standards are not available. Consultation with local health officials is then advisable. Provision for maximum rather than minimum loads is recommended in view of future expansion.

The general architectural plan can now take shape in a schematic drawing showing the arrangement and relationship of the five main areas of a health center. These are:

1. Waiting, including the main entrance.
2. Administration, including offices and record space.
3. Clinic, including sub-waiting, exam, treatment and consultation rooms.
4. Assembly, including storage for projector, film, etc.
5. Service, including heating, storage and maintenance rooms.

The size of the health center laboratory will be determined by the size of the community and the amount of work done by other laboratories in the area or at the state level. The laboratory serves the clinician, the epidemiologist, the nurse, the milk inspector or the sanitary engineer, in examining submitted specimens. Today's standards indicate about 6000 such examinations a year per 100,000 population. Space and equipment for conducting bacteriological, microscopic, physical and chemical examinations and analyses must be calculated, keeping in mind possible expansion of services in these fields. Proper storage space for biological products, drugs, and antibiotics, to be drawn upon by private physicians and by disease prevention services, should be studied and provided. The laboratory is usually located adjacent to the sanitary engineers, as it largely serves them.

In designing the clinic area a certain freedom of use of some areas should be considered. Most of the services provided in health center clinics today may safely share common areas and facilities. Multi-use of clinic space should be exploited in the interest of economy, not only of expensive space but of valuable personnel. Careful scheduling can accomplish much in this direction. In small health centers, general clinics are not uncommon.

The specialized rooms such as dental and X-ray rooms, are not adaptable to use by other clinics. Crippled children, multiple screening programs, cardiac or cancer clinics, are some which might use the X-ray room. The dental room might also serve cancer clinics or multiple-screening programs for oral inspections.

It is suggested that a type of examination-consultation room be developed wherein the physician can do a complete examination, consultation and write-up on each patient. This is facilitated if the usual dressing cubicle is replaced simply by a draw curtain about the examination area of the room. Concern over the safety of their belongings is relieved and any tendency to dawdle is discouraged.

Such exam-consultation rooms should be arranged in groups of two or more intercommunicating rooms to permit the physician to work most efficiently. While the patient prepares for examination behind the curtain, the physician can be checking his medical record or attending the patient in the adjoining room. Consultation may proceed during examination and continue while the patient dresses.

It is possible then to place sub-waiting areas and nurses' work stations for one or more clinics with the bank of exam-consultation rooms. The nurses' work stations may be within the sub-waiting area, in the waiting room for maternal and child health or in a kind of utility-treatment room, set up for injections, in connection with venereal diseases and other contagious diseases and for minor emergency treatments, blood tests, etc. A toilet facility is also necessary in this area.

These exam-consulting rooms are adaptable to many uses by the nurses. Private consultations with patients, private phone calls in connection with patients, and write-up work can be done by them in these rooms. In case there is no room provided for venereal disease interviews one of these rooms might well be used.

Though separate interview and examination facilities are still desirable for the tuberculosis clinic, with proper scheduling and technique, these rooms could be utilized where space restrictions make it necessary.

Case-finding, diagnostic and post-hospital cases comprise the bulk of the tuberculosis clinic work. Pneumotherapy requires weekly treatments, so special arrangements, such as referral to a specialist or to a hospital, may be expedient. Pneumotherapy in the health center is said to have diminished to an average of only 10 per cent of the regular tuberculosis clinic load today.

The tuberculosis clinic should provide facilities for at least 16 cases per session, to justify the mustering of the one medical specialist, one technician, two nurses experienced in interviewing, and one clerk-receptionist, needed to operate this clinic efficiently. The physician will need an exam-consultation room, with facilities for reading and interpreting X-ray films. The technician will operate the X-ray room where a combination unit for radiography and fluoroscopy should be provided. This will provide for 14 in. by 17 in. plates as well as a quick method of checking chest conditions with the fluoroscope. The fluoroscope is also needed for the pneumotherapy process.

If photo-fluorographic (35 and 70 mm. film) case-finding programs are planned for the health center for an average of 50 or more per session, they may warrant the increased cost of equipment and increased room size entailed in the more powerful unit and the supplemental equipment, such as a hood and camera. Usually case-finding is more economically provided by mobile X-ray units which visit schools, health centers and other local meeting places in most states. Many hospitals are also providing this service for each patient coming through their receiving departments.

Pneumotherapy will require a special treatment room, adjacent to the X-ray room. This room should provide a work counter with sink and cupboards under. At least three dressing cubicles between the X-ray room and sub-waiting are required in connection with this treatment, as well as for the regular radiographic work.

Two nurses will be needed to interview patients, to advise them, according to the physician's findings and to mobilize their courses of treatment, hospitalization, social welfare and rehabilitation. For this purpose, each nurse should have a small semi-private room or cubicle adjacent to sub-waiting and to the physician's exam-consultation room. The clerk-receptionist's station may

be set up adjacent to the sub-waiting area where control of the patients and their medical records will be maintained.

Demonstration work in the maternal and child health clinic has expanded to include fathers in many areas. This, coupled with crowded clinic sessions, has often resulted in formation of special instruction classes which must be held in the assembly room or other larger meeting places.

The provision of dental facilities in the health center is decided in the program. In a community of 50,000, for example, dental care for only those school children who cannot pay will justify a full-time dentist and a fully equipped dental facility. Dental examination of school children is provided in most of the schools of the nation. The large majority of those needing care are referred to family dentists. Indigent cases, through local dental societies, are cared for in private offices, hospital clinics, health centers, etc. Many health departments are also providing dental care for pre-natal, pre-school, venereal disease and tuberculosis patients and these clinics are very often synchronized in health center schedules.

Nutrition programs will seldom require space in the average health center. They are usually part of the health education program and are integrated into the work of the health educator, the public health nurses and the clinic physicians. In a large urban or district health department, office space should be provided for a nutritionist or nutrition supervisor. This specialist will inform and train the nurses in good nutrition for use in their everyday field work.

It is estimated that one full-time mental health clinic per 50,000 population should be provided as a minimum need. Mental health programs are still in an early developmental state and standards are quite undetermined. A full-time clinic is defined as one with at least one professional staff member on duty 35 hours or more per week. A fully effective mental health service should have the skills of a multi-discipline team, made of a psychiatrist, a clinical psychologist, two psychiatric social workers and a clerk-typist.

In the average health center, where a part time mental health clinic might be set up, common use areas and multi-purpose examination rooms might suffice, with careful scheduling. A mental health clinic should hold at least two sessions per week, preferably three. Although child guidance predominates in these clinics it is recognized that mental hygiene has much to contribute in the field of chronic diseases and geriatrics.

In the field of chronic diseases the efforts of health departments are still concentrated on education of the public in improved health habits, leading to prevention or early diagnosis of heart disease, cancer, diabetes or other similar long term incapacitating diseases. Mass case-finding programs seem not far in the future. The health center should be planned accordingly, for adaptation of existing space and coördination of extensions.

# Check List on Health Center Planning

Multiple use of clinic rooms is considered practical if proper technique is enforced. General clinics, wherein a variety of health services are rendered in one area at one session, are common. However, where certain individual clinic loads are heavy, it is practical to limit the clinic use to that one health service.

Dressing cubicles for examination rooms are not recommended. If draw curtains are provided around the examination table area, dressing and undressing is expedited.

Assignment of patients to several sub-waiting areas reassures the patient of more personal and prompt attention. Location of these areas on an exterior wall makes them more cheerful and inviting. Lightweight metal armchairs permit a variety of arrangement. They are more comfortable than fixed or built-in benches.

Counters and cabinets are not feasible in examination rooms. Rooms equipped with a lavatory, an examination table, an instrument table or cabinet and an examination light are adequate. Examination rooms should be at least 9 ft wide, however.

Toilets should always be provided within or directly accessible to the clinic area.

The dental clinic should be located close to the main lobby to minimize interference with other clinics. It should be arranged as an optional area, readily omitted as the program dictates.

The pneumotherapy room should also be planned as an optional area.

Photofluorography (small-film mass case finding) should be provided in the X-ray room only if 50 or more cases are processed per clinic session. This entails extra space and cost to provide for the more powerful unit and supplemental camera, hood, etc.

X-ray film files for 5 years are usually stored in the tuberculosis interview room. Dark rooms are often too small even for occasional use. A minimum inside dimension of 6 ft by 6 ft is recommended. The door width should be determined by the size of the dark room equipment.

Outdoor play area, located off the clinic wing, should be enclosed and a portion of it covered and screened.

Provide appropriate and properly sized storage closets in convenient locations in the clinic wing.

In the nurses' workroom instruments and materials used in the clinics are cleaned, sterilized and set up. Here, also, blood samples and smears are taken and stored or examined. Injections and immunizations are given and entries are made on patients' record cards. This room is also adaptable to use by diagnostic clinics for cardiacs, diabetes, arthritis, etc.

Assembly rooms are valuable not only for providing health education programs but for other community use. Facilities for movies, microphones and storage of supplementary equipment such as film projectors, film, display racks, folding chairs and tables as well as posters, pamphlets and other printed matter should be provided. Air conditioning will also increase the value of the assembly room. A built-in kitchenette including a range, a sink and cupboards is often provided for demonstration work in connection with some clinics.

Staff toilets should provide a few lockers to accommodate the volunteer workers. Rest rooms are also recommended at least for the female members of the staff.

The offices of the health officer and his staff are preferred at a distance from the public lobby and near a separate staff entrance.

The laboratory is equipped to serve the clinic and the sanitary engineers in performing bacteriological, microscopic, physical and chemical examinations and analyses of specimens submitted or collected. It is located adjacent to the sanitary engineers, whom it largely serves. Proper storage space is provided for fresh supplies of biological products, drugs and antibiotics, which are distributed to physicians and disease prevention services, according to policy established by the State Agency supplying them.

Where play areas are assigned in waiting rooms, a cabinet for storage and display of toys should be provided.

A covered terrace for parking of perambulators is much appreciated.

Avoid entering public toilet rooms directly from waiting areas. Water closets should be separated from lavatories by stall partitions wherever possible.

Future extensions to all wings should be considered in anticipation of new health programs and added services.

It is suggested that high window sills be avoided in administrative offices and waiting areas, in the interest of better ventilation and view.

Air conditioning of the entire health center building is desirable, wherever possible.

Acoustical treatment of ceilings to reduce sound transmission must be considered, especially in clinic examination and interview rooms and in conference or assembly rooms. Better insulation against transmission of heat should be provided in roof spaces, especially where flat roofs are used.

The nurses' work room should be located adjacent to the medical records for convenient reference. Where space permits, the area should be subdivided into rooms of four nurses each.

# Mechanical and Electrical Systems for Health Centers

THE mechanical work consisting of: plumbing, heating, ventilation, and in the warmer climates, cooling systems, requires careful study to achieve efficient service at a minimal operating cost.

**Plumbing.** Fixture placement and service piping should be so planned as to permit future room changes with a minimum of disturbance. The selection of fixtures and fixture trim for the clinical areas is of particular importance. Hand washing facilities used by doctors and nurses in the examination and treatment areas should be trimmed with elbow, knee action or foot action valves as required.

Non-corrosive water heater storage tanks and hot water piping systems are recommended.

**Heating.** Hot water heating with thermostatically controlled zones provides an economical system for this type of structure where intermittent use of the clinical section may occur and where evening meetings utilizing the assembly room are not uncommon.

In warmer climates where air cooling is essential, a warm air heating and cooling system utilizing the same duct system may reduce installation costs.

Where a separate air cooling system is contemplated, consideration should be given to individual systems for administrative and clinical areas.

Automatic firing is recommended to provide for weekend and unsupervised heating service.

**Ventilation.** As mass clinics are the order rather than the exception, ample ventilation is recommended for assembly and waiting rooms which will often be overcrowded. Ample ventilation is also required for the X-ray rooms which may be tight areas because of light proof shades and ray protection required. The exhaust from film dryer and the dark room should be discharged to the outside.

**Electrical.** The minimum standards recommended for electrical work in health centers is that of the National Electrical Code. Where movable partitions are installed, wiring should be arranged for minimum interruption of service when such partitions are relocated.

X-ray equipment and wiring should conform with the applicable requirements of article 660 of the National Electrical Code, and the National Electrical Manufacturers Association's "wiring data and minimum power requirements." As a minimum, the power feeder to the X-ray unit should be direct from the main distribution panel or from a separate transformer. Where portable X-ray is used, polarized receptacles on one circuit are recommended to minimize the probability of other loads being plugged in on the circuit and causing voltage fluctuations while the X-ray unit is being operated. Rooms or areas containing fixed (nonportable) X-ray equipment should have ray protection as recommended in National Bureau of Standards' Handbook 41. (See also Handbook 50, "X-ray Protection Design.")

For supplying power to mobile or ambulatory bus X-ray units, two weather resistant (raintight) receptacles on separate circuits, located outside the building convenient to parking area are recommended: One 60A., 220 V., 1-phase, 3-wire, 3-pole for X-ray, and one 30A., 110 V., 1-phase, 2-wire, 3-pole for lighting, heating and other utilities.

*Proper lighting* is conducive to efficient work, influences better housekeeping, accentuates architectural beauty and is economical. Fixtures should be of a type, or so located, as to avoid objectionable glare. To encourage proper maintenance, fixtures should be easy to clean and to relamp. Parking lots should be lighted.

A signal system, either buzzer or intercommunication type, should be provided which will permit the health officer to originate calls to other principal areas.

**Catastrophes.** In case of a major disaster such as that of enemy use of nuclear weapons and biological warfare, health centers located in or near target areas would be vitally needed to relieve overcrowded hospitals of some of the ambulant casualties. This would involve treatment and facilities somewhat different from those commonly required in health centers. As an example, decontamination would become an important and serious problem in treating people who have radioisotopes or deleterious biologicals on their person or clothing. For this service, washing or shower facilities would be needed at some segregated location so as to minimize the possibility of scattering these contaminants in other parts of the building. Disposal of contaminated clothing and a supply of other clothing should also be considered.

In view of the remote possibility, or infrequency, of such a disaster and the high cost of construction, it is recommended that health centers be designed to meet ordinary peacetime needs but that in probable target areas consideration be given to an arrangement whereby certain areas may be easily converted to such emergency use, either inside or outside the building.

# Type Plans for Health Centers

*Possible clinic-use schedules based on analyses of clinic loads in public health centers (revised)*

In determining space requirements for health centers a clinic schedule and personnel roster will be found helpful. Case loads and personnel requirements may be estimated according to standard practice and local vital statistics. In view of possible expansion, maximum rather than minimum standards should be used.

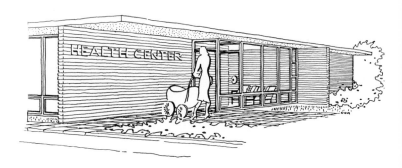

| Session / Clinic | Type A (Revised) 35,000 Pop. Visits | Type B-1 60,000 Pop. Visits | Type C (Revised) 100,000 Pop. Visits |
|---|---|---|---|
| **Monday** | | | |
| A.M. Prenatal | 10 | 12 | — |
| Dental | 7 | 7 | — |
| Mental Hygiene (Child Guidance) | — | — | 20 |
| P.M. Prenatal | — | 12 | 12 |
| Child Health | — | — | 16 |
| Venereal Disease | 22 | — | — |
| Eve. Venereal Disease | — | 25 | 25 |
| Mental Hygiene | — | — | 20 |
| **Tuesday** | | | |
| A.M. Prenatal | — | — | 12 |
| Dental | 7 | 7 | 14 |
| Child Health | 16 | 16 | 16 |
| P.M. Prenatal | 10 | — | — |
| Dental | — | — | 14 |
| Child Health | — | 16 | 16 |
| Eve. Dental | — | — | 14 |
| Venereal Disease | — | — | 25 |
| **Wednesday** | | | |
| A.M. Dental | — | 7 | 14 |
| Child Health | — | 16 | 16 |
| P.M. Prenatal | — | 12 | 12 |
| Child Health | — | 16 | 16 |
| **Thursday** | | | |
| A.M. Prenatal | — | — | 12 |
| Dental | — | 7 | — |
| Child Health | 16 | 16 | 16 |
| P.M. Prenatal | — | — | 12 |
| Child Health | 16 | — | 16 |
| Mental Hygiene (Child Guidance) | — | 20 | — |
| Eve. Venereal Disease | — | — | 25 |
| Mental Hygiene | — | 20 | 20 |
| **Friday** | | | |
| A.M. Dental | 7 | 7 | — |
| Child Health | — | — | 16 |
| Tuberculosis | 16 [1] | 20 [2] | — |
| P.M. Dental | — | — | 14 |
| Venereal Disease | — | 25 | 25 |
| Mental Hygiene | — | 20 | — |
| Tuberculosis | — | — | 23 |
| Eve. Venereal Disease | 22 | 25 | 25 |
| Tuberculosis | 16 [3] | 20 [4] | 23 [5] |
| Total visits per week | 145 | 306 | 477 |
| Total visits per year | 7,540 | 15,912 | 24,830 |
| Total sessions per week | 10.75 | 20 | 27.5 |
| Total sessions per year | 559 | 1,140 | 1,430 |

[1] (2/mo.)  [3] (3/mo.)
[2] (1/mo.)  [4] (1/mo.)  [5] (2/mo.)

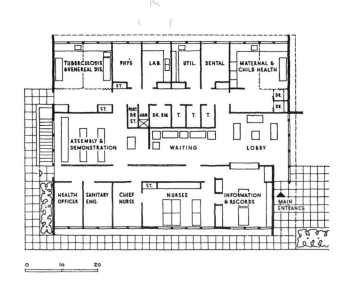

## TYPE A HEALTH CENTER

This basic one-story health center, with floor area of 3000 sq ft, is designed for a community of approximately 35,000 population.

Two clinic rooms are supplemented by a utility room, a laboratory, a consultation room and a dental room along one side of an extra wide corridor, which serves as lobby, waiting and assembly room.

On the opposite side of this light and open corridor are the administrative offices. The staff will include 1 health officer, 1 chief nurse, 6 public health nurses, 1 or 2 sanitary engineers and 2 clerks.

A part basement (not shown) contains storage for equipment, supplies and dead records, a maintenance room and the boiler and fuel room.

About 7600 patient-visits can be handled per year.

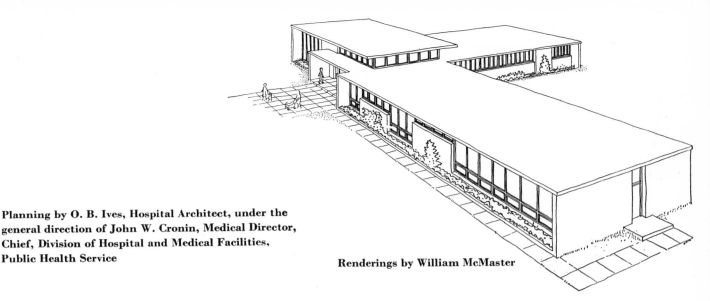

Planning by O. B. Ives, Hospital Architect, under the general direction of John W. Cronin, Medical Director, Chief, Division of Hospital and Medical Facilities, Public Health Service

Renderings by William McMaster

# TYPE B-1 HEALTH CENTER

For a community with a maximum population of about 60,000, this one-story facility with floor area of 5960 sq ft, provides separate sections for clinics, administration and assembly, all opening off a main waiting room. The clinic wing provides facilities for tuberculosis control (including X-ray), dental hygiene and a multiple purpose area. Prenatal and child health clinics, immunizations, venereal disease treatments and test and diagnostic clinics for some chronic diseases can make use of this multiple purpose area.

The administration wing contains information counter, records room, laboratory and offices for public health nurses, health officer, health educator, medical social service worker and secretaries, plus staff toilets.

The assembly room has been provided for meetings,

conferences, educational lectures and demonstration classes. This wing can be locked off separately.

A part basement (not shown) contains storage for equipment, supplies and dead records, a maintenance room and the boiler and fuel room.

Minimum full-time staff includes 1 health officer, 1 chief nurse, 1 assistant chief nurse, 12 public health nurses, 4 sanitary engineers (including the chief engineer), 1 health educator, 1 medical social service worker, 1 laboratory technician, 2 secretaries and 3 clerks.

Part time staff may include clinic physicians, a venereal disease investigator, mental hygiene personnel, dentists, and volunteer clerks and aides.

Some 16,000 patient-visits can be handled per year.

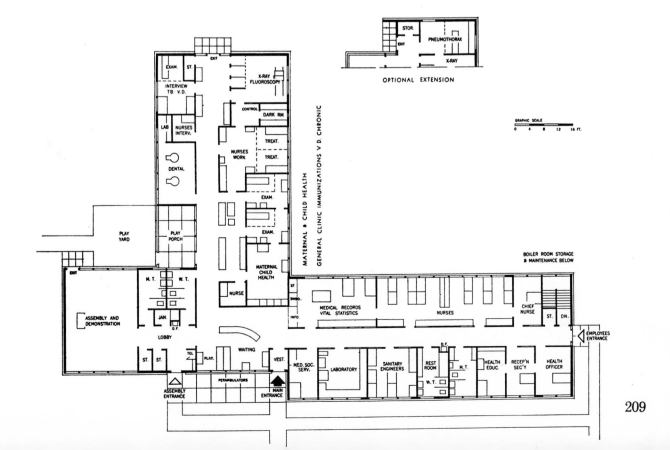

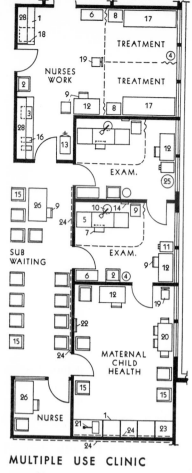

## MULTIPLE USE CLINIC

GRAPHIC SCALE
0  2  4  6  8 FT.

# EQUIPMENT LEGEND

*Plans of Principal Departments of the Type B Public Health Center, with Equipment Indications*

1. Work counter with cabinets below
2. Lavatory with gooseneck spout and knee or elbow control
3. Sink with gooseneck spout and knee or elbow control
4. Sanitary waste receptacle
5. Examination table
6. Instrument cabinet
7. Operator's footstool
8. Instrument table
9. Straight chair
10. Gooseneck examination light
11. Mayo table
12. Nurses' flat top desk, 20″ x 36″
13. Pressure sterilizer on stand, 12″ x 20″
14. Hook strip
15. Armchair
16. Microscopes, 1 ordinary and 1 dark field
17. Treatment table
18. Refrigerator, under counter
19. Clinical scale
20. Children's table and chairs
21. Infant scale
22. Pamphlet rack
23. Baby dressing bins
24. Educational display
25. Laundry hamper
26. Single pedestal desk
27. Executive chair
28. Wall cabinet
29. Clothes locker, 15″ x 15″ x 60″
30. Wastepaper receptacle
31. Filing cabinet, letter size, 4 drawer
32. Film filing cabinet, 3 drawer
33. Control unit
34. Film storage bin
35. Developing tank, with thermostatic mixing valve
36. Film loading counter, 36″ high, cabinets, cassette bins and film storage bins below
37. Wall hung film drier, water cooler below
38. Towel bar
39. Safe light
40. Timer
41. Mirror
42. Executive type desk
43. Combination radiographic, fluoroscopic unit
44. Cassette changer
45. Lead lining (size and extent varies)
46. Leaded glass view window
47. X-ray film illuminator
48. Lightproof shade

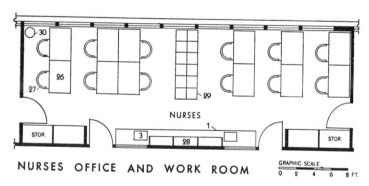

## NURSES OFFICE AND WORK ROOM

GRAPHIC SCALE
0  2  4  6  8 FT.

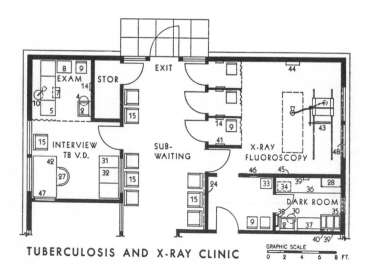

## TUBERCULOSIS AND X-RAY CLINIC

GRAPHIC SCALE
0  2  4  6  8 FT.

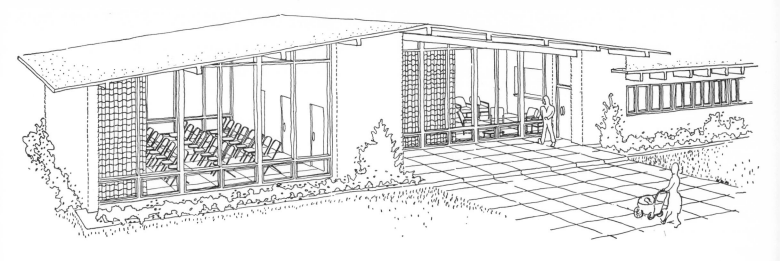

## TYPE C HEALTH CENTER

For a community with a maximum population of about 100,000, this one-story facility, with floor area of 9570 sq ft, provides separate sections for clinics, administration and assembly, all opening off a main waiting room. The clinic wing has facilities for tuberculosis control, including X-ray, dental hygiene, and a multiple purpose area. Prenatal and child health clinics, immunizations, venereal disease treatments and tests and diagnostic clinics for some chronic diseases can use this area.

The administration wing contains separate counters for clinic information and for health certificates or vital statistics in the records room. Offices for public health nurses, health officers, sanitary engineers, health educator, medical social service worker and secretaries, as well as a staff room and library and a laboratory are also provided. A rest room for female staff, staff toilets and necessary storage closets complete this wing.

The assembly room has been provided for meetings, conferences, educational lectures and demonstration classes. This wing can be locked off from the rest of the building.

A part basement (not shown) contains storage for equipment, supplies and dead records, a maintenance shop and the boiler and fuel room.

Minimum full-time staff includes 1 health officer, 1 assistant health officer, 1 chief nurse, 1 assistant chief nurse, 20 public health nurses; 1 chief engineer, 7 sanitary engineers, 1 health educator, 1 medical social service worker, 1 laboratory chemist, 1 laboratory technician, 1 laboratory clerk, 3 secretaries and 6 clerks.

Part time staff may include clinic physicians, venereal disease investigators, mental hygiene personnel, dentists and volunteer clerks and aides.

About 25,000 patient-visits can be handled per year.

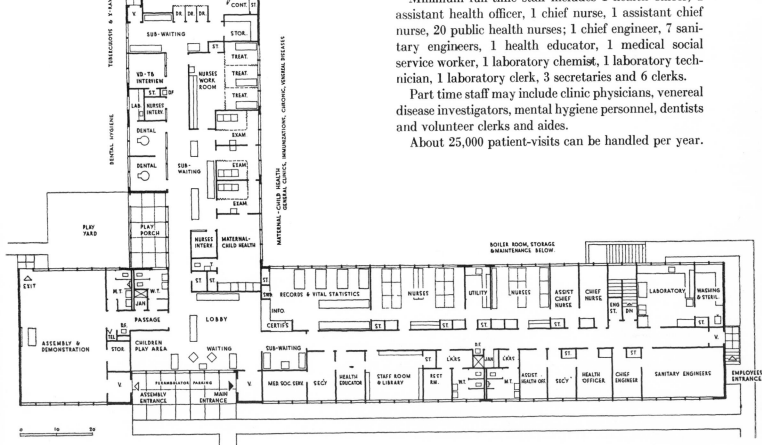

## PUBLIC HEALTH CENTER
## COST INFORMATION

National average cost figures for Public Health Centers participating in the Hospital and Medical Facilities Survey and Construction Program, U. S. Department of Health, Education and Welfare:

| Building and Fixed Equipment | Project Cost |
|---|---|
| $15.98 per Sq. Ft. | $19.02 Sq. Ft. |

The cost information that follows is also derived from the same source material. Additional cost information may be obtained from The Division of Hospital and Medical Facilities, Public Health Service, U. S. Department of Health, Education and Welfare, Washington 25, D. C.

Expressed as A Percentage of Average Project Cost.

General Construction............................ 60.8%
Mechanical...................................... 15.1%
Electrical...................................... 6.2%
Contingency..................................... 2.3%

Total Construction Contracts................... 84.4%
Group II & III Equipment....................... 9.2%*
Site Survey and Soil Investigation.............. .2%
Architect's fee................................. variable
Supervision & Inspection at Site................ 1.2%

* In many projects this equipment cost figure represents only the cost of equipment purchased to augment serviceable equipment on hand. Public Health Centers equipped with new Group II and III Equipment may be as much as 100% higher than this figure.
† variable.

## PRELIMINARY COST ESTIMATES

| Public Health Center Type | A | B-1 | C |
|---|---|---|---|
| for community with a maximum population of.............. | 35,000 | 60,000 | 100,000 |
| Approximate Gross Floor Areas: | | | |
| Basement S. F............... | 692 | 1,840 | 2,550 |
| 1st Floor S. F.............. | 3,008 | 5,960 | 9,570 |
| Total S. F............. .. | 3,700 | 7,800 | 12,120 |
| **Project Cost:** | | | |
| Construction Contract........ | $59,130 | $125,070 | $194,395 |
| Equipment (Group II & III)*.. | 6,500 | 13,630 | 21,185 |
| Site Survey & Soil Investigation | 150 | 300 | 400 |
| Architect's fee†.............. | 3,500 | 7,400 | 11,500 |
| Supervision & Inspection...... | 840 | 1,600 | 2,550 |
| Acquisition of Site........... | variable | variable | variable |
| Other....................... | 180 | 200 | 250 |
| **Total** | **$70,300** | **$148,200** | **$230,280** |

Project cost per S. F. (site not included) $19.00.

NOTE: The Construction Contract figures include an amount normally required for contingencies and Group I Equipment.

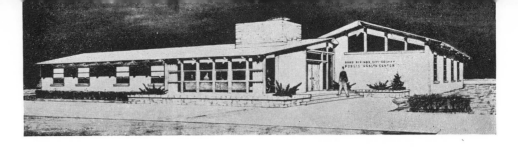

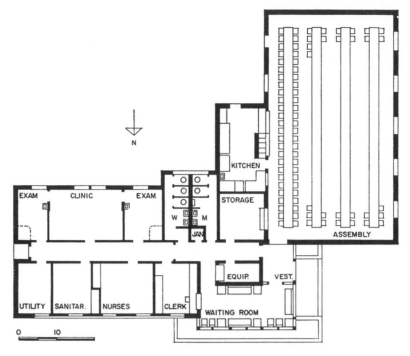

# Tulsa Builds Several Health Centers

*Outlying Health Centers*
*for Tulsa County*
*Tulsa, Oklahoma*
*McCune, McCune & McCune*
*Architects and Engineers*

HERE are three of five outlying public health centers, by the same architects, for a forward-looking program by Tulsa County. All five have similar plans (the one above is typical), and all were designed for a friendly, residential character. Health education is strongly stressed hence the larger assembly room, with kitchen for demonstrating food handling techniques. These facilities prove useful also for group luncheons and conferences in connection with health programs. The clinic department works on daily schedules for different health problems. The outlying centers operate in conjunction with a large downtown center, from which the program is administered.

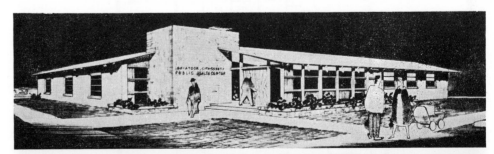

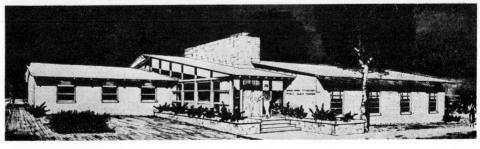

This one-story health center serves a county with a population of approximately 20,000. It is conveniently located within one block of the Jackson Hospital. The plan separates offices from clinic areas, with storage space between them. There are the usual offices for health officer, dental officer, nurses and sanitary engineer. The clinic serves for venereal disease, tuberculosis, maternity and child health. VD and TB clinics use the spaces nearest the X-ray department; maternity and child health are isolated in separate rooms.

Construction is concrete slab on grade. Exterior walls are brick, with aluminum awning type windows. Tile wainscots are used on walls of clinics, examining rooms, utility rooms, darkrooms; other interior walls are of plaster. Summer-winter air conditioning is used throughout the building. The building contains 5000 sq ft; cost something less than $75,000.

*1. Jackson County Health Center*
*Marianna, Florida*
*Sherlock, Smith & Adams*
*Architects and Engineers*

# Two Public

*2. Montgomery County*
*Health Center*
*Montgomery, Alabama*
*Sherlock, Smith & Adams*
*Architects and Engineers*

One of the larger county health centers, this one goes to two stories, contains 24,000 sq ft, and cost almost $500,000.

It houses the usual public health activities and facilities plus some of those not found in smaller centers. There is a mental health clinic, and clinics also for polio therapy and immunization. Educational sessions are correspondingly increased, X-ray facilities are more comprehensive, and the work and activities of many charitable organizations are accommodated in the building.

The general office quarters are on the second floor, clinics and related activities on the first.

Construction uses aluminum wall panels with tile back-up at spandrels, and porcelain enamel panel inserts. Windows are of heat resisting glass, and the building is fully air conditioned.

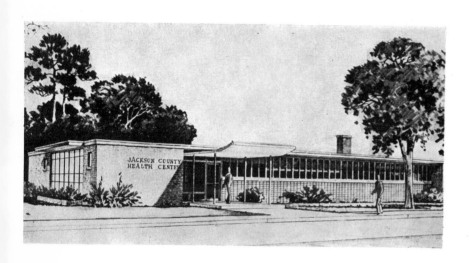

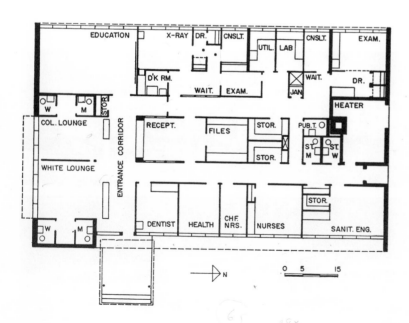

214

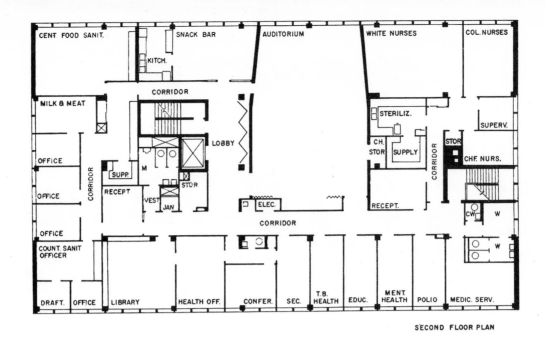

SECOND FLOOR PLAN

# Health Centers for Counties in the South

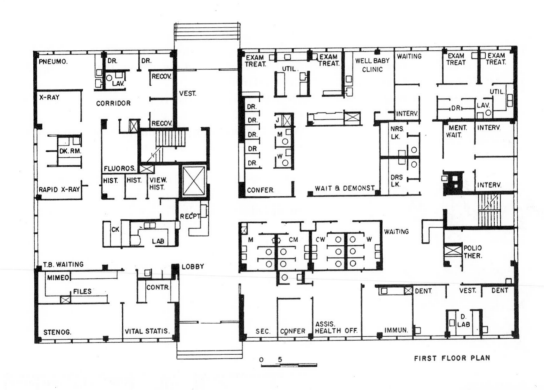

FIRST FLOOR PLAN

0   5

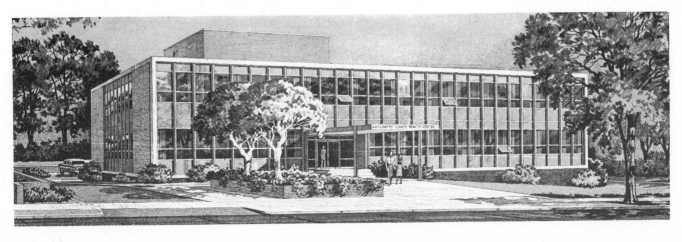

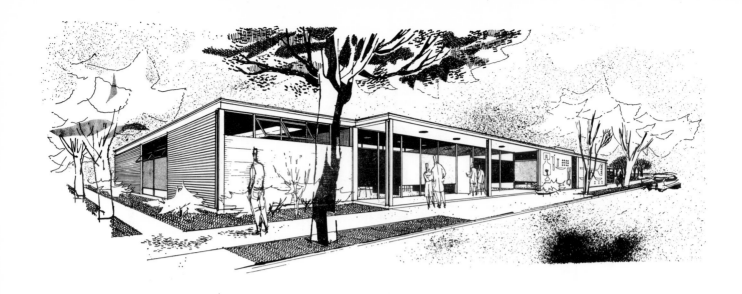

# Small Health Center for a Rural Town

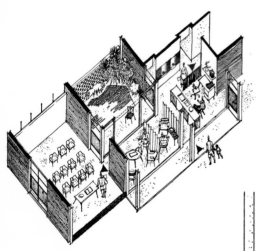

*Washington Parish Health Clinic*
*Bogalusa, Louisiana*
*Burk, Le Breton and Lamantia*
*Architects and Engineers*

HERE is another health center built close to (two blocks from) the local hospital, which can readily extend its diagnostic work. So the center's functions are on the minimal side — offices for the sanitarians and nurses, who really occupy the building only for report-writing and conferences; and clinic space for shots and vaccinations and pre- and post-natal care to mothers. Again the principal planning precepts are observed — separate entrance for staff, public, and for the auditorium. The building is air conditioned by a heat pump installation. Construction is light steel frame on concrete spread footings; exterior walls of 10-in hollow tile, exposed brick on two sides, steel sash and enameled steel panels. Floor is concrete slab on fill. A nice feature is a small controlled courtyard at the waiting room, which offers both a pleasant view and a place for children to play.

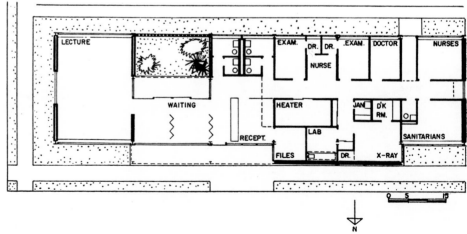

216

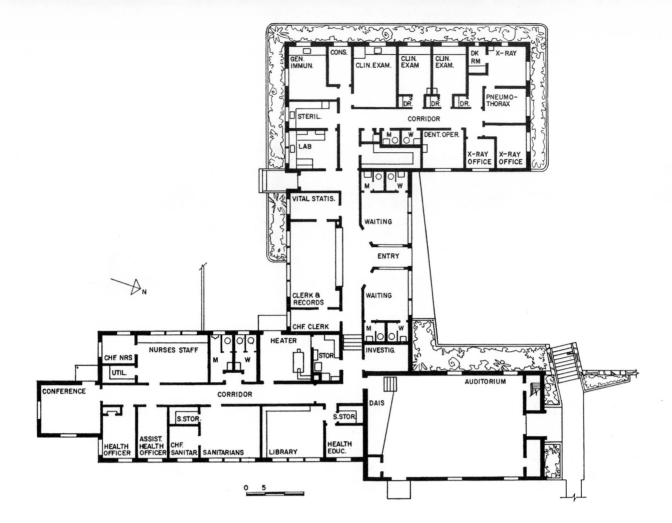

# Medium-Sized Health Center for the South

*Laurens County Health Center*
*Laurens, South Carolina*
*Lyles, Bissett, Carlisle & Wolff*
*Architects and Engineers*

IT HAS often been observed that the preventive techniques of the modern public health center are especially useful where a large proportion of the people are by no means wealthy, it being good economics to minimize the need for full hospital treatment. This health center is rather typical in that respect — good diagnostic, immunization and educational facilities, good quarters for the official guardians of local food, water and sanitation, a large auditorium for health programs. The building separates the two classes of space by taking natural advantage of a sloping site, with the office space in a separate wing at a level a bit lower than that of the clinic portion. The auditorium has its own entrance, can be shut off from the rest of the building.

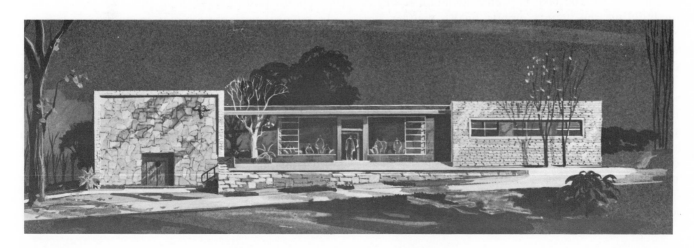

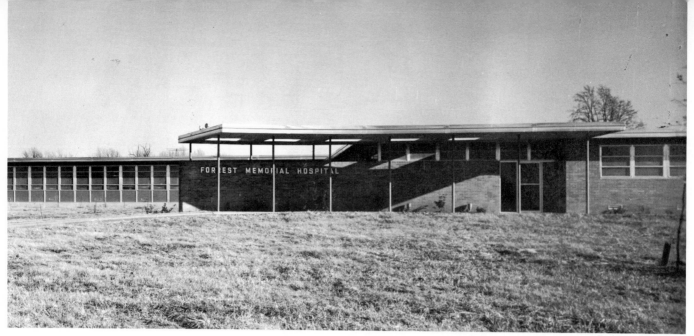

# 65-Bed General Hospital and County Health Center

*Forrest Memorial Hospital, Forrest City, Ark.; Erhart, Eichenbaum, Rauch and Blass, Architects; Edgar K. Riddick, Jr., Mechanical Engineer; H. Price Roark, Structural Engineer; J. E. Pyle, General Contractor*

## COST TABULATION

| | |
|---|---:|
| Square feet—First Floor | 36,610 |
| Square feet—Basement | 2,020 |
| **TOTAL SQUARE FEET** | **38,630** |
| **TOTAL CONSTRUCTION COST**<br>Includes all Group I Equipment—$19.25 per sq ft | **$744,196.00** |
| GENERAL CONSTRUCTION COST<br>Includes Case and Cabinet Work<br>Includes Site Work ($24,351.00) | $412,981.00 |
| PLUMBING, HEATING AND AIR CONDITIONING (100%)<br>Includes all Sterilizers, 100% Oxygen and Vacuum System | 241,233.00 |
| ELECTRICAL AND FIXTURES<br>Includes Surgical Lights | 78,165.00 |
| KITCHEN EQUIPMENT | 11,767.00 |
| ARCHITECT'S FEE | 44,650.00 |
| SURVEY AND BORINGS | 1,500.00 |
| LAND COST | 10,000.00 |
| GROUP II AND III EQUIPMENT | 113,000.00 |
| **TOTAL PROJECT COST** | **$913,346.00** |
| TOTAL USABLE BEDS | 68 |
| **TOTAL COST PER BED** | **$ 13,431.00** |

This project was partially financed with Hill-Burton funds administered by the Division of Hospitals, Arkansas State Board of Health

This hospital, at present a 65-bed general facility expandable to 100-bed capacity, combines within the building the county public health center. The health center has its separate entrance and in fact its own wing so that its operation can be kept isolated from the main building.

With a nine-acre site the building could afford to spread out in a one-story scheme. The nursing portion of the hospital is in effect two nursing units in line. There are two nurses' stations, so placed that either can be closed down during the night hours, or in case the hospital load is unexpectedly light. Major adjunct facilities are in separate wings, the operating suite having the cul de sac location at the end of one wing, the obstetrical suite a similar placing in another. Kitchen and service are together in another separate wing, placed at the central point in the long nursing section.

In general patients are not in private rooms, although there are a dozen or so one-bed rooms in the general nursing units, and a few more in the maternity section. There are two four-bed wards and 17 semi-private rooms. All patient rooms have their own toilet and bath facilities, or share a bath with the adjoining room.

The building is completely air conditioned, with a chilled water and hot water system. There is a central oxygen system, and a central vacuum system also. Doctors' and nurses' call systems are of audio variety.

The building was completed and put into operation within the past year.

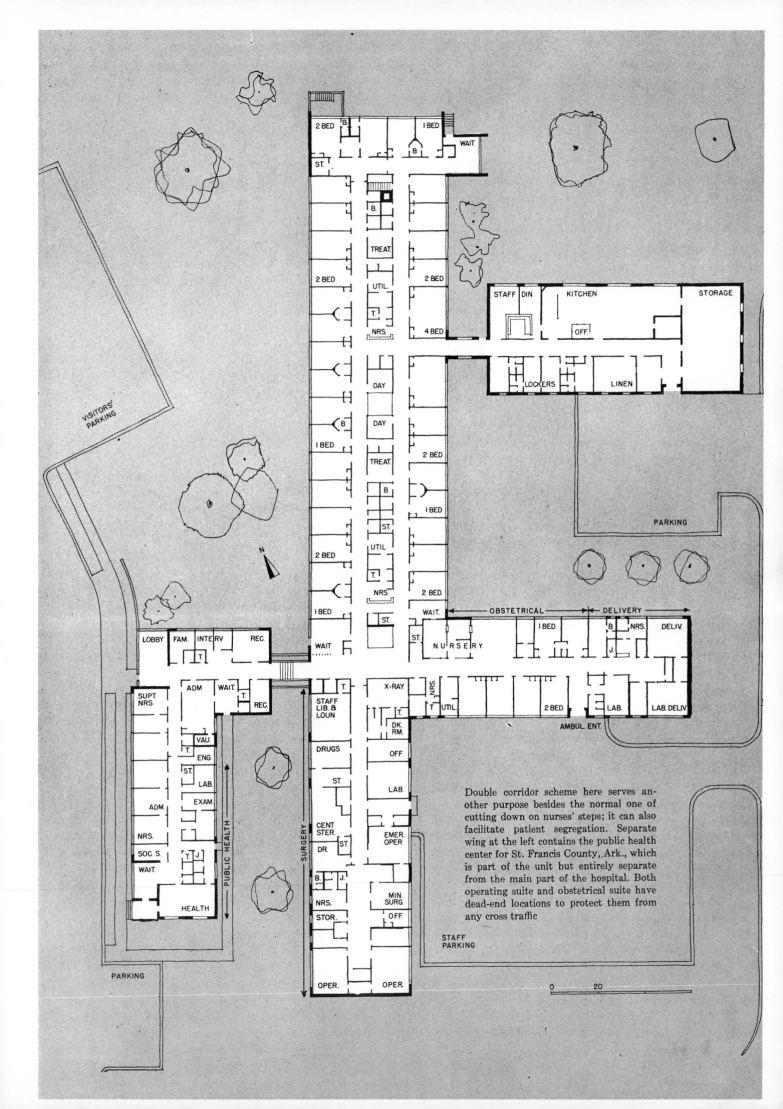

2 BED · B. · 1 BED · WAIT.
ST.
B.
TREAT.
2 BED · UTIL. · 2 BED
T.
NRS. · 4 BED

STAFF · DIN. · KITCHEN · STORAGE
OFF.
LOCKERS · LINEN

DAY
DAY
1 BED · B. · 2 BED
TREAT.
B
1 BED
ST.
2 BED · UTIL · PARKING
T.
NRS. · 2 BED
ST.
1 BED

WAIT. · OBSTETRICAL · DELIVERY
ST. · 1 BED · B. · NRS. · DELIV.
NURSERY · J.

LOBBY · FAM. · INTERV · REC.
T.
WAIT

ADM · WAIT · T. · NRS. · X-RAY · T · UTIL. · 2 BED · LAB. · LAB. DELIV.
REC. · T. · STAFF LIB. & LOUN · AMBUL. ENT.

SUPT. NRS.
VAU. · T. · DK. RM.
T. · ENG. · DRUGS · OFF
ST. · LAB. · ST. · LAB.
ADM. · EXAM.
NRS. · CENT STER. · EMER. OPER.
SOC. S. · T. J · DR. · ST.
WAIT · B. · J.
HEALTH · NRS. · MIN. SURG.
STOR. · OFF.

VISITORS' PARKING

N

PUBLIC HEALTH

SURGERY

Double corridor scheme here serves another purpose besides the normal one of cutting down on nurses' steps; it can also facilitate patient segregation. Separate wing at the left contains the public health center for St. Francis County, Ark., which is part of the unit but entirely separate from the main part of the hospital. Both operating suite and obstetrical suite have dead-end locations to protect them from any cross traffic

STAFF PARKING

OPER. · OPER.

PARKING

0 · 20

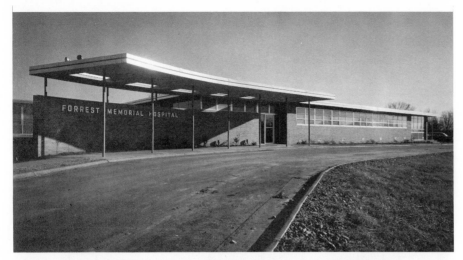

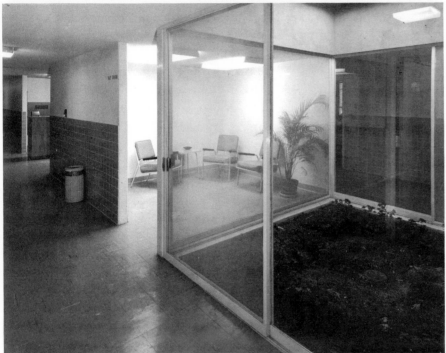

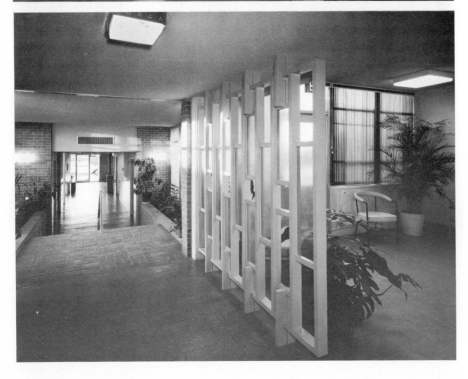

*Upper left:* main entrance to hospital is at one end of the separate wing that contains the public health center; special entrance for center at far end. *Left center:* small courtyard at the juncture of the cruciform plan. *Lower left:* view down main corridor looking toward main entrance; visitors' waiting room is shown at the right

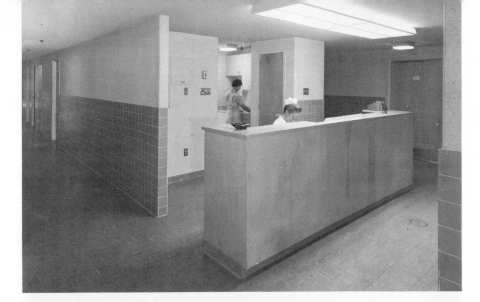

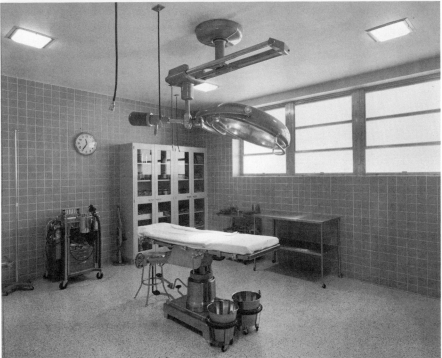

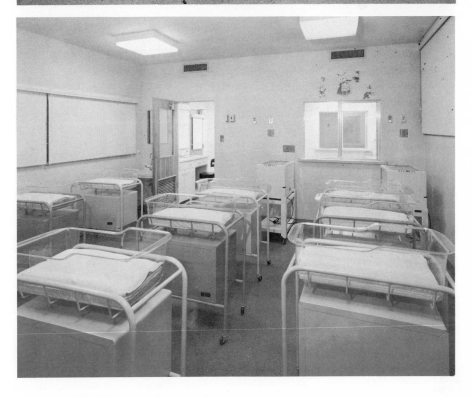

*Upper right:* one of the nurses' stations between the two corridors. Nurses' stations, two in a long line, can be activated or closed down as load or hours may indicate. *Right center:* one of the main operating rooms. *Lower right:* one of the nursery rooms; these are located in the separate wing, going off to the right in the plan, for maternity section

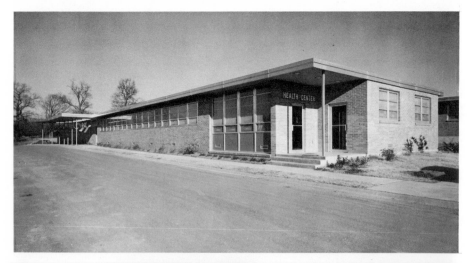

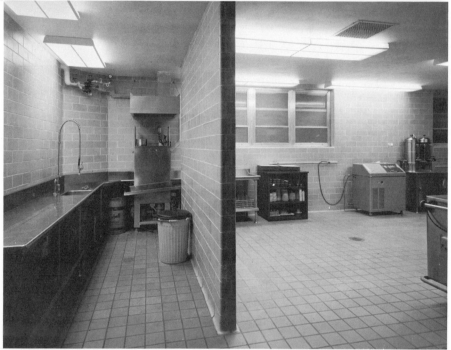

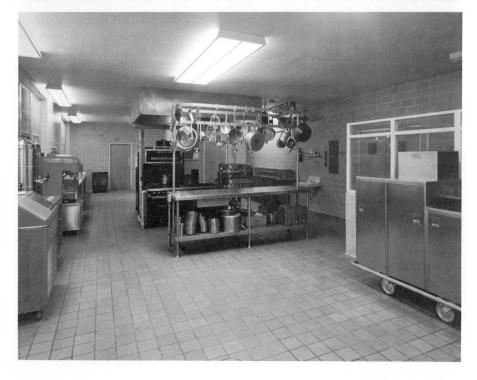

*Upper left:* separate entrance in the public health center wing permits use of the facility, especially its auditorium, during evening hours. *Left, lower and center:* kitchen and dishwashing area have tile floors, concrete block walls. Block walls are standard in service area; exterior walls are of pink brick, with block backup, plastered in bed rooms

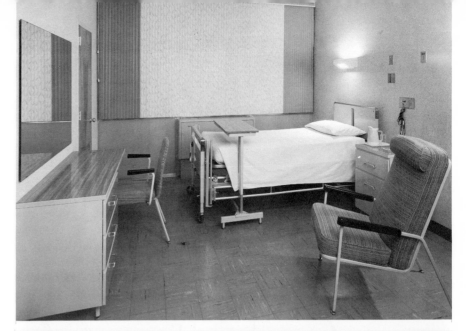

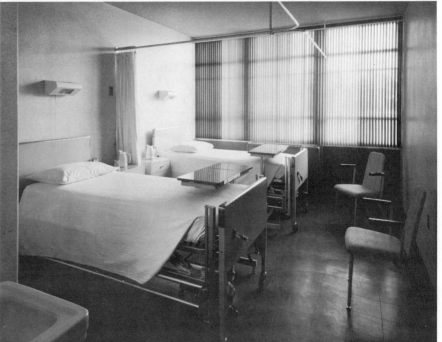

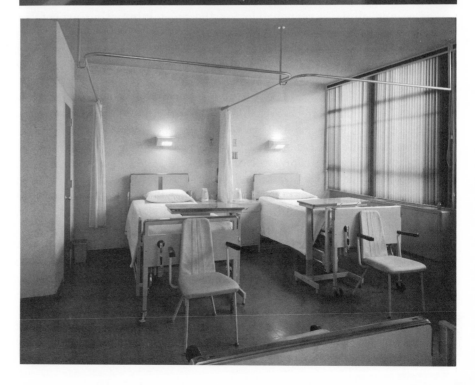

*Right, top to bottom:* private room, semi-private room and four-bed ward. In the main portion of the hospital the beds are distributed as follows: 12 private rooms, two single rooms for isolation use, two four-bed wards and 17 semi-private rooms. In maternity sections there are two private rooms, four semi-private and nursery bassinets for 12, plus premature nursery

*Forrest Memorial Hospital*

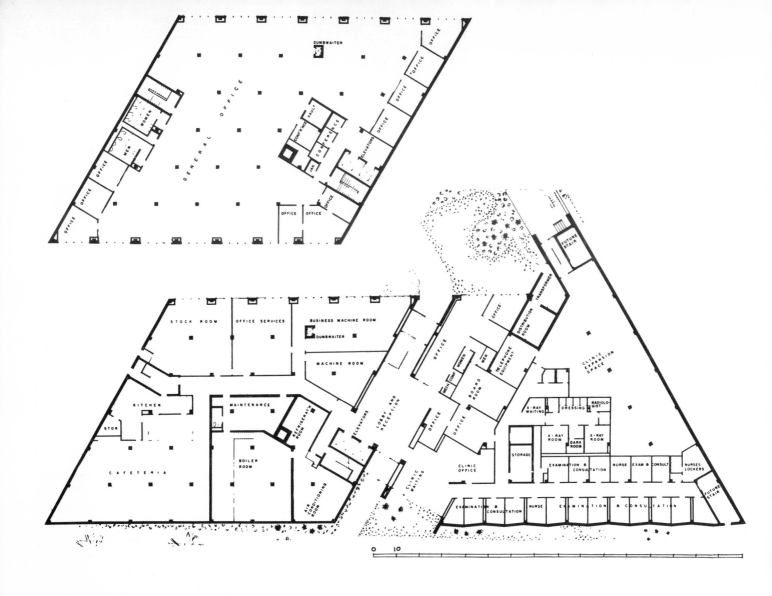

# Health Insurance and Outpatient Clinic

The triangular lot utilized for the site of the Group Health home office and clinic is responsible for the most interesting aspects of this building's design. A significant geometrical pattern, dictated by the equilateral dimensions and angles of the property, is evident in the plan view, where two separate functions within the building are represented by two different geometrical shapes—a parallelogram and a triangle. The restrictions imposed by the site were turned to advantage in creating a natural, though arbitrary division of space utilization. The wedge-shaped elements of structural design are subtly transferred to other parts of the building, as in the undulating exterior wall of the clinic, the triangular shaped reception desk, the bent angle of the free standing wall in the lobby, the "flying wedge" shape of the clinic office desk and the clean, simple interpretation of pine trees in the firm's symbol over the doorway.

The building is of reinforced concrete construction with exterior of brick, alumilited silicone panels and insulated glass. Walls are plaster except in special areas, such as toilets, where glazed structural tile is used, and in mechanical areas where lightweight concrete blocks are left exposed. Ceilings in all work and public areas are acoustical plaster with the exception of the large general office which is sound conditioned with a fiberglass insulated, perforated metal acoustical ceiling.

*Group Health Office
and Clinic Building
St. Paul, Minn.*

*Architects and Engineers:
Haarstick Lundgren
and Associates, Inc.*

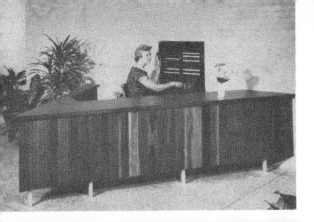

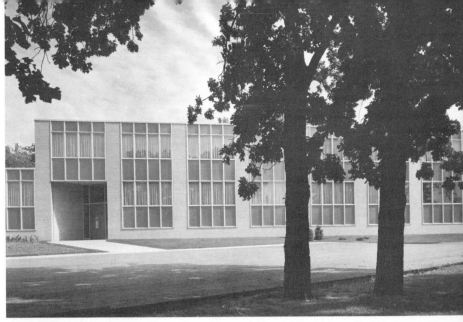

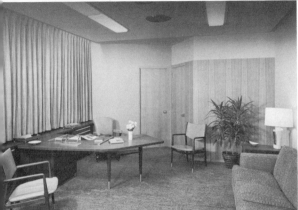

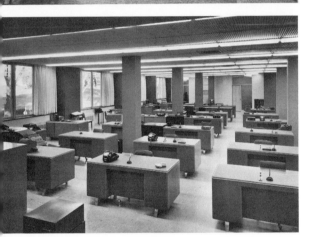

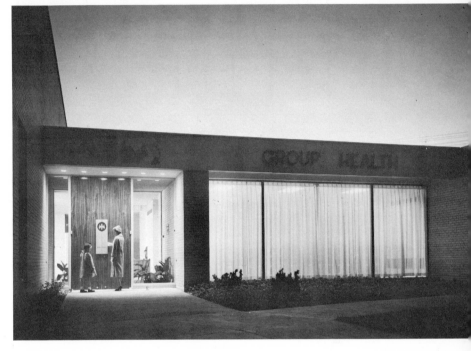

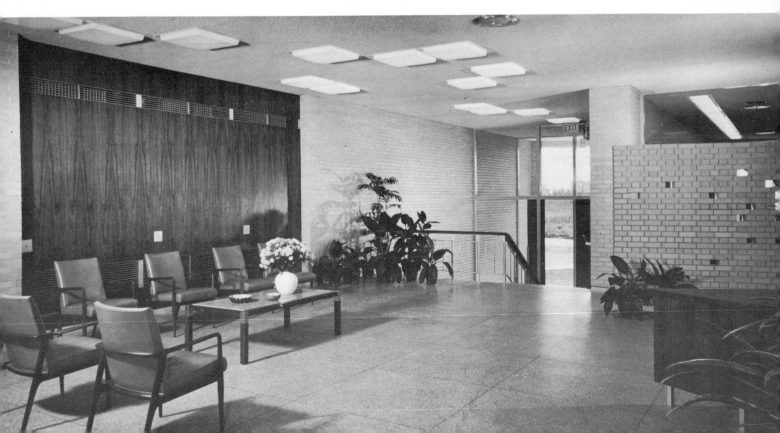

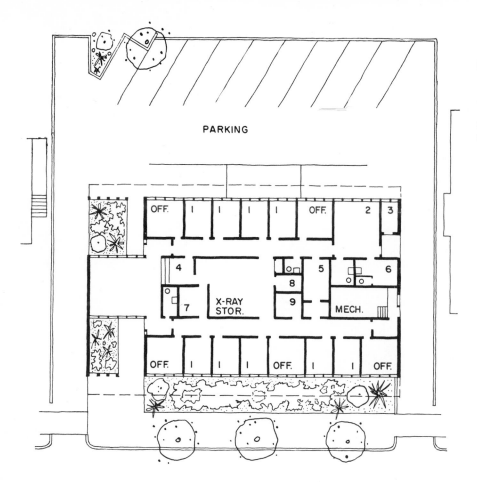

PARKING

1. Examination
2. Lounge
3. Storage
4. Reception
5. Laboratory
6. Nurses
7. Consultation
8. Fluor.
9. EKG.

# Medical Clinic with Non-Medical Look

A nice bit of gospel is expressed in this little building for a group of doctors: a medical-oriented building doesn't have to express the more hygienic aspects of the association; it might emphasize more human ones. The program here called for "clinic space for five doctors on an interior lot in a residential district, with a maximum amount of off-street parking, and avoid a sterile, clinical appearance and create a building with an intimate and inviting atmosphere." The waiting room was developed to create that inviting note; the fireplace provides a center of interest and was designed with a minimum mass to give the receptionist a good view into the room. The building was placed on the front of the lot, to minimize the prominence of the parking facility.

The building is a wood frame structure on concrete perimeter foundation. There is a four-foot crawl space under the entire building to permit easy access to piping. Materials were selected to minimize medical suggestions: natural woods and gay colors wherever possible. Walls are vertical grain hemlock in interiors; exterior siding 1 by 4 cedar; cabinet work natural birch.

*Hoyt Street Clinic*
*Portland, Ore.*

*Architects:*
*Skidmore, Owings & Merrill*

*Mechanical Engineers:*
*J. Donald Kroeker*

*Electrical Engineers:*
*Grant Kelley & Associates*

*Landscape Architects:*
*Florence and Walter Clarke*

*Dearborn-Massar*

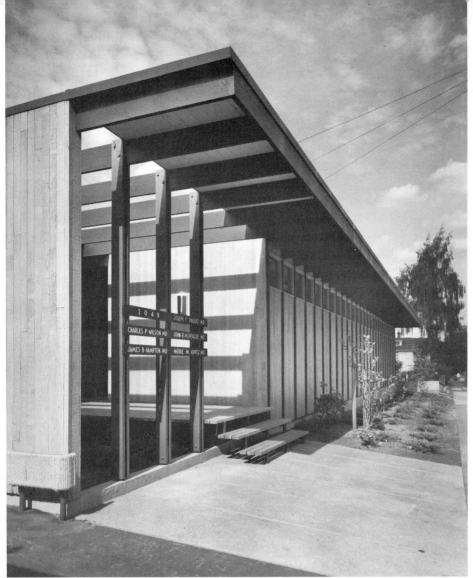

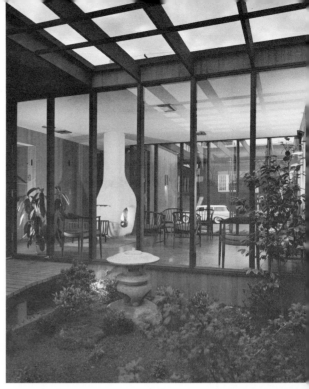

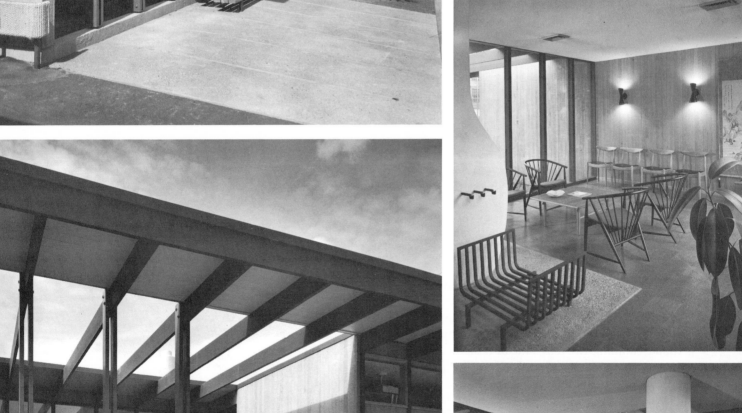

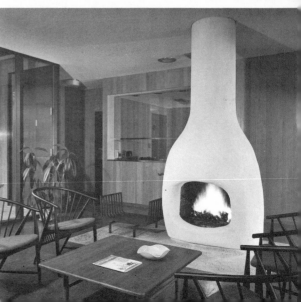

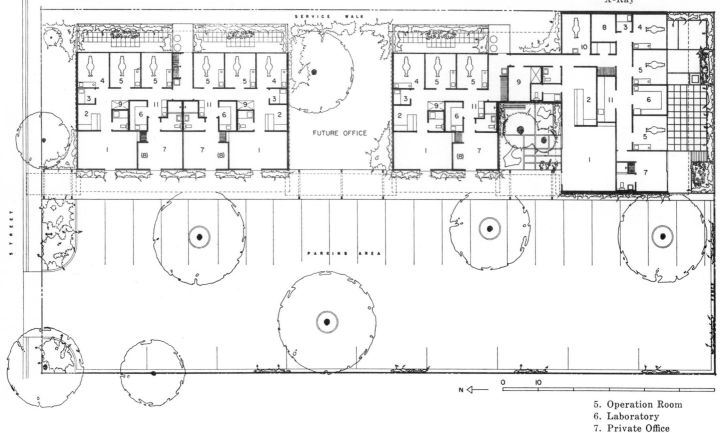

1. Reception
2. Business Office
3. Dark-Room
4. Examination &
   X-Ray

5. Operation Room
6. Laboratory
7. Private Office
8. Recovery
9. Mechanical
   Equipment
10. Hygienist
11. Sterilization

# Prestige Values in a Dental Clinic

This is a dental clinic building with a considerable quantity of built-in appeal to patients as well as doctors. It has actually contributed to doctors' work by permitting them to do a larger volume of work with less effort, and patients have commented that the building takes some of the pain out of dental visits. Since some of the dentists are tenants, the result is particularly happy, and the prestige value noticeable. The building (actually two buildings) is disposed along the long side of a narrow deep lot, allowing the parking to be in "front" of each office. For privacy the "fronts" are relatively closed, the operating rooms having a full wall of glass overlooking a landscaped court. These rooms are aligned for great convenience, and are well separated from waiting rooms. The courts were designed to enchance the open feeling in what is really a tight plot. Buildings are connected with covered walks, the design of which was intended to produce sufficient interest to tie together visually the three façade elements of the buildings. Framing is light steel columns and beams, with steel bar joists. Exterior walls for the most part are non-load-bearing curtain walls; floor is concrete slab on grade, independent of roof framing; thickened edges support the walls. Interiors are a collaboration between the owner-dentist and the architect, in a generally Mayan note. The mural was designed and executed by this owner-architect team.

*Dental Arts Building*
*Gainsville, Fla.*

Owner:
*Dr. Lewis J. Marchand*

Architect:
*David Reaves*

Landscape Architect:
*J. M. Crevasse, Jr.*

*Wm. Amick photos*

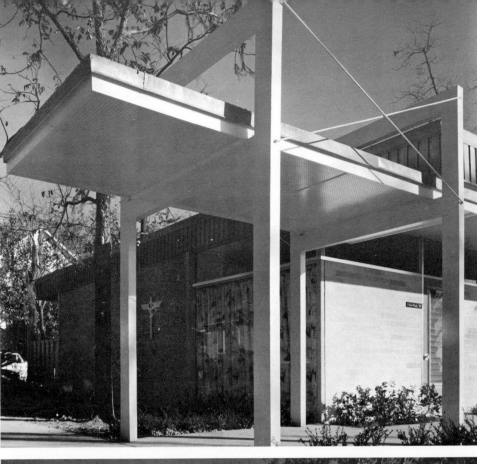

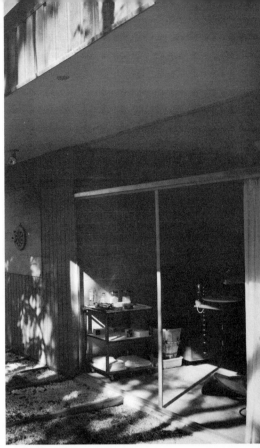

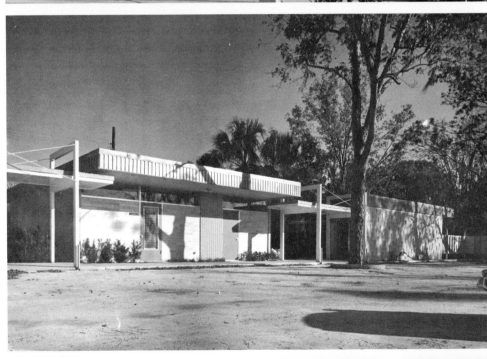

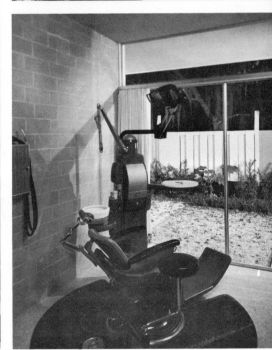

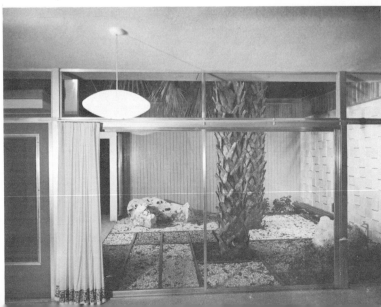

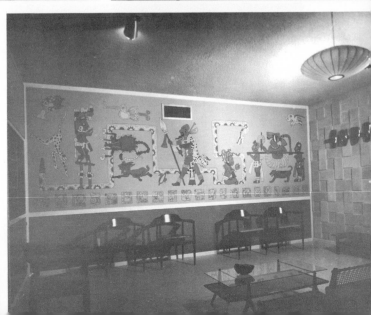

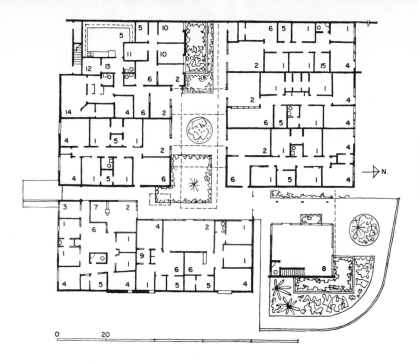

1. Exam
2. Reception
3. Contagious
4. Consultation
5. Lab
6. Nurse
7. Child
8. Pharmacy
9. Fluor.
10. Operatory
11. Recovery
12. Basal
13. Blood Test
14. X-Ray
15. Audio

# Large Clinic Screened from Traffic Noise

Medical concept for the clinic group is the now familiar one of several doctors banding together to provide a comprehensive medical service. Architecturally, the concept takes off from a desire to produce amenity values for a site on a noisy, heavy-traffic boulevard. The medical services include: internal medicine, gynecology, chest and general surgery, general practice, ear, nose and throat, psychiatry and dentistry, with supplementary services including laboratory, radiology, pharmacy. The site is on Ventura Boulevard, with heavy noisy traffic. For a visual and acoustic barrier the architect placed most of the building behind a concrete block screen wall, with an enclosed landscaped patio area. The wall and the courts are relied upon for the adornment of a very simple building. The separate office units are fairly large, the largest of 1100 sq ft. Some of the suites are combined, with two doctors sharing reception space. The doctors have a get-together lounge, actually a penthouse. The building is of stud and plaster construction, concrete slab on grade. Ceilings have acoustical tile and treatment room walls are soundproofed. Square foot cost was under $15.

*Woodley Medical Center*
*Los Angeles, Cal.*

*Architect:*
*Victor Gruen*

*Partner in Charge:*
*Ben Southland*

*Engineer:*
*Dan Alvy*

*Gordon Sommers photos*

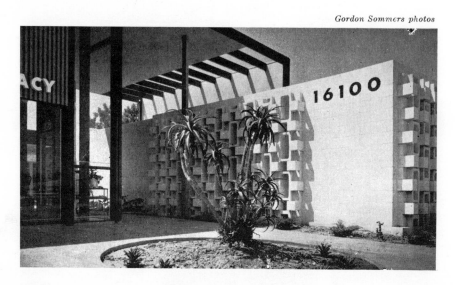

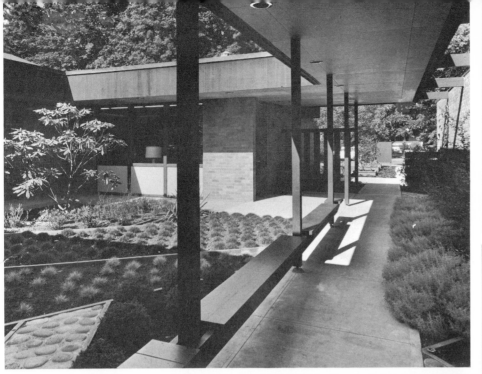

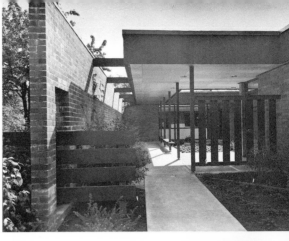

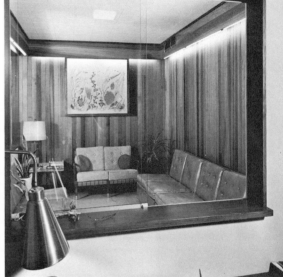

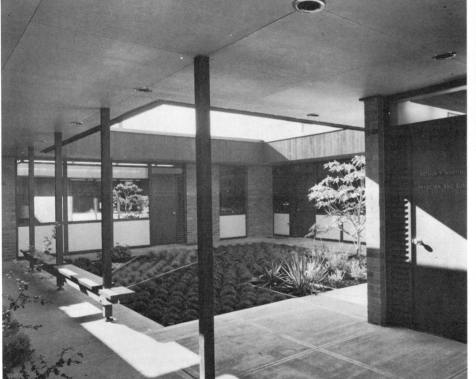

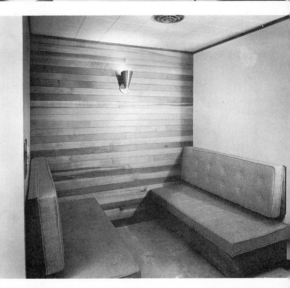

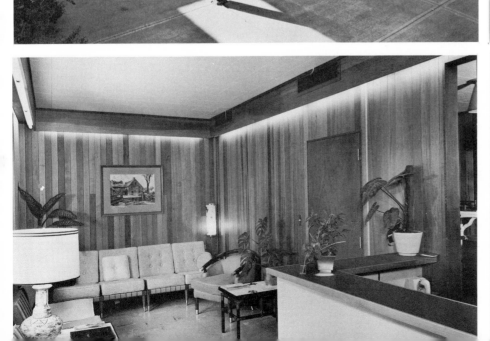

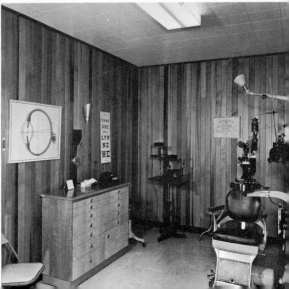

# Doctors' Offices for Group Practice

*Doctors' Clinic*

*Lake City, Washington*

*Paul H. Kirk, Architect*

WHEN doctors want their own buildings, for a more or less clinical type of practice, they commonly pose just such a problem as this one. In this instance two doctors wanted accommodations for themselves and two additional doctors to be brought in as assistants. The strip of four examining rooms separates the two principals on opposite sides. Common facilities — X-ray, laboratory and surgery — form a sort of mechanical core. Rooms for BMR, therapy and shots by nurses are grouped along the front. Patients in the waiting room do not see other patients enter or leave, an idea of the doctors

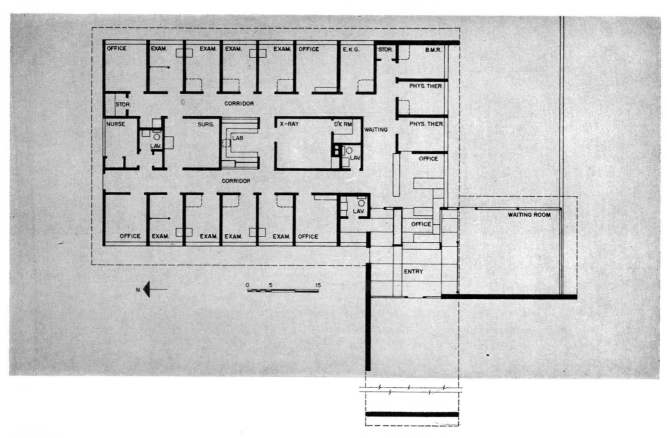

Dearborn-Massar

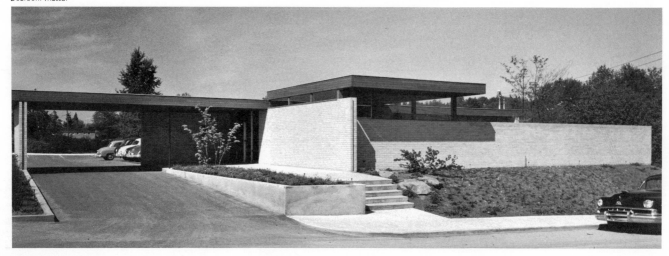

234

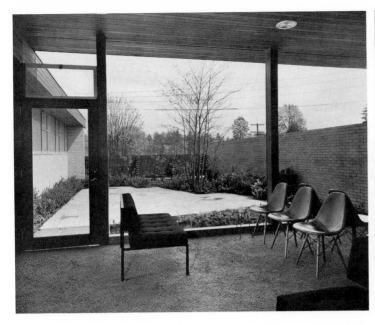
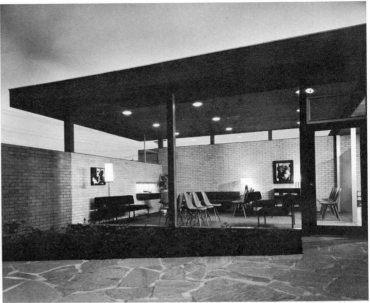

to obviate impatience in case some patients, say for shots, are ushered in and out quickly. One of the nicest features is the open court beside waiting room (picture *upper left*) which is bound to induce some relaxation in patients waiting.

The exterior is of smooth "clinical" face brick in a light cream color with dark manganese spots, this brick setting the color note for the whole building. Interior woodwork is walnut, matching the dark of the brick. Corridors were painted a brownish-beige. Even the landscaping was chosen to contribute bronze-green or copper tones.

Dearborn-Massar

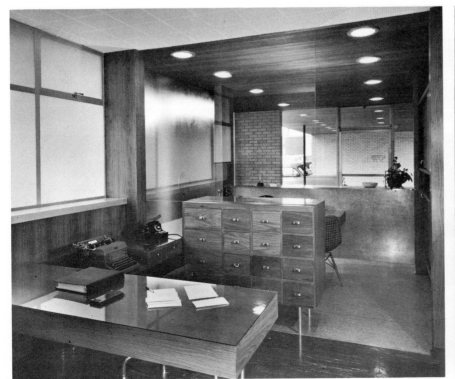
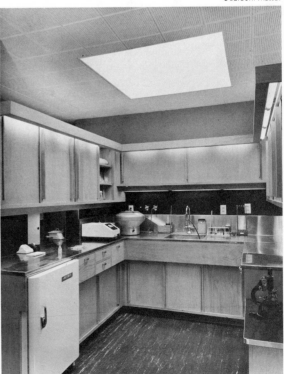

*Children's Clinic*

*Dallas, Texas*

*Wiltshire and Fisher, Architects*

PERHAPS the nicest thing about this children's clinic, though the architect doesn't mention it, is the scaling of the building for its small patients, plus the quiet sheltered note its roof lines achieve. The architect stresses three principal planning points: (1) the arrangement of the doctors' suites so that each has a sub-corridor connecting two examining rooms and private office, making it possible for the doctor to circulate without appearing in the public corridor; (2) a back waiting room for the reception of children with a temperature, where they can be kept isolated until a doctor has examined them for contagious disease; (3) the air conditioning system, which circulates hot or chilled water to individual cabinet units in the various rooms, making

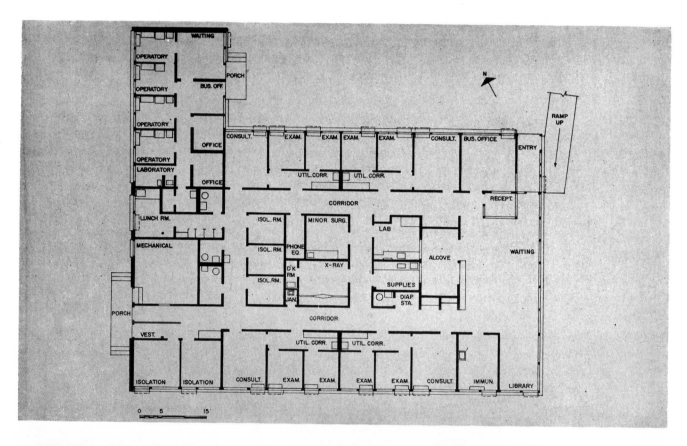

Ulric Meisel

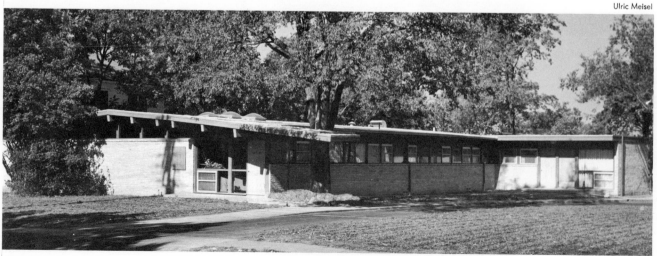

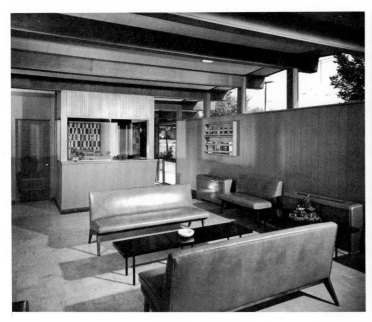 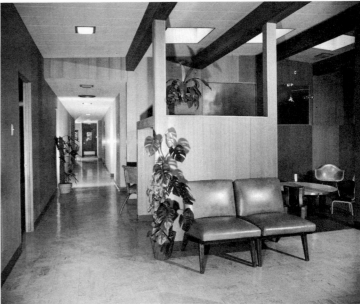

it possible to control each room to the needs of unclothed children, if that should be advisable, rather than a set temperature which might be harsh for the sick child.

The building is occupied by four pediatricians and two pediodontists, the latter occupying the rear wing shown on the plan, with separate entrance. Each doctor in each group practices independently, but each has use of common facilities in the two sections of the building.

After the building had been in operation for a couple of years a questionnaire was circulated among the staff people which asked for recommended changes in case the building were to be rebuilt, but the results turned up only two minor suggestions for changes.

Ulric-Meisel

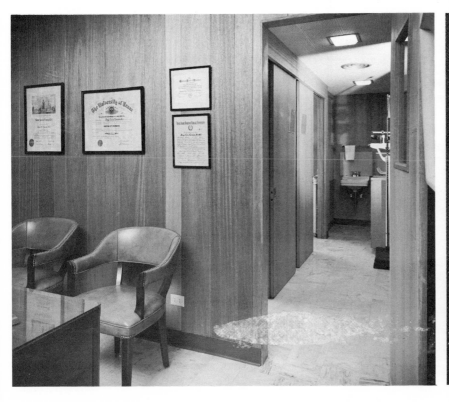 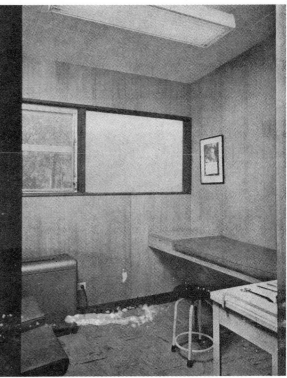

*Dr. Clifford M. Bassett Clinic*

*Cushing, Oklahoma*

*Coston-Frankfurt-Short,*

*Architects and Engineers*

THOUGH a single doctor built this extensive office building, it was designed for an essentially staff operation with the addition of two or more doctors as assistants. The building probably sets some sort of record for its facilities and equipment. The X-ray installation runs to deep therapy; there is television in the waiting room; piped music; extensive signal system; full air conditioning; piped oxygen; not to mention the diet kitchen. Indeed the good doctor told the architects that he wanted to equal or surpass the facilities available to big-city doctors. Red brick and redwood give the building its main color scheme, though heavy use of tinted

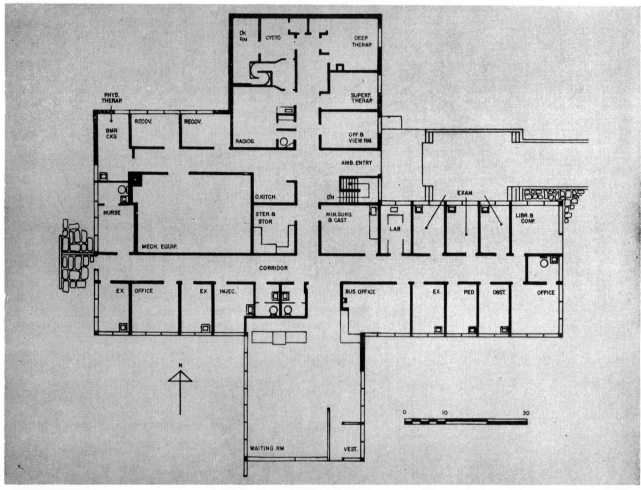

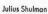
Julius Shulman

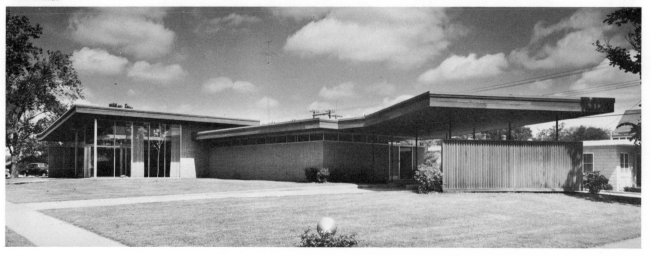

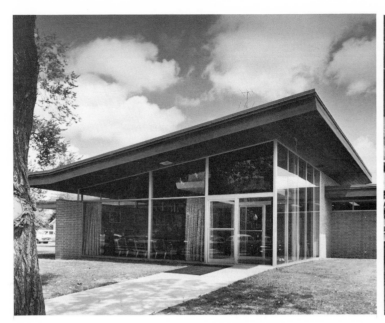

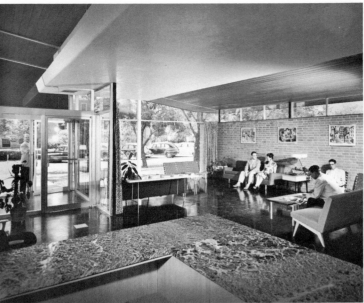

glass produces some strong contrasts. Inside the color schemes are fairly lively, and according to the local newspaper, there is "modern art with just enough whimsy and humor to contribute toward mental therapy of patients."

Ceramic tile was used for all corridor walls; here the color is gray. In examining rooms, however, and generally throughout the interior, the colors are anything but "medical," with greens, suntan, blues and a cocoa brown for the fabric wall covering that has been extensively used in many of the rooms. Woodwork is mainly walnut, in blonde finish. Even the metal cabinets avoid the clinical white, with lively color schemes. All ceilings are of acoustic tile.

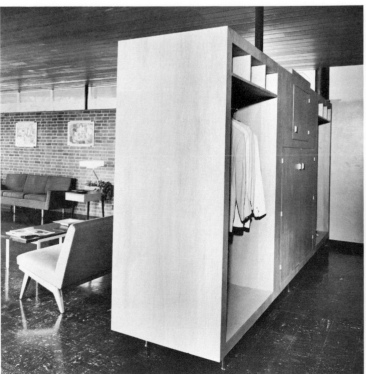

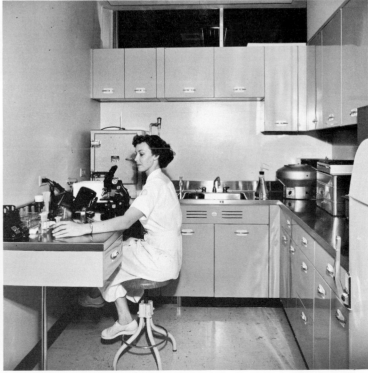

*Mahorner Clinic*

*New Orleans, Louisiana*

*Curtis & Davis, Architects*

IT HAS been said rather frequently of late that a few purely nostalgic touches in decoration might not be amiss, and it has been implied that architects who indulged in something of that sort would not be stricken from the favored lists, but it still is worthy of note when one does nerve himself to do it. As a matter of fact, these architects are inclined to point with pride to the little New Orleans patio in this building, and to the decorative wrought iron balcony railing, adding that this softening of their contemporary leanings has produced much favorable comment. The patio should be especially commendable for a doctors' clinic in a busy city neighborhood, establishing a note of calm and quiet, and the balcony "has proven very useful in our climate." However pleasant the shaded balcony, it probably proves useful in the strict functional sense, for

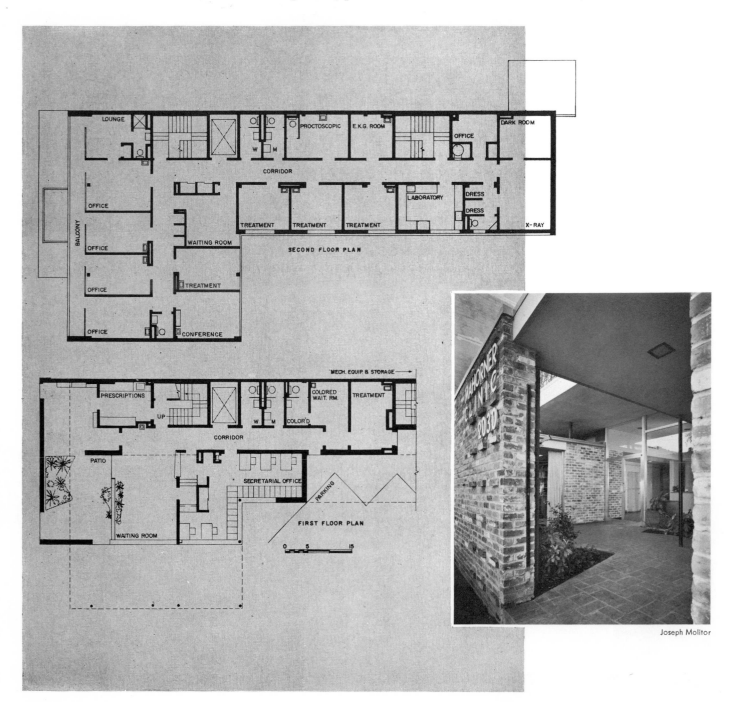

SECOND FLOOR PLAN

FIRST FLOOR PLAN

Joseph Molitor

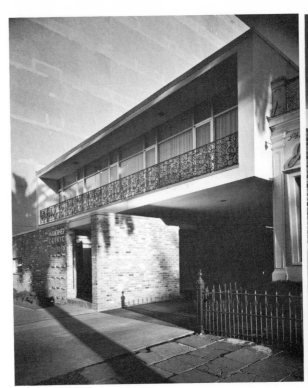

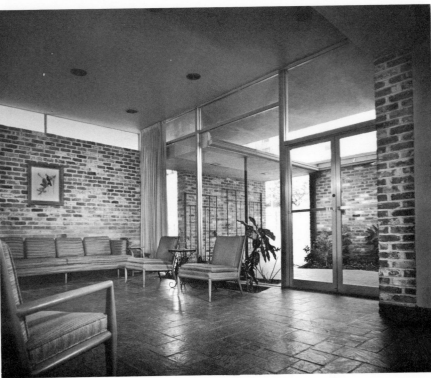

one can imagine the doctors using it as a private passage when some particularly garrulous client is known to be in the corridor.

The structural system consists of a rigid steel frame and bar joists. Roof and floor decks are lightweight concrete. Exterior walls are second-hand common brick, concrete block and stucco. The brick walls and slate floor of the patio extend into the waiting room on the ground floor. The entire building is fully air conditioned.

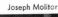
Joseph Molitor

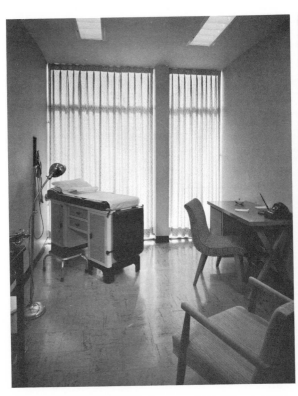

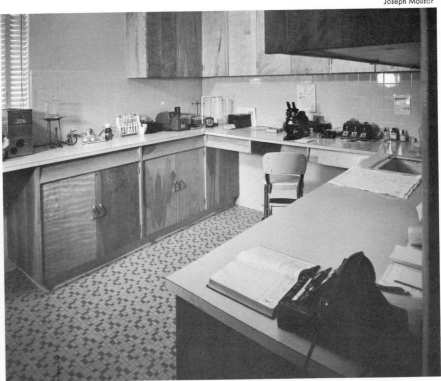

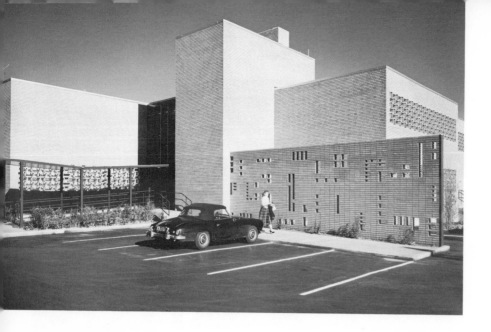
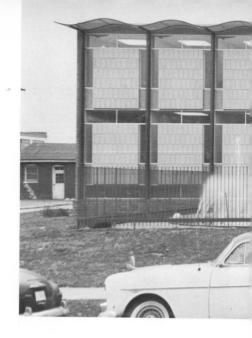

# Examination and Treatment Center for a Union

Medical Institute of Local 88, Meat and Related Industries Health and Welfare Fund; St. Louis, Mo.; Harris Armstrong, Architect; Leslie J. Bergmeier, Structural Engineer; Belt & Given, Mechanical Engineers; G. Carl Cooper, Jr., Electrical Engineer; C. Rallo Contracting Company, Contractors

This building houses a highly complex and complete medical service for the members of a labor union and their families. It is the first new building to be designed and constructed for such a purpose.

Located on a city lot, the building has been conceived by the architect as a three-level structure, oriented to take advantage of sunlight when desired and to control it when necessary. Major problems were the location and planning of the building and related parking on the available ground and the extremely complicated circulation necessary for the many functions to be housed. By placing parking and main entrance on one side of the building with the service entrance facilities nearby (the two are screened from each other by a wall), the architect devised simple, workable traffic patterns.

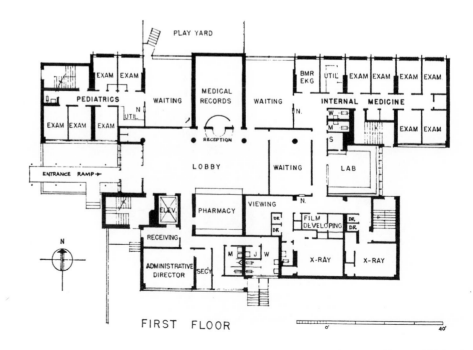

FIRST FLOOR

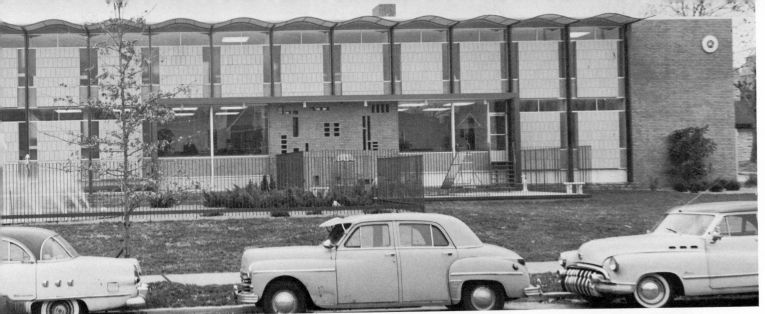

*All photos: Art Fillmore*

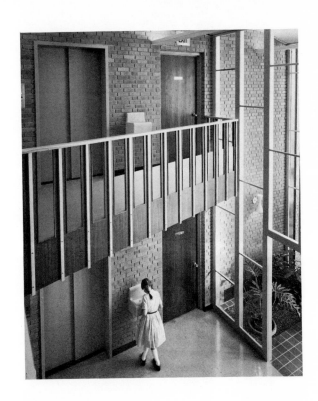

The control center of the building is the two-story-high lobby. Patients are received at a reception desk near the records storage area. From this point, patients are routed to various departments of the building according to their specific needs.

Each department has its own waiting room and all departmental facilities are closely related to this area. Relationships between departments were closely studied. As a result, circulation patterns between them are free of confusion and highly efficient. Room sizes most suitable for the various specialties were meticulously studied. Desirable optimums were established and used. One result of this care is the provision of internal medicine and obstetrics examining rooms sizable enough for placement of tables lengthwise or crosswise in the rooms.

The main lobby (above) has balconies at the second level, contributing to an open and spacious feeling. As may be seen in the major floor plans shown, the facilities are extraordinarily complete. These include necessary spaces for physical examinations, preventive medicine, and treatment for approximately 7500 people (union members and their families attached to this local). Only hospital inpatient care and major surgery require performance elsewhere. The facilities provided are strictly departmentalized. An additional floor, located partially below grade, contains service equipment, offices, and an auditorium for staff meetings and similar purposes

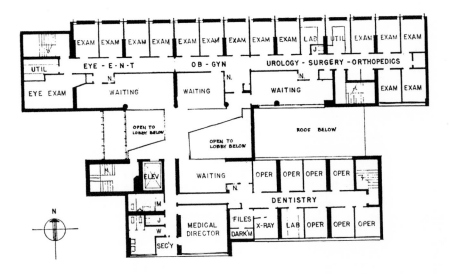

SECOND FLOOR

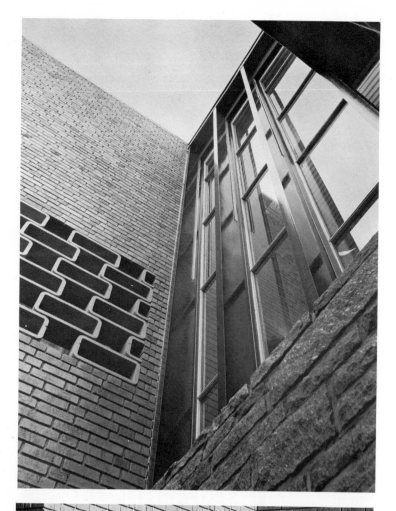

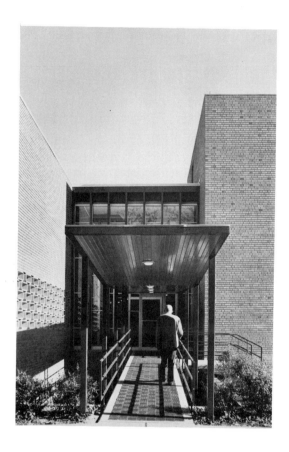

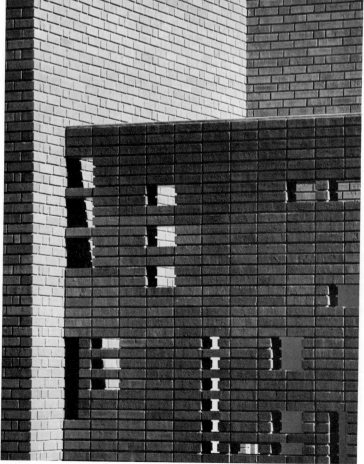

The careful study made by the architect of the masses of the building and their relationships to each other is indicated in the illustrations (left). The care used in the selection of the great variety of coordinated materials (including brick, pierced brick, tile grilles, granite, and glass curtain walls on the exterior) may also be seen. These are used in conjunction with a reinforced concrete frame structure. Some of the exterior feeling is translated to the inside spaces by the continuation of brick walls into the interior. The main entrance (above) is reached via a ramp designed for easy access by patients in wheel chairs or otherwise handicapped. The ramp passes over a landscaped entrance courtyard adjacent to the building

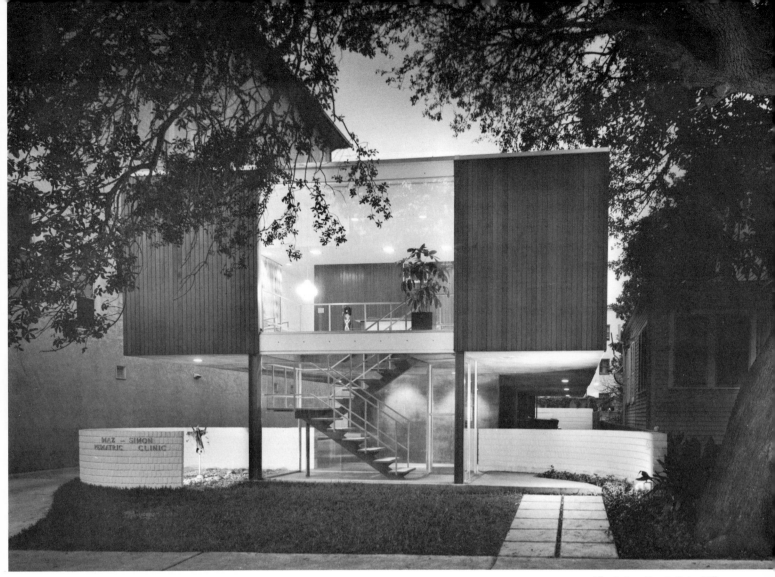

# Pediatric Clinic for Four Doctors

*Diaz-Simon Pediatric Clinic, New Orleans, La.; Colbert and Lowrey and Associates, Architects; Ogle-Rosenbohm & Associates, Structural Engineers; John W. Waters, Contractor*

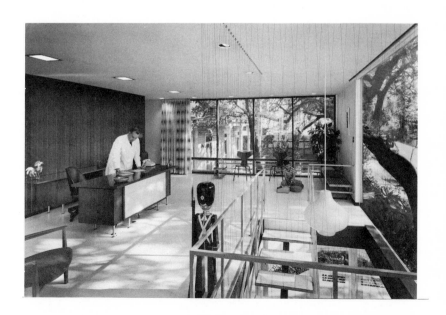

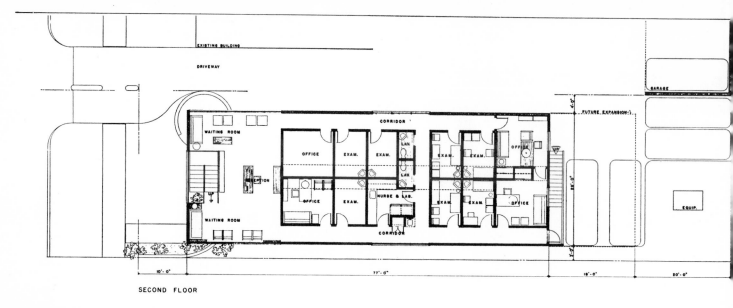

SECOND FLOOR

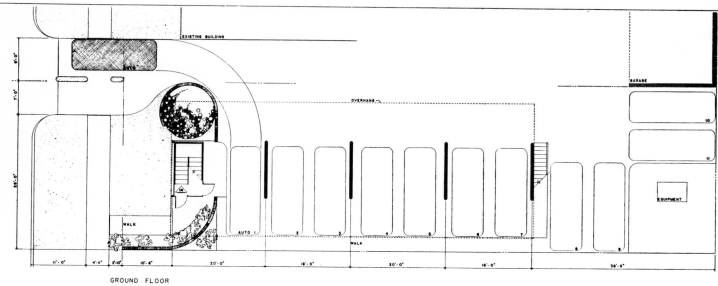

GROUND FLOOR

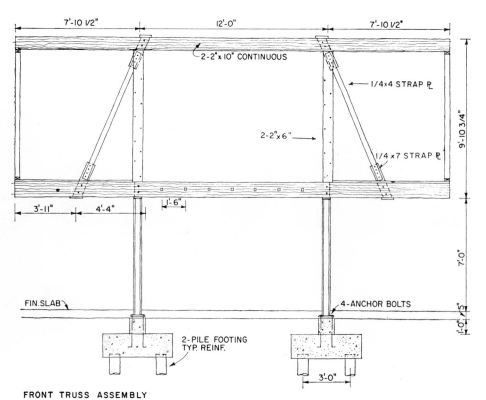

FRONT TRUSS ASSEMBLY

Because of the limited size of the site and zoning restrictions, the ground floor is used only for parking, stairwells, entrance foyer, and equipment spaces. The second floor contains all medical spaces including a small laboratory for routine work. As shown in the section, the structure at the front of the building consists of steel columns supporting wood frames. The remainder of the upper floor is supported on concrete piers located under the upstairs walls, which are designed to act as conventional (story high) wood truss members. These are cantilevered both sides by means of metal straps anchored near the heads of columns and at the top chord of the trusses as shown

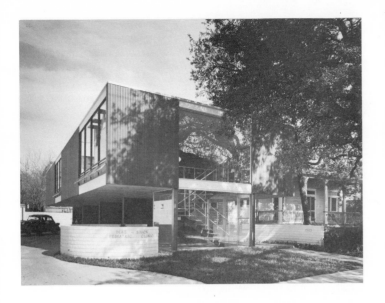

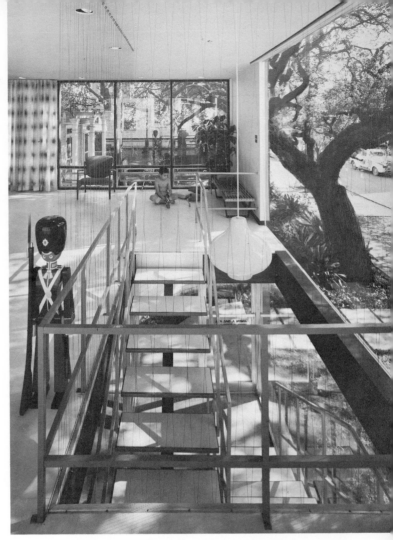

From the waiting room on the second level, the views are toward a large live oak tree and the surrounding residential neighborhood. The open stair leads down to a glass-enclosed entrance foyer on the ground floor

The architects for this small, four-doctor pediatric clinic have achieved an economical and efficient solution to a difficult problem. For their accomplishments, they have received a 1959 A.I.A. National Honor Award.

Located on a limited-size urban site, severely restricted as to allowable lot coverage by zoning regulations and requirements for off-street parking, the clinic has been raised off the ground. In this way, maximum space was provided for required medical functions while the ground floor was essentially preserved for parking. Circulation was planned for reducing steps between consultation and examining rooms for the staff, to reduce congestion to a minimum, and to provide for easy patient access, traffic, and egress. The last was accomplished by providing for an entrance at the front with traffic flow around the central rooms and an exit at the rear. Incidentally, this scheme allows injections to be given at the last possible moment, after which children may depart without disturbing incoming patients.

A concentrated effort was made to keep the entire building as comfortable and simple as possible, yet retain a childlike and playful atmosphere. This has been accomplished through the use of natural materials such as the stained redwood exterior panels in conjunction with clean interior surfaces. Accents are provided by the contemporary Scandinavian furniture (which one doctor collects), playful wood sculpture, and other carefully planned details.

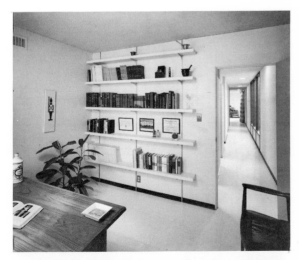

The doctor's consultation room-office shown indicates the simplified treatment used in the interior. Gypsum board walls, painted or covered with vinyl, are used with vinyl floors and acoustical plaster ceilings

*Diaz-Simon Pediatric Clinic*

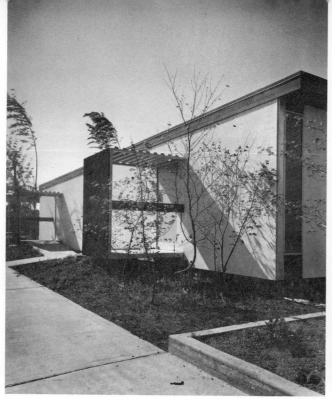 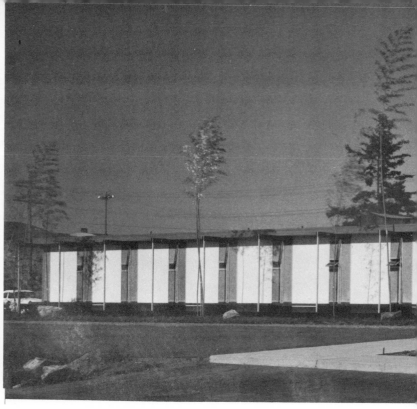

# Pleasant Atmosphere for Group Medicine

*Group Health Cooperative Northgate Clinic, Seattle, Washington; Paul Hayden Kirk & Associates (Don S. Wallace & David A. McKinley, Jr.) Donald G. Radcliffe, Structural Engineer; Stern and Towne, Mechanical Engineers; William G. Teufel, Landscape Architect*

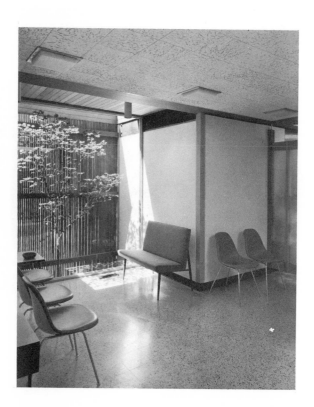

In this rather large clinic (10 doctors), the architect has created an efficient and functional layout, a pleasant and skillfully detailed building. Not the least of its virtues is the feeling of relaxation and well-being engendered in patients through its design and detailing.

The clinic was established as a branch of the downtown Seattle Group Health Cooperative Hospital in order to relieve over-crowding and to provide more easily accessible medical facilities for the residents of Northgate community. Circulation of staff and patients is initially separated through the use of two parking lots, one for each group. Entry for the staff is at the end of the building, while patients enter from the front. From the control receptionist's station, patients are directed to the various waiting rooms, from which they are controlled and routed from the nurses' stations nearby. Throughout the entire building, an effort has been made to open up interior spaces to the outdoors and to obtain an appearance as opposite to the institutional character of many such buildings as possible. The use of simple surfaces and natural wood contributes to this purpose. Colored plastic panels and other spots of color combined with extremely well thought out planting do much toward achieving this end.

The structure of the building is wood frame with laminated beams. The exterior is finished with stucco. Windows are aluminum, glazed with translucent plastic panels and clear glass. Interior walls are finished with hardwood plywood and painted gypsum wallboard. Ceilings are fiberboard acoustical tile and floors are covered with vinyl-asbestos tile.

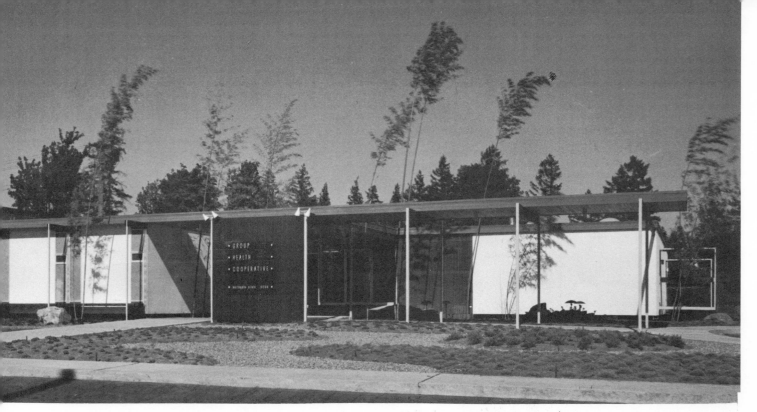

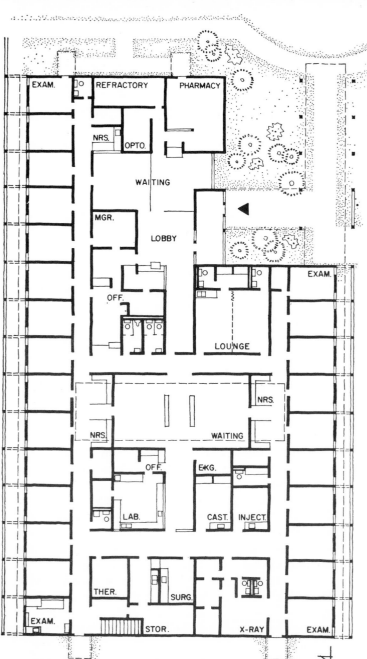

Patients enter the building from a covered walkway passing through the landscaped entrance court. The unclinical appearance of the building entrance contrasts with the ordered look of the examining rooms

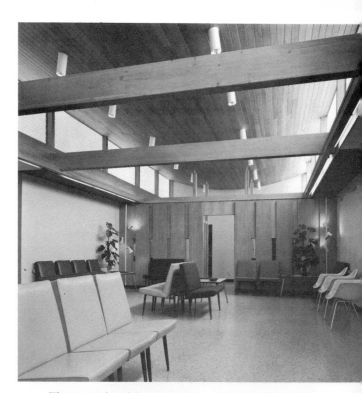

The central waiting room is located for efficient handling of patients bound for various departments. A pleasant feeling is achieved by the use of clerestory windows, exposed beams, and the reverse-curve roof

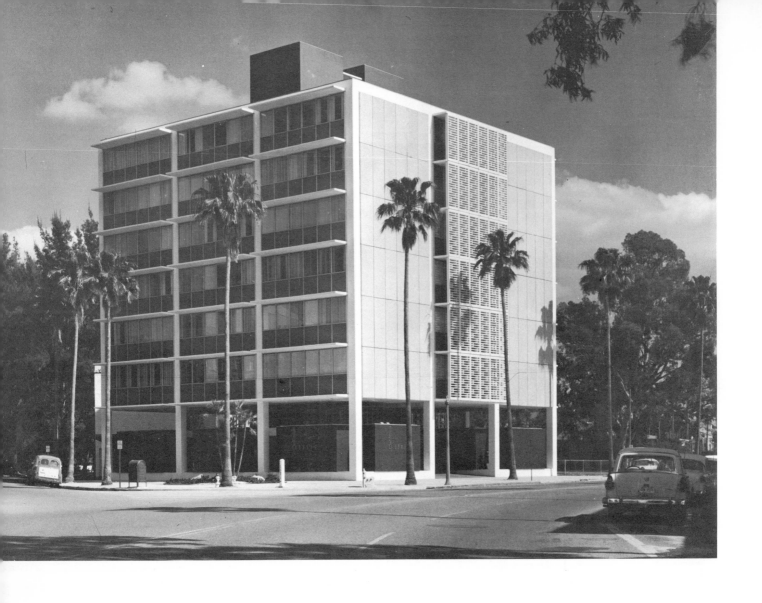

# Medical Building with Rental Offices

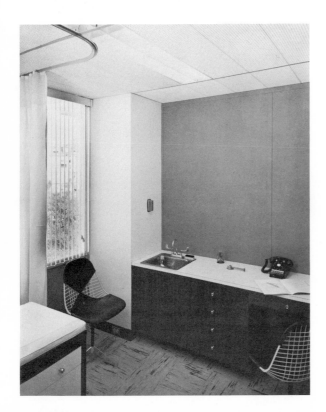

This building was designed by the architect to satisfy the complex and somewhat indeterminate requirements involved in providing flexible space for a number of individual medical practices.

Owned by a corporation formed by a group of doctors, the building is located on an island near the heart of the Tampa business district. It commands a view of the bay and the bridge to the mainland. Nearby is the newly enlarged and remodeled Municipal Hospital. Parking is handled by an existing garage adjacent to the building. This was altered to provide a sheltered entry connecting the two. The ground floor contains a pharmacy, laboratory, and X-ray department available for use by all building occupants. The six upper floors were constructed with their entire areas completely open except for the fixed central service cores which contain elevators, stairs, and toilets. Movable partitions are used for subdividing these spaces as required.

The building frame is of reinforced concrete with lightweight concrete floors. Exteriors are aluminum curtain walls with porcelain enamel panels and lightweight, gravel-surfaced precast concrete panels.

*Number One Davis Medical Office Building; Davis Island, Tampa, Florida; Mark Hampton, Architect; Russello & Barker, Structural Engineers; Charles T. Healy, Mechanical Engineer; DeWitt, Furnell & Spicer, Inc., Contractors*

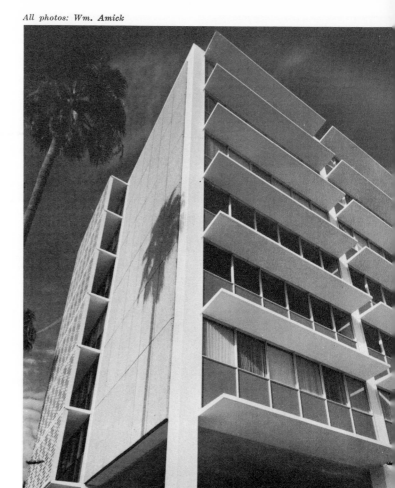

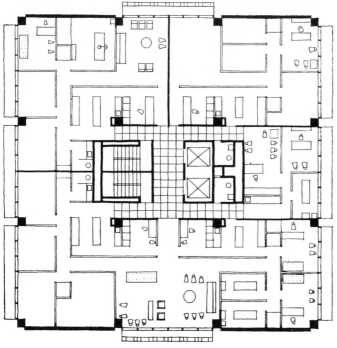

UPPER LEVEL

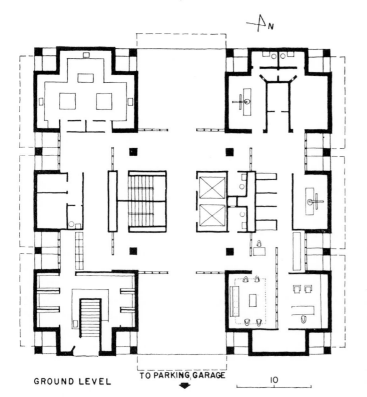

GROUND LEVEL      TO PARKING GARAGE          10

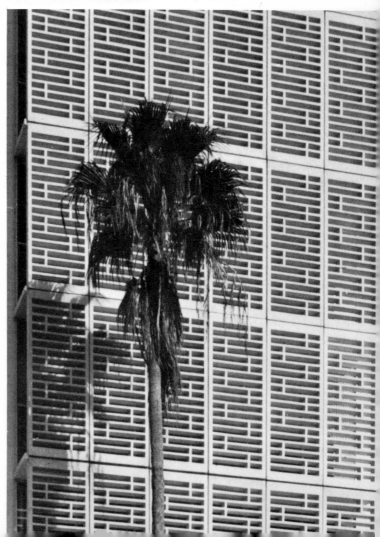

Cantilevers on north and south sides (right, above) act as sun controls and as platforms for window washing. Precast concrete grilles on east and west (right, below) were omitted on other sides for budgetary considerations

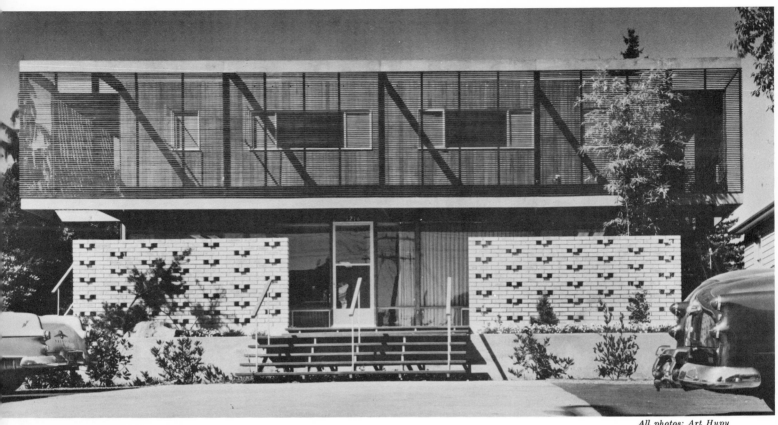

# Dental Clinic Combined with Apartments

*Clinic and Duplex Building for Dr. K. M. Robertson; Seattle, Washington; Bystrom and Greco, Architects; Stern and Towne, Mechanical Engineers; Tom Paulsen, Contractor*

Second-floor rental apartments have been combined with a ground floor dental clinic by the architects of this building, resulting in a friendly, residential atmosphere for two widely-varied functions.

Located on the fringes of a neighborhood business district, the site is quite small. This consideration primarily dictated the two-story scheme. The building was placed near the rear lot line in order to provide on-site parking at the front and to create an attractive foreground. Since the lot slopes up about seven feet from front to rear, terracing was used to minimize grading and to provide some separation between the parking area and the building. Louvered wood screens are used at the second level on three sides for sun control and preservation of privacy in the apartments. These also serve to considerably lighten the appearance of the upper story. Both floors have a shallow, planted area on the north side. The apartments have balconies on this side, accessible through sliding glass doors.

The structure is wood frame on a concrete foundation and slab. Exterior walls are finished with natural finish T & G cedar siding. Interior walls are painted gypsum board. Floors are vinyl-asbestos in the clinic, asphalt tile in the apartments. Ceilings of the clinic are fiberboard acoustical tile, while those in the apartments are gypsum board.

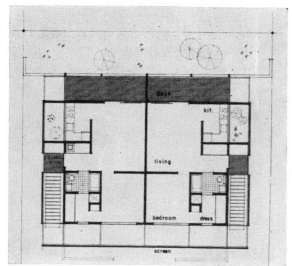

Duplex Level

Clinic Level

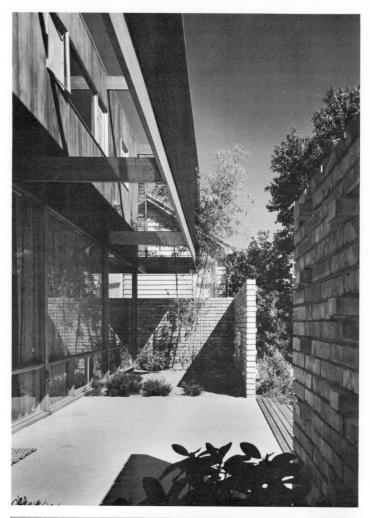

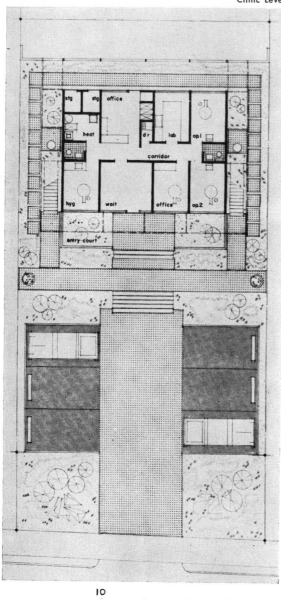

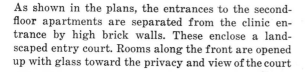
10

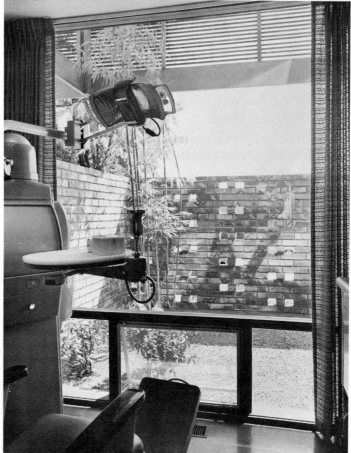

As shown in the plans, the entrances to the second-floor apartments are separated from the clinic entrance by high brick walls. These enclose a landscaped entry court. Rooms along the front are opened up with glass toward the privacy and view of the court

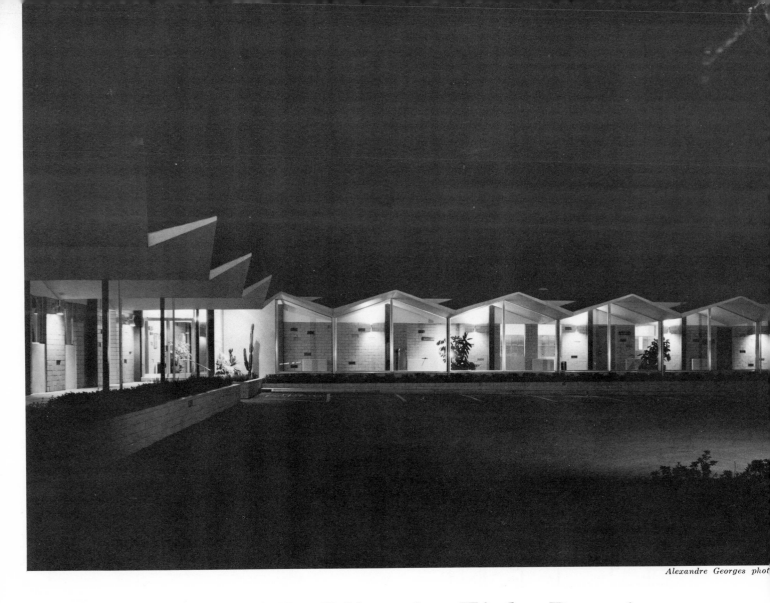

# Co-op Medical Building for Eight Practices

*The 1661 Building*
*Jacksonville, Florida*

*Hardwick and Lee, Architects*
*Gomer E. Kraus, Structural Engineer*
*Van Wagenen, Taylor, and Van Wagenen,*
*Mechanical and Electrical Engineers*
*The Auchter Company, Contractors*

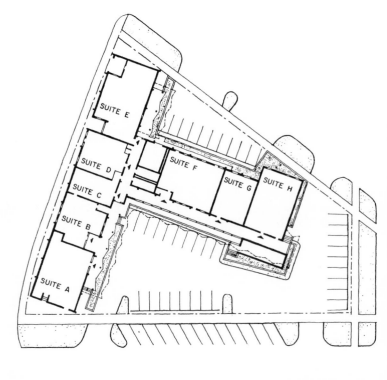

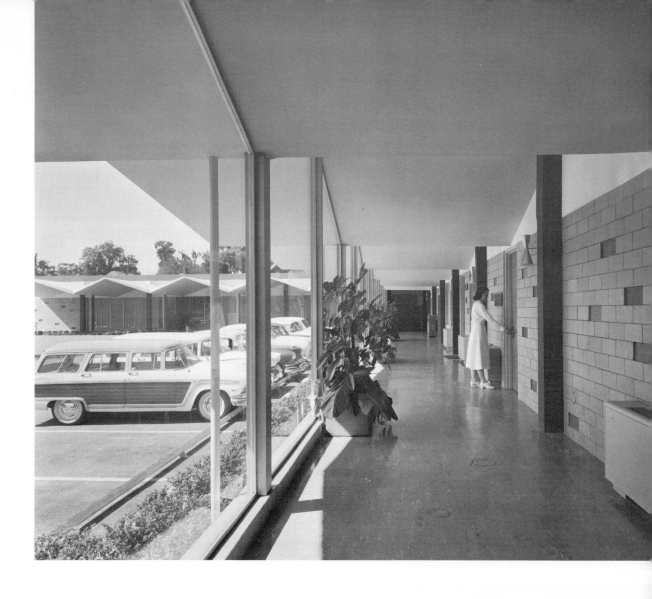

This building is owned jointly by 16 doctors in eight separate practices. A one-story scheme to house these practices—yet avoid the appearance of a group practice—was the major requirement of the owners. The irregularly shaped site was also a limiting factor of some importance. Regarding the design principles followed, the architects say, "conferences were conducted with each practice as if it were a separate client. When all schemes had been developed, their integration into an intelligent whole began. We believe this was preferable to the adoption of an arbitrary structural system of module and then developing suite schemes."

The structural frame is reinforced concrete. A portion of the space under the folded-plate concrete canopy is glazed to form a protected corridor. Exterior walls are structural tile with inserts of Italian glass.

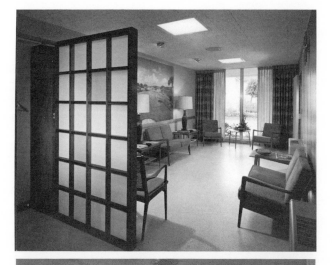

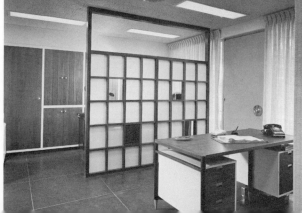

# Small Medical Clinic
# on a Sloping Site

*for Dr. Robert E. Reagan,*
*Benton Harbor, Michigan*

*George Fred Keck-William Keck, Architects*
*Pearson Construction Co., Inc., Contractor*

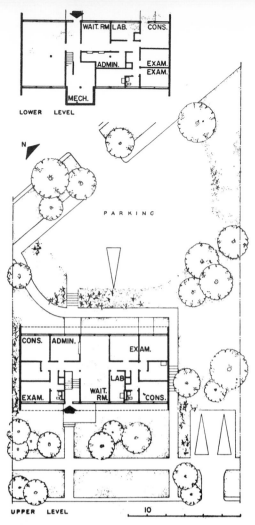

*Hedrich-Blessing photos by Hube Henry*

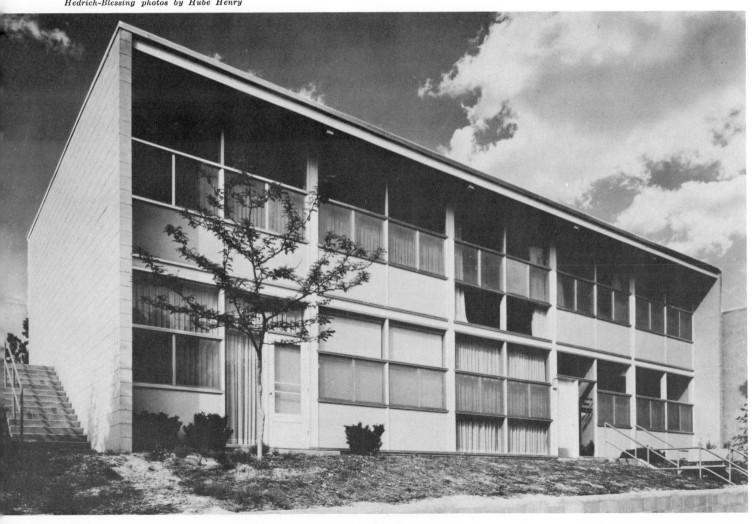

256

Reduced to its simplest elements, the program for the building required provision for the practice of the owner (a physician-surgeon), his assistant, and rental space for a cardiologist and an otolaryngologist, with off-street parking for the staff and patients. For maximum economy, the form of the building is a simple rectangle.

Structure is fireproofed steel frame with precast concrete floor and roof decks. Concrete block (8 in.) bearing walls are used on the ends of the building.

Interior partitions are exposed concrete block (4 in.). Floors and ceilings are concrete. Carpet is used in the waiting rooms and offices. Waiting rooms have acoustical tile ceilings applied directly on the concrete. Central heating and air conditioning is used. Electrical conduit is located in the wood door jambs (extra wide for this purpose).

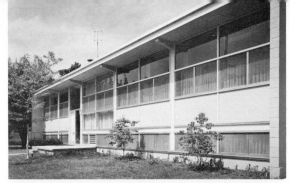

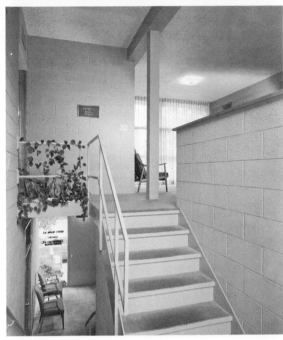

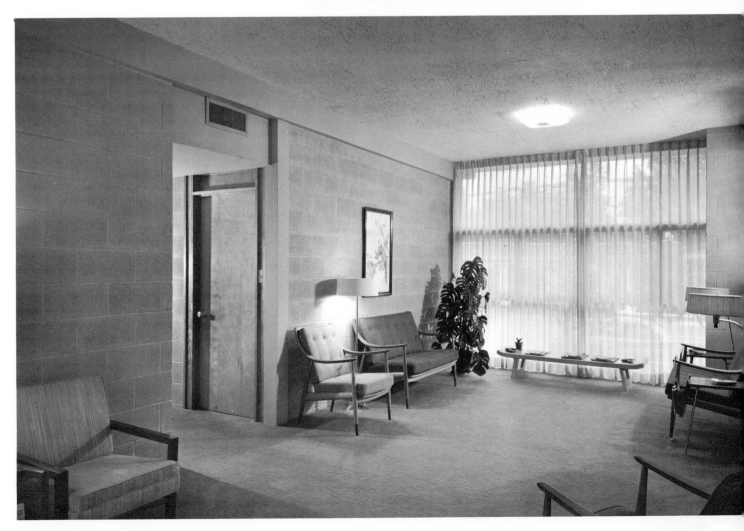

# INDEX

## A

Abramson, Louis Allen, 119
Acoustics; speech center, 190
Adams, Bruce, 72-77
Administrative department; location of, 6-7
Agnew, Peckham & Assoc., 56-60
Air conditioning; physical therapy department, 175
    rehabilitation center, 198
Air distribution; operating room, 134-136
Alabama Society for Crippled Children and Adults, 192-195
Alvy, Dan, 230-231
Ambulatory diagnostic facilities, 74-75
American Academy of Pediatrics, 137-139
American Psychiatric Association, 111
Anchorage, Alaska; Elmendorf Hospital, 61-67
Anderson, M.D., Hospital and Tumor Inst.; Houston, Tex., 132-133
Apartments combined with clinic, 252-253
Arcadia, Calif.; Methodist Hospital of Southern California, 103-106
Architects Collaborative, The, 78-85
Army, United States; Alaska Dist. Office, Corps of Engineers, 61-67
Ashdown, Ark.; Little River Memorial Hospital, 23-25
Assembly rooms, 206
Associated Architects and Engineers, 201-202
Aucher Co., The, 254-255
Aydellot, A. L., and Assoc., 26-31

## B

Balconies; indoor, 243
    for observation of patients, 199
Barge, Waggoner & Sumner, 190-191
Bassett Clinic; Cushing, Okla., 238-239

Beling Engineering Consultants, 32-35
Benesch, Alfred, and Assoc., 32-35, 78-85
Benson, Robert W., 190-191
Benton Harbor, Mich.; clinic for Dr. Robert Reagan, 256
Berwick Hospital; Berwick, Pa., 36-38
Bethesda, Md.; National Institutes of Health, 120-121, 134-136
Biggs, Wir & Chandler, 186-188
Bill Wilkerson Hearing and Speech Center; Nashville, Tenn., 190-191
Blaylock, Rawland, E., & Assoc., 23-25
Blytheville Air Force Base Hospital; Memphis, Tenn., 26-31
Boespflug, J. C., 61-67, 180-185
Bogalusa, La.; Washington Parish Health Clinic, 216
Bolt, Beranek, and Newman, 134-136
Bond, Lloyd, 232-233
Boner and Lane, 86-93
Bors, Ernest, 178-180
Bradshaw, Richard R., 166-172
Bronx, N. Y.; Misericordia Hospital, 94-99
Brown, John L., 8
Brush, Hutchinson & Gwinn, 190-191
Built-in toilet-lavatory, 77
Buonaccorsi & Murray, 20-22
Burk, Le Breton, and Lamantia, 216
Bush-May & Assoc., 190-191
Bystrom and Greco, 252-253

## C

Caldwell, George B., 8
Call system; nurses', 155
Cardiovascular surgical suite, 120-121
Carolyn Rose Strauss Rehabilitation Center; Monroe, La., 201-202

Carroll County General Hospital; Westminster, Md., 40-42
Cedercreutz, Jonas, 100-102
Central Hospital for Middle Finland; Jyväskylylä, Finland, 100-102
Cerebral palsy facilities, 186-188
    *see also* Rehabilitation facilities
Chicago, Ill.; Michael Reese Hospital, 78-85
Children's Clinic; Dallas, Tex., 236-237
Children's medical facilities; clinics, 236-237, 245-247
    hearing and speech clinic, 190-191
    pediatric nursing unit, 137-139
    physical therapy department, 182
    rehabilitation hospital school, 186-188
Chronic disease hospitals; Mt. Sinai Hospital, 166-172
    U.S. Public Health Service plan, 161-163
Chuquicamata Hospital; Chuquicamata, Chile, 131-132
Circular surgical suite, 120-121
Circulation; core-plan hospital, 25
    planning, 2-6
    surgical suite, 115
    Temple University Medical Center, 118
Clarke, Florence, 226-227
Clatworthy, R. N., 43-48
Cleaner, ultrasonic; *see* Ultrasonic cleaner
Clerestory windows, 249
Clinics; Bassett Clinic, 238-239
    Children's Clinic, 236-237
    Cleveland Clinic Hospital, 130-131
    Clinic and Duplex Building, 252-253
    dental clinic, 228-229
    Diaz-Simon Clinic, 245-247
    Doctors' Clinic, 234-235
    Group Health Cooperative Northgate Clinic, 248-249
    Hoyt Street Clinic, 226-227
    Mahorner Clinic, 240-242
    Rotary Foundation Clinic, 192-195
    Washington Parish Health Clinic, 216
    Woodley Medical Center, 230-231
Coddington Co., 92-97
Colbert and Lowrey and Assoc., 245-247
Commons rooms in hospitals, 75
Communication systems, 155
Connor, Paul J., 8
Consultation-examination room, 139, 174, 204-205
Cooling panels; radiant, 120
Co-op medical building, 254-255
Cooper, Dan S., and Assoc., 196-200
Core-planned hospital, 23-25
Coston-Frankfurt-Short, 238-239
Courts; garden, 109, 249, 253
Crevasse, J. M., 238-239
Cronin, John W., 209
Cubicles; dressing, 206
    pediatric department, 138
    physical therapy department, 174
Curtis & Davis, 201-202, 240-241
Cushing, Okla.; Bassett Clinic, 238-239

# D

Dallas, Tex.; Children's Clinic, 236-237
Dark room, 116
David Wohl Health Inst. of St. Louis University; St. Louis, Mo., 107-112

Davis Medical Foundation; Marion, Ind., 72-77
deLaureal and Moses, 201-202
Dental Arts Building; Gainsville, Fla., 228-229
DeVan, Edward A., 134
DeWitt, Furnell & Spicer, 250-251
Diagnostic facilities; *see* X-ray department
Diaz-Simon Pediatric Clinic; New Orleans, La., 245-247
Dinkeloo, John, 72-77
Di Stasio & Van Buren, 94-99
Doctors' Clinic; Lake City, Wash., 234-235
Doctors' collaborative, 232-233
Doctors' offices; *see* Clinics; Medical office buildings
Doors; physical therapy department, 176
Double corridor, 219
Dressing cubicles, 206
Drought, Frank T., 68-77

# E

Eason, F. C., Construction Co., 201-202
Eason, Thompson, and Assoc., 107-112
Electrical facilities, 152-156, 207
Elevators, 156
Ellerbe and Co., 125-126, 130-131
Ellison and King, 72-77
Elmendorf Hospital; Anchorage, Alaska; 61-67
Emergency facilities, 52-55
Entrances, 2-3
    glass enclosed, 247
Equipment; Public Health Center, 211
Erhart, Eichenbaum, Rauch, and Blass, 218-223
Erick, Murray, and Assoc., 178-180
Eugene, Ore.; McLymar Medical Building, 232-233
Examination-consultation room, 139, 174, 204-205
Exercise area; 175

# F

Faucets; electrically controlled, 122
Finland; Jyväskylylä; Central Hospital for Middle Finland, 100-102
Fisher and Davis, 180-185
Floorspace; operating room, 115
Forrest Memorial Hospital; Forrest City, Ark., 218-223
Friesen, Gordon, and Assoc., 36-38, 40-41, 43-48, 86-93
Frozen section laboratory, 116

# G

Gainsville, Fla.; Dental Arts Building, 228-229
Galbraith, Thomas, 158-160
Garden courts, 109

Goble, Emerson, 2
Golub, Jacob, 78-85
Good, Edmund George, 32-38
Goshen, Charles E., 111
Gottsche Rehabilitation Center; Thermopolis, Wyo., 181-185
Grace-New Haven Community Hospital; New Haven, Conn., 126-127
Greater Niagara General Hospital; Ontario, Canada, 56-60
Griffenhagen, Paul F., 8-19
Gritschke, E. R., and Assoc., 8-19
Group Health Cooperative Northgate Clinic; Seattle Wash., 248-249
Gruen, Victor, 230-231

# H

Haarstick Lundgren and Assoc., 224-225
Hampton, Mark, 250-251
Harlan Memorial Hospital; Harlan, Ky., 117
Harris, Julian, 190-191
Hartman, Gerhard, 32-35
Harwick and Lee, 254-255
Hattis, Robert E., 78-85
Health centers; Forrest Memorial Hospital, 218-223
    Medical Inst. of Local 88, 242-244
    see also Public health centers
Health insurance clinic, 224-225
Healy, Charles T., 250-251
Hearing and speech center, 190-191
Heating systems, 207
Hellmuth, Obata, and Kassabaum, 107-112
Hewitt and Royer, 52-55
Hexagonal patient-rooms, 77
Hill-Burton funds, 53, 55, 180, 198, 201
Holy Cross Hospital; San Fernando, Calif., 43-48
Hospital-school, 186-188
Hot Springs Memorial Hospital; Thermopolis, Wyo., 181-185
Houston, Tex.; M. D. Anderson Hospital and Tumor Inst., 132-133
    Texas Inst. for Rehabilitation and Research, 196-200
Hoyt Street Clinic; Portland, Ore., 226-227
Hubbard & Hyland, 8-19
Hydrotherapy unit, 179-180
    see also Swimming pools

# I

"Instrumentation" room; surgical suite, 115
Insulation of Alaskan hospital, 63
Interior finishes, 175-176
Investment; doctors' collaborative for, 232-233
Isolation rooms; pediatric unit, 138-139
Ives, O.B., 137-139, 209

# J

Jackson, Miss.; Mississippi Hospital School for Cerebral Palsy, 186-188
Jackson County Health Center; Marianna, Fla., 214-215
Jacksonville, Fla.; The 1661 Building, 254-255
Jamieson, Thomas C., 232-233
Jensen, Peter, 161-163
Johnson, Frank B., 86-93
Jones, Everett W., 8
Jyväskylylä, Finland; Central Hospital for Middle Finland, 100-102

# K

Kaplan Pavilion, Michael Reese Hospital; Chicago, Ill., 78-85
Keck and Keck, 256-257
Keller & Gannon, 61-67
Kelley, Grant, & Assoc., 226-227
Kiff, Aaron N., 115
    Colean, Voss & Souder, 94-99, 120-121, 124, 131-132, 134-136
Kirk, Paul H., 234-235, 248-249
Kitchen; location of, 7
Klawa, Fritz, 232-233
Knutson Construction Co., 196-200
Koenig, August W., 49-51
Kornacker, Frank J., 72-77
Kraus, Gomer E., 254-255
Kroeker, J. Donald, 226-227
Krey & Hunt, 134-136

# L

Laboratory; lighting of, 153
Lake City, Wash.; Doctors' Clinic, 234-235
Lankton, Ziegele-Terry, and Assoc., 32-35
Laredo, Tex.; Mercy Hospital, 68-71
Laurens County Health Center; Laurens, S.C., 217
Levine & McCann, 103-106
Lighting; operating room, 122
    recommended foot-candles, 153-154
    surgical suite, 118
Lindstrom, McLendon & Holbrook, 190-191
Little River Memorial Hospital; Ashdown, Ark., 23-25
Loebl, Schlossman & Bennett, 78-85
Long Beach Veterans Administration Hospital; Long Beach, Calif., 178-180
Long Island Jewish Hospital; New Hyde Park, N. Y., 119

Longwood, James C., 232-233
Los Angeles, Calif.; Mt. Sinai Hospital, 166-172
    Woodley Medical Center, 230-231
Lyles, Bissett, Carlisle & Wolff, 217

# M

Maas, Hendrik P., 8-19
McCune, McCune & McCune, 213
McDonough Dist. Hospital; Macomb, Ill., 32-35
MacKie and Kamrach, 132-133
McKinley, David A., 248-249
McLymar Medical Building; Eugene, Ore., 232-233
Macomb, Ill.; McDonough Dist. Hospital, 32-35
Maguolo and Quick, 72-77
Mahorner Clinic; New Orleans, La., 240-241
Marchand, Lewis, 228-229
Marianna, Fla.; Jackson County Health Center, 214-215
Marion, Ind.; Davis Medical Foundation, 72-77
Marshall and Johnson, 180-185
Masur, Jack, 134-136
Mechanical and electrical systems, 207
Medical office buildings; Dental Arts Building, 229-229
    McLymar Medical Building, 232-233
    Number One Davis Medical Office Building, 250-251
    The 1661 Building, 254-255
Mendocino County Hospital; Ukiah, Calif., 20-22
Mercy Hospital; Laredo, Tex., 68-71
Methodist Hospital of Southern California; Arcadia,
    Calif., 103-106
Meyer, Strong & Jones, 94-99
Mezger, W. J., 166-172
Michael Reese Hospital; Chicago, Ill.; Kaplan Pavilion,
    78-85
Military and civilian hospital, 61-67
Minasian, John, 103-106
Misericordia Hospital; Bronx, N. Y., 94-99
Mississippi Hospital School for Cerebral Palsy; Jackson,
    Miss., 186-188
Mobile, Ala.; Rotary Foundation Clinic and Rehabilita-
    tion Center, 192-195
Modern Hospital, The, 8
Moeller, H. H., 69
Moffitt, Herbert C., Hospital; San Francisco, Calif.,
    128-129
Monroe, La.; Carolyn Rose Strauss Rehabilitation Center,
    201-202
Montgomery & Williams, 86-93
Montgomery County Health Center; Montgomery, Ala.,
    214-215
Moore, Walter P., 196-200
Morris, Edwin B., 164-165
Motel-like diagnostic unit, 77
Mt. Sinai Hospital; Los Angeles, Calif., 166-172

# N

Nashville, Tenn.; Bill Wilkerson Hearing and Speech
    Center, 190-191
National Institutes of Health; Bethesda, Md., 120-121,
    134-136

Neptune and Thomas, 103-106
Neurological surgery; facilities for, 120-121
New Hyde Park, N. Y.; Long Island Jewish Hospital, 119
New Orleans, La.; Diaz-Simon Pediatric Clinic, 245-247
Newberg, Gust K., 178-180
Noakes, Edward H., & Assoc., 40-42
Noakes & Neubauer, 36-38, 196-197
Noel, James A., 118
Noise control, 230-231
North Kansas City Memorial Hospital; North Kansas
    City, Mo., 52-55
Number One Medical Office Building; Davis Island, Fla.,
    250-251
Nurseries; location of, 5
Nurses' call system, 155
Nurses' station; location of, 3-4
    in pediatric unit, 137-139
Nurses' workroom, 206
Nursing home, 164-165
Nursing school in Misericordia Hospital, 94

# O

Observation dome; cardiac operating room, 134
Obstetrics department; location of, 5
Ochsner Foundation Hospital; New Orleans, La.; 125-126
O'Connor, A. C., 72-77
Ogle-Rosenbohm & Assoc., 245-247
Ollinkari, Lasse, 100-102
Ontario, Canada; Greater Niagara Hospital, 56-60
Operating rooms; air distribution in, 134-136
    equipment in, 115
    lighting of, 118, 134
Orr, Douglas, 126-127
Ouachita Parish Society for Crippled Children and Adults,
    201
Outlying Health Centers for Tulsa County; Tulsa County,
    Okla., 213

# P

Page, Southerland & Page, 86-93
Päivärinne, Esko, 100-102
Palmer, Krisel & Lindsay, 166-172
Parking facilities, 242, 247, 250
Partitions; movable, 250
    in pediatric unit, 138
Patti, S., Construction Co., 32-35
Paulsen, Tom, 252-253
Pearson Construction Co., 256-257
Pediatric clinic, 236-237, 245-247
Perkins & Will, 8-19
Pfleuger, Milton T., 128-129
Philadelphia, Pa.; Temple University Medical Center,
    118
Phillips, Ralph E., 166-172
Photo-flurography, 206
Physical therapy department; Mt. Sinai hospital, 166
    planning of, 173-177

Pinckney, V. H., 103-106
Platt Roberts & Company, 192-195
Playroom; pediatric, 139
Plumbing fixtures, 207
Pneumotherapy, 205
Portland, Ore.; Hoyt Street Clinic, 226-227
Post, Howard L., 94-99
Post and Witty, 186-188
Providence, R. I.; Rhode Island Hospital, 122-123
Psychiatric units, 20-22, 106
Public health centers; mechanical and electrical systems, 207
   planning, 204-206
   southern health centers, 214-217
   type plans, 208-212
Public Health Service, U. S.; *see* United States Public Health Service
Pyle, J. E., 218-223


# R

Radcliffe, Donald G., 248-249
Railo, Helge, 100-102
Reagan, Robert E.; clinic for, 256-257
Reaves, David, 228-229
Recovery room, 115, 116
Redondo Beach, Calif.; South Bay Hospital, 49-51
Rehabilitation facilities; Bill Wilkerson Hearing and Speech Center, 190-191
   Carolyn Rose Strauss Rehabilitation Center, 201-202
   Gottsche Rehabilitation Center, 181-185
   Long Beach Veterans Administration Hospital, 178-180
   Mississippi Hospital School for Cerebral Palsy, 186-188
   for multiple disability, 158-160
   Rotary Foundation Clinic and Rehabilitation Center, 192-195
   Texas Inst. for Rehabilitation and Research, 196-200
   U. S. Public Health Service plans, 158
   vocational, 178
   *see also* Physical therapy department
Reinheimer & Cox, 23-25, 86-93
Research facilities; Davis Medical Foundation, 72-77
   Texas Inst. for Rehabilitation and Research, 196-200
Reverse-curve roof, 249
Rhode Island Hospital; Providence, R.I., 121-123
Riddick, Edgar K., 218-223
Roark, H. Price, 218-223
Robertson, K. M.; Clinic and Duplex Building for, 252-253
Rockford Memorial Hospital; Rockford, Ill., 8-19
Rotary Foundation Clinic and Rehabilitation Center; Mobile, Ala., 192-195
Russello & Barker, 250-251


# S

St. Louis University; David Wohl Health Inst., 107-112
St. Luke's Hospital; New York, N. Y.; Stuyvesant Pavilion, 124

San Fernando, Calif.; Holy Cross Hospital, 43-48
San Francisco, Calif.; Herbert C. Moffitt Hospital, 128-129
St. Paul, Minn.; Group Health Office and Clinic Building, 224-225
Sasaki & Novak, 78-85
Schedule; health center clinic, 208
Schmidt, Garden & Erickson, 132-133
School combined with hospital, 186-188
Screens; louvered wood, 252
Seattle, Wash.; Clinic and Duplex Building, 252-253
   Group Health Cooperative Northgate Clinic, 248-249
Segal, B., 86-93
Severud-Elstad-Kreuger, 190-191
Shefferman and Bigelson, 36-38
Shellhorn, Ruth, 178-180
Sherlock, Smith & Adams, 117, 214-215
Showers, 48
Sinks, 175
1661 Building, The; Jacksonville, Fla., 254-255
Skidmore, Owings & Merrill, 61-69, 118, 226-227
Shuler, F. W., 52-55
Smith, Art, 20-22
Smith Brothers Construction Co., 56-60
Snedeker, Lendon, 137-139
Snow, D. L., 134-136
South Bay Hospital; Redondo Beach, Calif., 49-51
Southland, Ben, 230-231
Speech and hearing center, 190-191
Starr, B. E., 40-42
Steed Brothers Construction Co., 43-48
Sterilizing equipment, 116
Stern and Towne, 248-249, 252-253
Stoley, Martin, 68-71
Stone, Marracini & Patterson, 20-22
Storage facilities, 175
   surgical suite, 116
   pediatric unit, 139
Supply system; Berwick Hospital, 36-39
   Carroll County General Hospital, 40-42
   Holy Cross Hospital, 43-48
   South Bay Hospital, 51
Surgical suites; examples, with evaluation, 117-133
   general planning, 114-117
Swanson and Rink, 180-185
Swimming pool for paraplegics, 180,


# T

T-shaped hospital, 8-19
Television; closed circuit, 122
Temperature control; Childrens' Clinic, 236-237
Temple University Medical Center, Philadelphia, Pa., 118
Teufel, William G., 248-249
Texarkana Construction Co., 23-25
Texarkana, Tex.; Wadley Hospital, 86-93
Texas Inst. for Rehabilitation and Research; Houston, Tex., 196-200
Thompson, Isadore, 61-67
Toilet facilities, 175
   built-in toilet-lavatory, 77

Tuberculosis; facilities for treating, 205
Thermopolis, Wyo.; Gottsche Rehabilitation Center, 180-185
   Hot Springs Memorial Hospital, 180-185
Transformers; electrical, 152
Tulsa County, Okla.; outlying health centers for, 213

# U

Ukiah, Calif.; Mendocino County Hospital, 20-22
Ultrasonic cleaner, 45, 116
Underwater exercise area, 174
United Mine Workers hospitals, 36, 43-48
United States Army; Alaska Dist. Office, Corps of Engineers, 61-67
United States Public Health Service, 137-139, 158-165
University of California Medical Center; San Francisco, Calif., 128
University of Texas; Houston, Tex., 132-133
Utah Construction Co., 20-22
Utility room; pediatric department, 139

# V

Van der Meulen, John, 72-77
Van Wagenen, Taylor, and Van Wagenen, 254-255
Ventilation; physical therapy department, 175
Verge, Gene, 43-48
Vermilya-Brown Co., Inc., 94-99
Vernor, Tom A., 68-71
Vocational rehabilitation, 178-180

# W

Wade, Gibson, Martin, 68-71
Wadley Hospital; Texarkana, Tex., 86-93
Wagner, Harry L., 52-55
Walker, Kalionzes, and Klingerman, 49-51
Walkway; covered, 249
Wallace, Don S., 248-249
Walter, Carl W., 72-77
Washington Parish Health Clinic; Bogalusa, La., 216
Waters, John, 245-247
Watson and Boaler, 78-85
Wedge-shaped clinic, 224-225
Welton Becket & Assoc., 166-172, 178-180
Westminster, Md.; Carroll County General Hospital, 40-42
White, Ken, Assoc., 180-185, 190-191
Wiltshire and Fisher, 236-237
Windows for sun control, 63
Woodley Medical Center; Los Angeles, Calif., 230-231
Worthen, Mary, 115

# X

X-ray department, 141-146
   electricity in, 156, 207
   film files in, 206
   location of, 5
X-ray unit; portable, 117

# Y

York & Sawyer, The Office of, 94-99, 115, 120-121, 124, 131-132, 134